P9-DHP-585

HANDBOOK OF

Nursing
Diagnosis

8TH EDITION

HANDBOOK OF

Nursing
Diagnosis

8TH EDITION

LYNDA JUALL CARPENITO, R.N., M.S.N., CRNP
Nursing Consultant, Clarksboro, New Jersey
Family Nurse Practitioner
ChesPenn Health Services
Chester, Pennsylvania

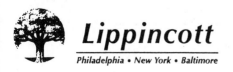

Lippincott

Philadelphia • New York • Baltimore

Acquisitions Editor: Ilze Rader   *Production Coordinator:* Nannette Winski
Assistant Editor: Dale Thuesen   *Art Director:* Doug Smock
Senior Project Editor: Tom Gibbons   *Indexer:* Ellen Brennan
Senior Production Manager: Helen Ewan

8th Edition

Carpenito Lynda Juall.
    Handbook of nursing diagnosis/Lynda Juall Carpenito—8th ed.
        p.   cm.
    Includes bibliographical references and index.
    ISBN 0-7817-1971-2 (pbk. : alk. paper)
    1. Nursing diagnosis–Handbooks, manuals, etc.   I. Title.
II. Title: Nursing diagnosis.
    [DNLM: 1. Nursing Diagnosis handbooks.   WY 49 C294h   1999]
RT48.6.C385   1999
616.07′5–dc21
DNLM/DLC
for Library of Congress   99-10471
9 8 7 6 5 4 3   CIP

Care has been taken to confirm the accuracy of the information presented and to describe generally accepted practices. However, the authors,
editors, and publisher are not responsible for errors or omissions or for
any consequences from application of the information in this book and
make no warranty, express or implied, with respect to the contents of the
publication.

The author, editors and publisher have exerted every effort to ensure
that drug selection and dosage set forth in this text are in accordance with
current recommendations and practice at the time of publication. However, in view of ongoing research, changes in government regulations,
and the constant flow of information relating to drug therapy and drug
reactions, the reader is urged to check the package insert for each drug for
any change in indications and dosage and for added warnings and precautions. This is particularly important when the recommended agent is a
new or infrequently employed drug.

Some drugs and medical devices presented in this publication have
Food and Drug Administration (FDA) clearance for limited use in restricted research settings. It is the responsibility of the health care provider
to ascertain the FDA status of each drug or device planned for use in his
or her clinical practice.

How to Use This Handbook

1. Collect data, both subjective and objective, from client, family, other health care professionals, and records. (Refer to Appendix: Adult Screening Admission Assessment.)
2. Identify a possible pattern or problem.
3. Refer to the medical diagnostic category in Section II, and review the possible associated nursing diagnoses and collaborative problems. Select the possibilities.
4. After you have selected what physiological complications or collaborative problems are indicated to be monitored for onset or status changes, label them Potential Complications: (specify).
5. After you have determined which functional patterns are altered or at risk of altered functioning, review the list of nursing diagnoses under that pattern and select the appropriate diagnosis (refer to Table I-1).
6. If you select an actual diagnosis:
   a. Do you have signs and symptoms to support its presence? (Refer to Section I, Nursing Diagnoses, under the selected diagnosis.)
   b. Write the actual diagnosis in three parts: Label related to contributing factors as evident by signs and symptoms
7. If you select a risk diagnosis:
   a. Are risk factors present? Is this person or group more vulnerable than others in the same or a similar situation?
   b. Write the risk diagnosis in two parts: Label related to risk factors
8. If you suspect a problem but have insufficient data, gather the additional data to confirm or rule out the diagnosis. If this additional data collection must be done later or by other nurses, label the diagnosis *possible* on the care plan or problem list.*

*Specific focus assessment criteria questions, outcome criteria, and interventions for each nursing diagnosis category can be found in Carpenito, L. J. (1999). *Nursing diagnosis: Application to clinical practice* (8th ed.). Philadelphia: Lippincott Williams & Wilkins.

Acknowledgments

1998 was the most difficult year of my life. In the midst of trying personal challenges and changes, this manuscript was due. A few friends rode an emotional roller coaster with me. Thank you, Ginny, Ros, Margo, Jamie, Donna, Stephen, and my dear sister Pati.

I would like to thank Pauline Elliot, at St. Francis Hospital, Cape Girardeau, Missouri, for coordinating the revisions of some care plans by staff nurses at St. Francis.

A sincere "thank you" to Lippincott's Susan Keneally and Tom Gibbons for help in this undertaking, and for their patience.

Please Note: In order to reflect a society where nurses are male and female and clients are male and female, the pronouns *she, her, he, his, him,* etc., will be used interchangeably throughout this book. The intent is to retain the use of gender pronouns without stereotyping.

Contents

MENTAL HEALTH DISORDERS 565

DIAGNOSTIC AND THERAPEUTIC PROCEDURES 572

Introduction

HOW TO MAKE AN ACCURATE NURSING DIAGNOSIS

In order to make an accurate nursing diagnosis the nurse must be able to do the following:

1. Collect data that is valid and pertinent
2. Analyze the data into clusters
3. Differentiate nursing diagnoses from collaborative problems
4. Formulate nursing diagnoses correctly
5. Select priority diagnoses

COLLECT DATA THAT IS VALID AND PERTINENT

Key Concepts

Nursing focused assessment
Screening versus focus
Significance of data
Evaluation of data

Nursing Focused Assessment

Nursing is defined as the diagnosis and treatment of human responses to actual or potential health problems and life situations (Nursing: A Social Policy Statement, 1985. NANDA, 1990). The assessment format the nurse utilizes must be able to direct data collection on human responses ranging from skin condition and urinary function to spiritual health and self-care abilities.

In other words, the nurses' knowledge of signs and symptoms for actual diagnoses, risk factors for risk diagnoses or possible physiological complications directs the data collection. This knowledge is also used to validate the accuracy of the diagnosis.

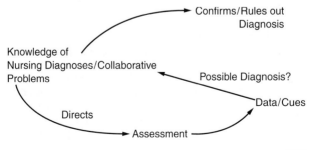

Screening Versus Focus

There are two types of assessments:

1. Screening: collection of predetermined data usually during initial contact
2. Focus: Collection of specific data as determined by the client, family, or situation

Frequently during first encounters with the individual, the nurse will focus on broad screening assessment questions to determine how the person is functioning in various areas. Such questions might include the following:

- Do you have a problem sleeping?
- Do you have a problem with eating?
- How often do you have a bowel movement?
- Is there a situation in your life that has been difficult for you to cope with?

The appendix provides screening assessment questions under Functional Health Patterns.

If the person is complaining of a certain problem or has a specific concern, the nurse would limit the assessment. A limited assessment focus might include the following questions:

- Now tell me about your pain (Onset? Location? Severity? Duration? What Helps? What aggravates?)
- What other symptoms do you have?
- How is this pain affecting sleep, eating, work, leisure?

In another situation, the nurse might be caring for a woman who has just had surgery, and complete a focus assessment of vital signs, wound appearance, intake, output, comfort level.

In many situations, the nurse would not be assessing for problem nursing diagnoses, but instead would be assessing wellness and healthy lifestyles. For example, a healthy 42-year-old woman may be assessed for fiber content in diet.

Significance of Data

Beginning students will need to learn to determine if data are significant or not in basic functional patterns or needs such as nutrition, safety, elimination, mobility, self-care. In order to recognize significant data, the nurse must first know what is expected or normal. For example, in order to determine if a person has a nutritional problem, the nurse must first understand the food pyramid of five food groups, normal weight for height, and food preparation. In addition the nurse needs to know that certain factors, such as nausea, poor dentures, sore mouth, or insufficient money, can interfere with food procurement, food preparation, eating, and metabolism.

Very simply, in order for assessment to be purposeful the nurse has to know the following:

- What is the range of normal?
- What is the range of abnormal?
- What are the risk factors?

Evaluation of Data

The evaluation of data involves:

- Differentiating cues from inferences
- Assuring validity
- Determining how much data is needed

Cues are facts that the nurse collects through interviewing, observing, examining, and reviewing the client record (eg, vital signs, feelings, laboratory results). Inferences are judgments that the nurse makes about cues, such as the following:

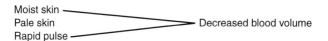

Validity is the extent to which data can be believed to be factual and true (Alfaro-Lefevre, 1999). Some data, such as decreasing blood pressure, are certain because there are agreed-upon standards. For situations where there are not clear-cut criteria, such as psychosocial responses, the nurse can increase the validity of the data or diagnosis by adding more evidence to support the inference.

The judgments nurses make are only as valid as the data used. The validity or accuracy of the data can be increased if the nurse verifies information.

Alfaro-Lefevre (1999) recommends several procedures to validate data:

- Recheck your own data
- Ask someone to check
- Compare subjective and objective data
- Ask the client to verify

ANALYZE THE DATA INTO CLUSTERS

Key Concepts

Knowledge of diagnostic categories
Sufficient number of cues
Differentiating one diagnosis from another
Tentative diagnosis (hypothesis)

Knowledge of Diagnostic Categories

Analysis of data is not possible unless you know which cues cluster or group to describe a diagnosis. In other words, you need to know which cues describe powerlessness before you can recognize the cluster. Some diagnoses are very easy to confirm, such as Constipation or Impaired Skin Integrity. Often a single cue, such as "I have leg pain," can confirm a diagnosis of pain.

Other diagnoses, especially more complex psychosocial diagnoses such as Body Image Disturbance, may necessitate several nurse–client interactions before the diagnosis can be confirmed or not. Table 1, at the end of this introduction, lists nursing diagnoses under Functional Health Patterns.

Sufficient Number of Cues

One of the most difficult aspects of making accurate diagnoses is determining if a sufficient number of cues are present to confirm an actual nursing diagnosis. The nurse should consult the list of defining characteristics for the diagnosis suspected. How many major characteristics are present? How many minor characteristics are present? Does the client confirm your suspected diagnosis? If you are still not confident, label the diagnosis Possible and collect more data.

Differentiating One Diagnosis From Another

Some diagnoses share some of the same defining characteristics as Activity Intolerance, Fatigue, and Sleep Pattern Disturbance. Review the definitions and the author's notes for help. Determine what the focus of the interventions would be for the problem, for example, energy conservation techniques (Fatigue), promotion of sleep (Sleep Pattern Disturbance) or increasing endurance (Activity Intolerance). Sometimes this technique helps to clarify the diagnosis.

Tentative Diagnosis (Hypothesis)

The last cognitive activity in data analysis is the proposal of one or more likely diagnostic explanations for the clustered data. Sometimes only one diagnosis is proposed because the clustered data clearly support its presence. When more than one diagnosis is likely, the nurse should review the defining characteristics (for actual) or risk factors (for risk) for the tentative diagnosis. Systematically, the nurse should compare these signs, symptoms, or risk factors to the data assessed. If more data collection is needed, the nurse can proceed to this focused assessment. Another option is for the nurse to label the tentative diagnosis Possible if additional data collection is not realistic or feasible at this time. For example, some of the coping diagnoses require repetitive interactions for confirmation of the diagnosis.

DIFFERENTIATE NURSING DIAGNOSES FROM COLLABORATIVE PROBLEMS

Key Concepts

Nursing diagnoses versus collaborative problems
Selection of collaborative problems

Nursing Diagnoses Versus Collaborative Problems

In 1983, Carpenito published the Bifocal Clinical Practice Model. In this model, nurses are accountable to treat two types of clinical judgments or diagnoses: nursing diagnoses and collaborative problems.

Nursing Diagnoses are clinical judgments about individual, family, or community responses to actual or potential health problems/life processes. Nursing diagnoses provide the basis for selection of nursing interventions to achieve outcomes for which the nurse is accountable (NANDA, 1990).

Collaborative problems are certain physiological complications that nurses monitor to detect onset or changes in status. Nurses manage collaborative problems using physician-prescribed and nursing-prescribed interventions to minimize the complications of the events (Carpenito, 1989)

Nursing interventions are classified as nurse-prescribed or physician-prescribed. Nurse-prescribed interventions are those that the nurse can legally order for nursing staff to implement. Nurse-prescribed interventions treat, prevent, and monitor nursing diagnoses. Nurse-prescribed interventions manage and monitor collaborative problems. Physician-prescribed interventions represent treatments for collaborative problems that the nurse initiates and manages. Collaborative problems require both nursing-prescribed and physician-prescribed interventions. Display 1 represents these relationships.

The following illustrates the types of interventions associated with the collaborative problem potential complications: Hypoxemia:

NP	1.	Monitor for signs of acid–base imbalance.
PP	2.	Administer low flow oxygen as needed.
NP	3.	Ensure adequate hydration.
NP	4.	Evaluate the effects of positioning on oxygenation.
NP/PP	5.	Administer medications as needed.

(NP: Nurse-prescribed   PP: Physician-prescribed)

Selection of Collaborative Problems

As mentioned earlier, collaborative problems are different from nursing diagnoses.

The nurse makes independent decisions regarding both collaborative problems and nursing diagnoses. The decisions differ in that, for nursing diagnoses, the nurse prescribes the definitive treatment for the situation and is responsible for outcome achievement; for collaborative problems the nurse monitors the client's condition to detect onset or status of physiological complications and manages the events with nursing and physician-prescribed interventions. Collaborative problems are labeled "Potential Complications" (specify).

Examples:

Potential Complication: Hemorrhage
Potential Complication: Renal Failure

The physiological complications that nurses monitor are usually related to disease, trauma, treatments, and diagnostic studies. The following examples illustrate some collaborative problems:

Situation	*Collaborative Problem*
Anticoagulant therapy	Potential Complication: Hemorrhage
Pneumonia	Potential Complication: Hypoxemia

DISPLAY 1. RELATIONSHIP BETWEEN NURSING-PRESCRIBED INTERVENTIONS AND PHYSICIAN-PRESCRIBED INTERVENTIONS

NURSING-PRESCRIBED INTERVENTIONS	NURSING DIAGNOSES	PHYSICIAN-PRESCRIBED INTERVENTIONS
• Reposition q2h • Lightly massage vulnerable areas • Teach how to reduce pressure when sitting	Risk for Impaired Skin Integrity related to immobility secondary to fatigue	Usually not needed

NURSING-PRESCRIBED INTERVENTIONS	COLLABORATIVE PROBLEMS	PHYSICIAN-PRESCRIBED INTERVENTIONS

• Maintain NPO state
• Monitor:
  Hydration
  Vital Signs
  Intake/output
  Specific gravity
• Monitor electrolytes
• Maintain IV at prescribed rate
• Provide/encourage mouth care
	Potential Complication: Fluid and Electrolyte Imbalances	• IV (type, amount)
		• Laboratory studies

DISPLAY 2. EVALUATION QUESTIONS

Is the diagnosis correct?

Has the goal been mutually set?

Is more time needed for the plan to work?

Does the goal need to be revised?

Do the interventions need to be revised?

Outcome criteria or client goals are used to measure the effectiveness of nursing care. When a client is not progressing to goal achievement or has worsened, the nurse must reevaluate the situation. Display 2 represents the questions to be considered. If none of these options is appropriate, the situation may not be a nursing diagnosis. For example:

Risk for Fluid Volume Deficit related to the effects of prolonged PTT secondary to anticoagulant therapy

Goal: The client will have hemoglobin >13

Examine the questions in Display 2. Which option is appropriate? The answer is none. The nurse would initiate physician-prescribed orders if the client presented signs of bleeding. This situation is a collaborative problem, not a nursing diagnosis. For example:

Potential Complication: Bleeding

Goal: The nurse will manage and minimize episodes of bleeding. Collaborative problems have nursing goals that represent the accountability of the nurse—to detect early changes and to co-manage with physicians. Nursing diagnoses have client goals that represent the accountability of the nurse—to achieve or maintain a favorable status after nursing care.

Table 1 includes frequently used collaborative problems.

Some physiological complications, such as pressure ulcers and infection from invasive lines, are problems that nurses can prevent. Prevention is different from detection. Nurses do not prevent paralytic ileus but, instead, detect its presence early to prevent greater severity of illness or even death. Physicians cannot treat collaborative problems without nursing knowledge, vigilance, and judgment.

FORMULATE NURSING DIAGNOSES CORRECTLY

Key Concepts

Types of nursing diagnoses
Diagnostic statements
Client validation
Clinical example

Types of Nursing Diagnoses

A nursing diagnosis can be actual, risk, or a wellness or syndrome type.

Actual: An actual nursing diagnosis describes a clinical judgment that the nurse has validated because of the presence of major defining characteristics.

Risk: A risk nursing diagnosis describes a clinical judgment that an individual/group is more vulnerable to develop the problem than others in the same or a similar situation.

Wellness: A wellness nursing diagnosis is a clinical judgment about an individual, family, or community in transition from a specific level of wellness to a higher level of wellness (NANDA).

Syndrome: A syndrome diagnosis comprises a cluster of actual or risk nursing diagnoses that are predicted to present because of a certain situation or event.

Possible nursing diagnosis is not a type of diagnosis as are actual, risk, and syndrome. Possible nursing diagnoses are a diagnostician's option to indicate that some data are present to confirm a diagnosis but are insufficient at this time.

Diagnostic Statements

The diagnostic statement describes the health status of an individual or group and the factors that have contributed to the status.

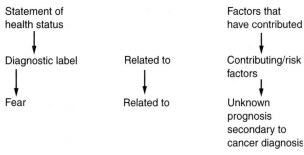

Statement of health status → Diagnostic label → Fear

Related to → Related to

Factors that have contributed → Contributing/risk factors → Unknown prognosis secondary to cancer diagnosis

One-Part Statements

Wellness nursing diagnoses will be written as one-part statements: Potential for Enhanced _____, eg, Potential for Enhanced Parenting. Related factors are not present for wellness nursing diagnoses because they would all be the same: motivated to achieve a higher level of wellness. Syndrome diagnoses, such as Rape Trauma Syndrome, have no "related to" designations.

Two-Part Statements

Risk and possible nursing diagnoses have two parts. The validation for a risk nursing diagnosis is the presence of risk factors. The risk factors are the second part, as in:

Risk nursing diagnosis related to risk factors

Possible nursing diagnoses are suspected because of the presence of certain factors. The nurse then either rules out or confirms the existence of an actual or a risk diagnosis.

The following are examples of two-part statements:

Risk for Impaired Skin Integrity related to immobility secondary to fractured hip
Possible Self-Care Deficit related to impaired ability to use left hand secondary to IV

Designating a diagnosis as possible provides the nurse with a method to communicate to other nurses that a diagnosis may be present. Additional data collection is indicated to rule out or confirm the tentative diagnosis.

Three-Part Statements

An actual nursing diagnosis consists of three parts.

Diagnostic label + contributing factors
+ signs and symptoms

The presence of major signs and symptoms (defining characteristics) validates that an actual diagnosis is present. It is not possible to have a third part for risk or possible diagnoses because signs and symptoms do not exist.

The following are examples of three-part statements:

Anxiety related to unpredictable nature of asthmatic episodes as evident by statements of "I'm afraid I won't be able to breathe"

Urge Incontinence related to diminished bladder capacity secondary to habitual frequent voiding evident by inability to
hold off urination after desire to void and report of voiding
out of habit, not need

The presence of a nursing diagnosis is determined by assessing
the individual's health status and ability to function. To guide the
nurse who is gathering this information, a Screening Assessment
Tool is included in the Appendix at the end of the book. This
guide directs the nurse to collect data according to the individual's functional health patterns. Functional health patterns and the
corresponding nursing diagnoses are listed in Table 1. If significant data are collected in a particular functional pattern, the next
step is to check the related nursing diagnoses to see if any of them
are substantiated by the data that are collected.

Client Validation

The process of validating a nursing diagnosis should not be done
in isolation from the client or family. Individuals are the experts
on themselves. During assessments and interactions, nurses are
provided a small glimpse of their clients. Diagnostic hunches or
inferences about data should be discussed with clients for their
input. Clients are given opportunities to select what they want assistance with, which problems are important to them, and which
ones are not.

Clinical Example

After the screening assessment has been completed, the nurse applies each of these questions to each functional or need area:

- Is there a possible problem in a specific area?
- Is the person at risk (or high risk) for a problem?
- Does the person desire to improve his/her health?

For example, after assessing a client's elimination pattern or
need, the nurse would then analyze the data. Does this person
have a possible problem with constipation or diarrhea? If yes, the
nurse would then ask the person more focused questions to confirm the presence of the defining characteristics of constipation or
diarrhea. If these defining characteristics are not present, then
there is no actual diagnosis of Constipation or Diarrhea. Is there a
risk diagnosis? To determine this, the nurse will assess for risk
factors of constipation or diarrhea (listed under related/risk factors). If none of these are present there is no risk for constipation
or diarrhea.

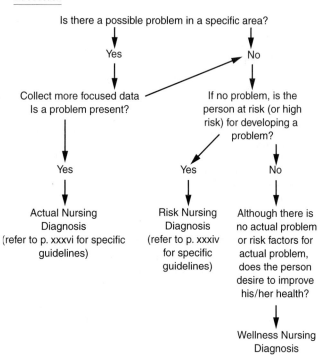

Is there a possible problem in a specific area?

Yes → No

Collect more focused data
Is a problem present?

If no problem, is the person at risk (or high risk) for developing a problem?

Yes → Yes → No

Actual Nursing Diagnosis (refer to p. xxxvi for specific guidelines)

Risk Nursing Diagnosis (refer to p. xxxiv for specific guidelines)

Although there is no actual problem or risk factors for actual problem, does the person desire to improve his/her health?

Wellness Nursing Diagnosis

Lastly, if there is no actual or at risk elimination nursing diagnosis, the nurse can ask if the individual would like to improve his or her elimination patterns. If the answer is yes, the wellness diagnosis Potential for Enhanced Elimination is the appropriate choice.

Actual Nursing Diagnoses

Actual nursing diagnoses are written in two or three part statements:

1st part	*2nd part*	*3rd part*
Diagnostic Label	related to *factors that have caused or contributed*	as evident by *signs & symptoms in the individual that indicate the diagnosis is present*

xxxvi

Now that the defining characteristics have been confirmed to be present in the individual, you have:

Label:	Constipation
Causative/contributing factors:	related to inadequate fiber and fluid intake
Signs/symptoms: (defining characteristics)	as evident from reports of dry, hard stools, q 3–4 days

Clinical Example

As part of the screening assessment under nutrition you elicit:

Usual food intake	Usual fluid intake
Weight/height ratio	Current weight
Appearance of skin, nails, hair	

You then analyze the data to determine which data are within a normal range, and which are not.

Are there sufficient servings of 5 food groups?
Is there sufficient intake of calcium, protein, and vitamins?
Is the fat intake <30% of total caloric intake?
Does the person drink at least 6–8 cups of fluid besides coffee or soft drinks?
Does the appearance of skin, hair, and nails reflect a healthy nutrition pattern?
Is the person's weight within normal limits for height?

For example, in a specific person, Mr. Jewel, you find there is:

Appropriate weight for height
Insufficient fluid intake (4-8 oz. glasses of water/juice)
Insufficient vegetable intake (2 servings)
Insufficient bread, cereal, rice, pasta intake (4 servings)
Dry skin and hair

From your assessment, you have confirmed that a nursing diagnosis is present because the person has signs or reports symptoms that represent those listed as defining characteristics under that specific diagnosis. These are usually the person's complaints.

At this point you have two parts of the diagnostic statement—the first and third but not the second:

Altered Nutrition: less than body requirement related to _____, as evident from dry skin and hair, dietary intake (low in fiber, vegetables, complex CHO and fluids)

Now you want to determine what has caused or contributed to Mr. Jewel's Altered Nutrition. Look at the list of related factors or risk factors under Altered Nutrition. Do any relate to Mr. Jewel's situation? Does Mr. Jewel think his diet is inadequate? If he says no, "lack of knowledge" would be the third part of your diagnostic statement. If he says yes, but it is not important to him to change his habits at his age, you will need to dialogue with him. Perhaps he has a problem with constipation or energy. Maybe a change of diet could help. When you are assured that Mr. Jewel understands the reasons for a balanced diet, but see that he has decided to continue his present diet, record his decision and your attempts to influence that decision.

SELECT PRIORITY SET OF DIAGNOSES

Key Concepts

Priority criteria
Use of consultants/referrals

Priority Criteria

Nurses cannot treat all the nursing diagnoses and collaborative problems that an individual client, family, or community has. Attempts to do this will result in frustration for the nurse and the client. By identifying a priority set—a group of nursing diagnoses and collaborative problems that take precedence over other nursing diagnoses or collaborative problems—the nurse can best direct resources toward goal achievement. It is useful to differentiate priority diagnoses from those that are important, but not priority.

Priority diagnoses are those nursing diagnoses or collaborative problems that, if not managed now, will deter progress to achieve outcomes or will negatively affect the client's functional status.

Important diagnoses are those nursing diagnoses or collaborative problems for which treatment can be delayed to a later time without compromising present functional status.

How does the nurse identify a priority set? In an acute-care setting, the client enters the hospital for a specific purpose, such as surgery or other treatments for acute illness.

- What are the nursing diagnoses or collaborative problems associated with the primary condition or treatments (eg, surgery)?
- Are there additional collaborative problems associated with coexisting medical conditions that require monitoring (eg, hypoglycemia)?
- Are there additional nursing diagnoses that, if not managed now, will deter recovery or affect the client's functional status (eg, High Risk for Constipation)?
- What problems does the client perceive as priority?

Use of Consultants/Referrals

How are other diagnoses not on the diagnostic cluster selected for a client's problem list? Limited nursing resources and increasingly reduced client care time mandate that nurses identify important nursing diagnoses that can be addressed at a later time and do not need to be included on the client's problem list. For example, for a client hospitalized after myocardial infarction who is 50 lbs. overweight, the nurse would want to explain the effects of obesity on cardiac function and refer the client to community resources for a weight reduction program after discharge. The discharge summary record would reflect the teaching and the referral; a nursing diagnosis related to weight reduction would not need to appear on the client's problem list.

SUMMARY

Making accurate nursing diagnoses takes knowledge and practice. If the nurse uses a systematic approach to nursing diagnosis validation, then accuracy will increase. The process of making nursing diagnoses is difficult because nurses are attempting to diagnose human responses. Humans are unique, complex, and ever-changing, thus attempts to classify these responses have been laborious.

References

Alfaro-LeFevre, R. (1999). *Applying nursing diagnosis and nursing process: A step-by-step guide* (4th ed.) Philadelphia: J.B. Lippincott.

American Nurse's Association (1985). *A Nursing Social Policy Statement*. Washington DC: ANA.

Carpenito, L.J. (1983). *Nursing diagnosis: Application to clinical practice*. Philadelphia: J.B. Lippincott.

Carpenito, L.J. (1999). *Nursing diagnosis: Application to clinical practice* (8th ed.) Philadelphia: Lippincott Williams & Wilkins.

North American Nursing Diagnosis Association (1998–1999). *Taxonomy I* (rev. ed.). Philadelphia: NANDA.

TABLE 1.
Conditions That Necessitate Nursing Care

NURSING DIAGNOSES*
1. **Health Perception–Health Management**
   Energy Field Disturbance
   Growth and Development, Altered
     Adult Failure to Thrive
     Growth, Risk for Altered
     Development, Risk for Altered
   Health Maintenance, Altered
   Surgical Recovery, Delayed
   Health Seeking Behaviors
   Injury, Risk for
     Risk for Suffocation
     Risk for Poisoning
     Risk for Trauma
   Injury, Risk for Perioperative Positioning
   Management of Therapeutic Regimen, Effective
   Management of Therapeutic Regimen, Ineffective
   Management of Therapeutic Regimen, Ineffective: Family
   Management of Therapeutic Regimen, Ineffective:
     Community
   Noncompliance
2. **Nutritional–Metabolic**
   Adaptive Capacity, Decreased: Intracranial
   Body Temperature, High Risk for Altered
     Hypothermia
     Hyperthermia
     Thermoregulation, Ineffective
   Breastfeeding, Effective
   Breastfeeding, Ineffective
   Breastfeeding, Interrupted
   Fluid Volume Deficit
   Fluid Volume Excess
   Fluid Volume Imbalance, Risk for
   Infection, Risk for
   ‡Infection Transmission, Risk for
   Latex Allergy
     Latex Allergy, Risk for
   Nutrition, Altered: Less Than Body Requirements
   Nutrition, Altered: More Than Body Requirements

(Continued)

TABLE 1. *(Continued)*

Nutrition, Altered: Potential for More Than Body
Requirements
Dentition, Altered
Feeding Pattern, Ineffective Infant
Swallowing, Impaired
Protection, Altered
Tissue Integrity, Impaired
Oral Mucous Membrane, Altered
Skin Integrity, Impaired

3. Elimination
Bowel Incontinence
Constipation
Constipation, Risk for
Perceived Constipation
Diarrhea
Urinary Elimination, Altered Patterns of
Urinary Retention
Total Incontinence
Functional Incontinence
Reflex Incontinence
Urge Incontinence
Urge Incontinence, Risk for
Stress Incontinence
‡Maturational Enuresis

4. Activity–Exercise
Activity Intolerance
Cardiac Output, Decreased
Disuse Syndrome
Diversional Activity Deficit
Home Maintenance Management, Impaired
Infant Behavior, Disorganized
Infant Behavior, Risk for Disorganized
Infant Behavior, Potential for Enhanced Organized
Mobility, Impaired Physical
Bed Mobility, Impaired
Walking, Impaired
Wheelchair Mobility, Impaired
Wheelchair Transfer Ability, Impaired
Peripheral Neurovascular Dysfunction, Risk for

(Continued)

TABLE 1. *(Continued)*

Respiratory Function, Risk for Altered
  Dysfunctional Ventilatory Weaning Response
  Ineffective Airway Clearance
  Ineffective Breathing Patterns
  Impaired Gas Exchange
  Ventilation, Inability to Sustain Spontaneous
‡Self-Care Deficit Syndrome (Specify): (Feeding, Bathing/
  Hygiene, Dressing/Grooming, Toileting, ‡Instrumental)
Tissue Perfusion, Altered: (Specify) (Cerebral,
  Cardiopulmonary, Renal, Gastrointestinal, Peripheral)

5. **Sleep–Rest**
   Sleep Pattern Disturbance
   Sleep Deprivation

6. **Cognitive–Perceptual**
   Aspiration, Risk for
   ‡Comfort, Altered
       Acute Pain
       Chronic Pain
       Pain
       Nausea
   ‡Confusion
       Acute Confusion
       Chronic Confusion
   Decisional Conflict
   Dysreflexia
       Dysreflexia, Risk for
   Environmental Interpretation Syndrome, Impaired
   Knowledge Deficit: (Specify)
   Risk for Aspiration
   Sensory–Perceptual Alteration: (Specify) (Visual, Auditory,
       Kinesthetic, Gustatory, Tactile, Olfactory)
   Thought Processes, Altered
   Unilateral Neglect

7. **Self-Perception**
   Anxiety
   Death Anxiety
   Fatigue
   Fear
   Hopelessness
   Powerlessness

(Continued)

TABLE 1. *(Continued)*

Self-Concept Disturbance
Body Image Disturbance
Personal Identity Disturbance
Self-Esteem Disturbance
Chronic Low Self-Esteem
Situational Low Self-Esteem

8. **Role–Relationship**
‡Communication, Impaired
Communication, Impaired Verbal
Family Processes, Altered
Family Processes, Altered: Alcoholism
Grieving
Grieving, Anticipatory
Grieving, Dysfunctional
Chronic Sorrow
Loneliness, Risk for
Parent/Infant/Child Attachment, Risk for Altered
Parenting, Altered
Parental Role Conflict
Role Performance, Altered
Social Interaction, Impaired
Social Isolation

9. **Sexuality–Reproductive**
Sexual Dysfunction
Sexuality Patterns, Altered

10. **Coping–Stress Tolerance**
Adjustment, Impaired
Caregiver Role Strain
Coping, Ineffective Individual
Defensive Coping
Ineffective Denial
Coping, Ineffective Family: Disabling
Coping, Ineffective Family: Compromised
Coping, Family: Potential for Growth
Coping, Ineffective Community
Coping, Potential for Enhanced Community
Post-Trauma Response
Post-Trauma Syndrome, Risk for
Rape Trauma Syndrome
Relocation Stress Syndrome

(Continued)

TABLE 1. *(Continued)*

    ‡Self-Harm, Risk for:
      ‡Self-Abuse, Risk for
       Self-Mutilation, Risk for
      ‡Suicide, Risk for
     Violence, Risk for

11. Value–Belief
    Spiritual Distress
     Spiritual Distress, Risk for
    Spiritual Well Being, Potential for Enhanced

§ COLLABORATIVE PROBLEMS

Potential Complication: Cardiac/Vascular

   PC: Decreased Cardiac Output
   PC: Dysrhythmias
   PC: Pulmonary Edema
   PC: Cardiogenic Shock
   PC: Thromboembolic/Deep Vein Thrombosis
   PC: Hypovolemia
   PC: Peripheral Vascular Insufficiency
   PC: Hypertension
   PC: Congenital Heart Disease
   PC: Angina
   PC: Endocarditis
   PC: Pulmonary Embolism
   PC: Spinal Shock
   PC: Ischemic Ulcers

Potential Complication: Respiratory

   PC: Hypoxemia
   PC: Atelectasis/Pneumonia
   PC: Tracheobronchial Constriction
   PC: Pleural Effusion
   PC: Tracheal Necrosis
   PC: Ventilator Dependency
   PC: Pneumothorax
   PC: Laryngeal Edema

(Continued)

TABLE 1. *(Continued)*

Potential Complication: Renal/Urinary

- PC: Acute Urinary Retention
- PC: Renal Failure
- PC: Bladder Perforation
- PC: Renal Calculi

Potential Complication: Gastrointestinal/Hepatic/Biliary

- PC: Paralytic Ileus/Small Bowel Obstruction
- PC: Hepatic Failure
- PC: Hyperbilirubinemia
- PC: Evisceration
- PC: Hepatosplenomegaly
- PC: Curling's Ulcer
- PC: Ascites
- PC: Gastrointestinal Bleeding

Potential Complication: Metabolic/Immune/Hematopoietic

- PC: Hypoglycemia/Hyperglycemia
- PC: Negative Nitrogen Balance
- PC: Electrolyte Imbalances
- PC: Thyroid Dysfunction
- PC: Hypothermia (Severe)
- PC: Hyperthermia (Severe)
- PC: Sepsis
- PC: Acidosis (Metabolic, Respiratory)
- PC: Alkalosis (Metabolic, Respiratory)
- PC: Hypo/Hyperthyroidism
- PC: Allergic Reaction
- PC: Donor Tissue Rejection
- PC: Adrenal Insufficiency
- PC: Anemia
- PC: Thrombocytopenia
- PC: Opportunistic Infection
- PC: Polycythemia
- PC: Sickling Crisis
- PC: Disseminated Intravascular Coagulation

(Continued)

TABLE 1. *(Continued)*

Potential Complication: Neurological/Sensory

- PC: Increased Intracranial Pressure
- PC: Stroke
- PC: Seizures
- PC: Spinal Cord Compression
- PC: Meningitis
- PC: Cranial Nerve Impairment (Specify)
- PC: Paralysis
- PC: Peripheral Nerve Impairment
- PC: Increased Intraocular Pressure
- PC: Corneal Ulceration
- PC: Neuropathies

Potential Complication: Muscular/Skeletal

- PC: Osteoporosis
- PC: Joint Dislocation
- PC: Compartmental Syndrome
- PC: Pathological Fractures

Potential Complication: Reproductive

- PC: Fetal Distress
- PC: Postpartum Hemorrhage
- PC: Pregnancy-Associated Hypertension
- PC: Hypermenorrhea
- PC: Polymenorrhea
- PC: Syphilis
- PC: Prenatal Bleeding
- PC: Preterm Labor

Potential Complication: Multisystem

- PC: Medication Therapy Adverse Effects
    - PC: Adrenocorticosteroids Therapy Adverse Effects
    - PC: Antianxiety Therapy Adverse Effects
    - PC: Antiarrhythmia Therapy Adverse Effects
    - PC: Anticoagulant therapy Adverse Effects
    - PC: Anticonvulsant Therapy Adverse Effects
    - PC: Antidepressant Therapy Adverse Effects

(Continued)

TABLE 1. *(Continued)*

PC: Antihypertensive Therapy Adverse Effects
   PC: Beta-Adrenergic Blockers Therapy Adverse Effects
   PC: Calcium Channel Blockers Therapy Adverse Effects
   PC: Angiotensin-Converting Enzyme Therapy Adverse Effects
PC: Antineoplastic Therapy Adverse Effects
PC: Antipsychotic Therapy Adverse Effects

---

* The Functional Health Patterns were identified in Gordon, M. (1982). *Nursing diagnosis: Process and application.* New York: McGraw-Hill, with minor changes by the author.

‡ These diagnoses are not currently on the NANDA list but have been included for clarity and usefulness.

§ Frequently used collaborative problem are represented on this list. Other situations not listed here could qualify as collaborative problems.

HANDBOOK OF

Nursing Diagnosis

8TH EDITION

Section I

Nursing Diagnoses

Activity Intolerance

DEFINITION

Activity Intolerance: A reduction in one's physiological capacity to endure activities to the degree desired or required (Magnan, 1987).

DEFINING CHARACTERISTICS

Major (Must Be Present, One or More) (Magnan, 1995)

During activity
  Weakness
  Dizziness
  Dyspnea
Three minutes after activity
  Dizziness
  Dyspnea
  Exertional fatigue
  Respiratory rate >24
  Pulse rate >95

Minor (May Be Present)

Pallor or cyanosis
Confusion
Vertigo

RELATED FACTORS

Any factors that compromise oxygen transport, lead to physical deconditioning, or create excessive energy demands that outstrip the person's physical and psychological abilities can cause Activity Intolerance. Some common factors are listed below.

Pathophysiological

Related to compromised oxygen transport system secondary
  to:
   (Cardiac)

Idiopathic hypertrophic subaortic stenosis	Dysrhythmias
	Angina
Congenital heart disease	Myocardial infarction
Cardiomyopathies	Valvular disease
Congestive heart failure	

   (Respiratory)

Chronic obstructive pulmonary disease	Atelectasis
	Bronchopulmonary dysplasia

   (Circulatory)

Anemia	Hypovolemia
Peripheral arterial disease	

Related to increased metabolic demands secondary to:
  (Acute or chronic infection)

Viral infection	Hepatitis
Mononucleosis	

  (Endocrine or metabolic disorders)
  (Chronic diseases)

Renal	Inflammatory
Hepatic	Musculoskeletal
Cancer	Neurological

Related to inadequate energy sources secondary to:

Obesity	Inadequate diet
Malnourishment	

Related to compromised oxygen transport secondary to
  Hypovolemia

Treatment-Related

Related to increased metabolic demands secondary to:

Surgery	Treatment schedule/
Diagnostic studies	treatments (frequency)

Situational (Personal, Environmental)

Related to the deconditioning effects of bed rest

Related to inactivity secondary to depression, lack of motivation, sedentary lifestyle

Related to increased metabolic demands secondary to:
    Assistive equipment (walkers, crutches, braces)
    Extreme stress
    Pain
    Environmental barriers (*e.g.*, stairs)
    Climatic extremes (especially hot, humid climates)

Related to decreased available oxygen secondary to atmospheric pressure (*e.g.*, recent relocation to high-altitude living)

Maturational

The elderly may experience decreased muscle strength and flexibility and sensory deficits. All of these can undermine body confidence and may contribute directly or indirectly to Activity Intolerance.

OUTCOME CRITERIA

The person will:

1. Identify factors that reduce activity tolerance
2. Progress to (specify the highest level of mobility possible)
3. Exhibit a decrease in hypoxic signs of increased activity (pulse, blood pressure, respirations)
4. Report a reduction of symptoms of Activity Intolerance

⊞ GENERIC INTERVENTIONS

1. Assess the individual's response to activity.
   a. Take resting pulse, blood pressure, and respirations.
   b. Consider rate, rhythm, and quality (if signs are abnormal—*e.g.,* pulse above 100—consult with physician about the advisability of increasing activity).
   c. Take vital signs immediately after activity; take pulse for 15 seconds and multiply by 4 instead of for 1 full minute.

      d. Have person rest for 3 minutes; take vital signs again.

      e. Discontinue the activity if the client responds to the activity with:

- Complaints of chest pain, dyspnea, vertigo, or confusion
- Decrease in pulse rate
- Failure of systolic rate to increase
- Decrease in systolic blood pressure
- Increase in diastolic rate 15 mm Hg
- Decrease in respiratory rate

      f. Reduce the intensity, frequency, or duration of the activity if:

- The pulse takes longer than 3 to 4 minutes to return within 6 beats of the resting pulse rate
- The respiratory rate increase is excessive after the activity
- Other signs of hypoxia are present (*e.g.*, confusion, vertigo)

2. Progress the activity gradually.

      a. For a person who is or has been on prolonged bed rest, begin range of motion (ROM) at least b.i.d.

      b. Plan rest periods according to the person's daily schedule (rest periods may occur between activities).

      c. Promote a sincere "can do" attitude to provide a positive atmosphere to encourage increased activity; convey to clients the belief that they can improve their mobility status. Acknowledge progress.

      d. Allow person to set activity schedule and functional activity goals (if the goal is too low, make a contract: *e.g.,* "If you walk halfway up the hall, I will play a game of cards with you.").

      e. Increase tolerance for the activity by having the client perform the activity more slowly, for a shorter period with more rest pauses, or with more assistance.

      f. Gradually increase exercise tolerance by increasing the time out of bed by 15 minutes each day, three times a day.

      g. Allow person to gauge the rate of the ambulation.

      h. Encourage person to wear comfortable walking shoes (slippers do not support the feet properly).

3. Teach energy conservation methods for activities.
   a. Take rest periods during activities, at intervals during the day, and 1 hour after meals.
   b. Sit rather than stand when performing activities, unless this is not feasible.
   c. When performing a task, rest every 3 minutes for 5 minutes to allow the heart to recover.
   d. Stop an activity if fatigue or signs of cardiac hypoxia are present (↑ pulse, dyspnea, chest pain).
4. Instruct the person to consult his or her physician and physiatrist for a long-term exercise program or to contact the American Heart Association for names of cardiac rehabilitation programs.
5. For persons with chronic pulmonary insufficiency:
   a. Encourage conscious controlled-breathing techniques during increased activity and times of emotional and physical stress (techniques include pursed-lip and diaphragmatic breathing).
   b. For pursed-lip breathing, the person should breathe in through the nose, then slowly breathe out through partially closed lips while counting to seven and making a "pu" sound (often this is learned naturally by person with progressive lung disease).
   c. Teach diaphragmatic breathing.
      • The nurse should place hands on the person's abdomen below the base of the ribs and keep them there while the client inhales.
      • To inhale, the person should relax the shoulders, breathe in through the nose, and push the stomach outward against the nurse's hands, holding breath for 1 to 2 seconds to keep the alveoli open.
      • To exhale, the person should breathe out slowly through the mouth while the nurse applies slight pressure at the base of the ribs.
      • Practice several times; then have the person place his or her own hands at the base of the ribs and practice independently.
      • Instruct to practice this exercise a few times each hour.
   d. Encourage gradual increase in daily activity to prevent "pulmonary crippling."
   e. Encourage person to use adaptive breathing techniques to decrease the work of breathing.

    f. Discuss physical barriers at home and at work (*e.g.*, number of stairs) and ways of alternating expenditure of energy with rest pauses (place a chair in bathroom near sink to rest during daily hygiene).

    g. Explain the importance of supporting arm weight to reduce the work of respiratory muscles (Breslin, 1992).

    h. Teach how to increase unsupported arm endurance with lower extremity exercises performed during exhalation phase of respiration (Breslin, 1992).

6. Refer to community nurse for follow-up if needed.

CHILD FOCUS INTERVENTIONS

1. Provide age-appropriate games and activities that are quiet and challenging:

    Sensory adventures (What does the hospital smell, sound, or look like?)

    Telling and writing stores, creating collages, playing with puppets, play acting

MATERNAL FOCUS INTERVENTIONS

1. Explain the causes of fatigue and dyspnea in mid to late pregnancy:

    Changes in center of gravity

    Increased weight

    Pressure of enlarged uterus on diaphragm

2. Teach energy conservation methods (refer to Generic Interventions).

Adaptive Capacity, Decreased: Intracranial

DEFINITION

Decreased Adaptive Capacity: Intracranial: A clinical state in which intracranial fluid dynamic mechanisms that normally compensate for increases in intracranial volumes are compromised, resulting in repeated disproportionate increases in intracranial pressure in response to a variety of noxious and non-noxious stimuli.

> **Author's Note:**
> This diagnosis represents increased intracranial pressure. It is a collaborative problem because it requires two disciplines to treat—nursing and medicine. In addition, it requires invasive monitoring for diagnosis. The collaborative problem, Potential Complication: Increased Intracranial Pressure, represents this clinical situation.

DEFINING CHARACTERISTICS

Major (Must Be Present)

Repeated increases in intracranial pressure (ICP) of >10 mm Hg for more than 5 minutes following any of a variety of external stimuli

Minor (May Be Present)

Disproportionate increase in ICP following a single environmental or nursing maneuver stimulus
Elevated P_2 ICP waveform
Volume pressure response test variation (volume–pressure ratio >2; pressure–volume index <10)
Baseline ICP ≥10 mm Hg
Wide-amplitude ICP waveform

Adjustment, Impaired

DEFINITION

Impaired Adjustment: The state in which an individual is unable to modify his or her lifestyle or behavior in a manner consistent with a change in health status.

Author's Note:
This diagnosis has presented problems in clinical use because of its lack of specificity. Generally speaking, are not most diagnoses a problem with adjustment? It is not clinically useful to have such a general diagnosis. The responses to illness and disabilities will be varied, and the nurse must clarify the response to be most helpful with treatment. Responses can be Grieving, Anxiety, Fear, and Ineffective Coping.

If a client is attempting to manage the changes the illness or disability has caused but is having difficulty, the diagnosis Ineffective Management of Therapeutic Regimen would be more useful.

DEFINING CHARACTERISTICS

Major (Must Be Present)

Verbalization of nonacceptance of health status change or inability to be involved in problem solving or goal setting

Minor (May Be Present)

Lack of movement toward independence; extended period of shock, disbelief, or anger concerning health status change; lack of future-oriented thinking

Anxiety

Death Anxiety

Anxiety

DEFINITION

Anxiety: The state in which an individual or group experiences feelings of uneasiness (apprehension) and activation of the autonomic nervous system in response to a vague, nonspecific threat.

Author's Note:
Anxiety is a vague feeling of apprehension and uneasiness due to a threat to one's value system or security pattern (May, 1987). The individual may be able to identify the situation (*e.g.*, surgery, cancer), but in actuality, the threat to self relates to the uneasiness and apprehension enmeshed in the situation. The situation is the source of the threats, but it is not the threat.

In contrast, fear is the feeling of apprehension to a specific threat or danger to which one's security patterns alert one (*e.g.*, flying, heights, snakes). When the threat is removed, the fearful feeling dissipates (May, 1987).

Fear can exist without anxiety, and anxiety can be present without fear. Clinically, both may coexist in a person's response to a situation. An individual who is facing surgery may be fearful of pain and anxious of a possible cancer diagnosis.

DEFINING CHARACTERISTICS

Major (Must Be Present)(Adams et al, 1997)

Manifested by symptoms from three categories: physiological, emotional, and cognitive; symptoms vary according to the level of anxiety.

Physiologic

Increased heart rate
Elevated blood pressure
Increased respiratory rate
Diaphoresis
Dilated pupils
Voice tremors/pitch changes
Trembling, twitching
Palpitations
Nausea or vomiting
Frequent urination
Diarrhea

Insomnia
Fatigue and weakness
Flushing or pallor
Dry mouth
Body aches and pains
 (especially chest, back, neck)
Restlessness
Faintness/dizziness
Paresthesias
Hot and cold flashes
Anorexia

Emotional

Person states that he has feelings of
 Apprehension
 Helplessness

Losing control
Tension or being "keyed up"

Nervousness
Lack of self-confidence
Person exhibits
Irritability/impatience
Angry outbursts
Crying
Tendency to blame others
Startle reaction

Inability to relax
Anticipation of misfortune

Criticism of self and others
Withdrawal
Lack of initiative
Self-deprecation
Poor eye contact

Cognitive

Inability to concentrate
Lack of awareness of
surroundings
Forgetfulness
Rumination
Orientation to past rather
than to present or future

Blocking of thoughts
(inability to remember)
Hyperattentiveness
Preoccupation
Diminished learning ability
Confusion

RELATED FACTORS

Pathophysiological

Any factor that interferes with the basic human needs for food,
air, comfort, and security

Situational (Personal, Environmental)

Related to actual or perceived threat to self-concept secondary
to:
Change in status and
prestige
Failure (or success)
Lack of recognition from
others

Loss of valued possessions
Ethical dilemma

Related to actual or perceived loss of significant others
secondary to:
Death
Divorce
Cultural pressures

Moving
Temporary or permanent
separation

Related to actual or perceived threat to biological integrity
secondary to:
Dying
Assault

Invasive procedures
Disease

Related to actual or perceived change in environment secondary to:

Hospitalization	Safety hazards
Moving	Environmental pollutants
Retirement	

Related to actual or perceived change in socioeconomic status secondary to: for example, unemployment, new job, promotion

Related to transmission of another person's anxiety to the individual

Maturational

Infant/child

Related to separation	Related to changes in
Related to unfamiliar	peer relationships
environment or persons	

Adolescent

Related to threat to self-concept secondary to: for example, sexual development, peer relationship changes

Adult

Related to threat to self-concept or role status secondary to:

Pregnancy	Career changes
Parenting	Effects of aging

Older adult

Related to threat to self-concept or role status secondary to:

Sensory losses	Financial problems
Motor losses	Retirement changes

OUTCOME CRITERIA

The person will:

1. Describe his or her own anxiety and coping patterns
2. Relate an increase in psychological and physiological comfort
3. Use effective coping mechanisms in managing anxiety, as evidenced by (specify)

⊞ GENERIC INTERVENTIONS

1. Assess level of anxiety: mild, moderate, severe, panic.
2. Provide reassurance and comfort.
   a. Stay with the person.

    b. Do not make demands or ask the person to make decisions. Sit in front of person.

    c. Emphasize that all people feel anxious from time to time.

    d. Speak slowly and calmly, using short, simple sentences. Sit in front of person.

    e. Be aware of your own concern and avoid reciprocal anxiety.

    f. Convey a sense of empathic understanding (*e.g.*, quiet presence, touch, allowing crying, talking).

3. Remove excess stimulation (*e.g.*, take person to quieter room); limit contact with others—clients or family—who are also anxious.

4. When anxiety is diminished enough for learning to take place, assist person in recognizing the anxiety to initiate learning or problem solving.

    a. Encourage the person to keep a diary (*e.g.*, when they felt anxious, what were they doing or thinking? Who was with them?)

    b. Assist to analyze diary to identify triggers.

    c. Explore what alternative behaviors might have been used if coping mechanisms were maladaptive (*e.g.*, assertiveness training).

5. Teach anxiety interrupters to use when stressful situations cannot be avoided (Grainger, 1990):

    a. Look up

    b. Control breathing

    c. Lower shoulders

    d. Slow thoughts

    e. Alter voice

    f. Give self-directions (out loud, if possible)

    g. Exercise

    h. "Scruff your face"—change facial expression

    i. Change perspective—imagine watching the situation from a distance

6. Assist person with anger (Thomas, 1989).

    a. Identify the presence of anger (*e.g.*, feelings of frustration, anxiety, helplessness, presence of irritability, verbal outbursts).

    b. Recognize your reactions to client's behavior; be aware of your own feelings when working with angry individuals.

    c. Do not interrupt; listen to grievance.

      d. Encourage alternative problem solving if expectations are not realistic or possible (*e.g.*, What can you do differently?).

      e. Provide positive validation if possible.

      f. Focus on what can be done, not what was not done.

      g. Explore consequences of explosive anger.

      h. Elicit alternative behavior to violent behavior (*e.g.*, What could you do instead of punching the wall?).

      i. Use "time-out" when needed (*e.g.*, "I can see that we are not accomplishing anything, let us try again when we are both less emotional.").

      j. State limits clearly; tell person exactly what is expected (*e.g.*, "I cannot allow you to scream" [throw objects, etc.]).

      k. When stating an unacceptable behavior, give an alternative (*e.g.*, suggest a quiet room, physical exertion, a chance for one-to-one communication).

      l. Develop behavior modification strategies; discuss with all personnel involved for consistency.

      m. Interact with the person when he or she is not demanding or manipulative.

7. Explore interventions that decrease anxiety (*e.g.*, music, aromatherapy, relaxation exercises, guided imagery, thought-stopping, massage)(Fishel, 1998).

8. If appropriate, provide activities that can reduce tension (*e.g.*, physical activity, games).

9. For persons identified as having chronic anxiety and maladaptive coping mechanisms, refer for psychiatric evaluation.

❧ CHILD FOCUS INTERVENTIONS

1. Explain events using simple, age-appropriate terms and illustrations, puppets, dolls, and sample equipment.

2. Allow child to wear underwear and have familiar toys or objects.

3. Assist parents or caregivers to manage their anxiety when with child.

4. Use the following nursing interventions to help children cope with anxiety:

      a. Establish a trusting relationship.

      b. Minimize separation from parents.

      c. Encourage expression of feelings.

    d. Involve the child in play.
    e. Prepare the child for new experiences (*e.g.*, procedures, surgery).
    f. Provide comfort measures.
    g. Allow for regression.
    h. Encourage parental involvement in care.
    i. Allay parental apprehension, and provide parents with information (Wong, 1999).

5. Assist child with anger.
    a. Encourage the child to share his or her anger (*e.g.*, "How did you feel when you had your injection?" "How did you feel when Mary would not play with you?").
    b. Tell the child that being angry is okay (*e.g.*, "I sometimes get angry when I can't have what I want.").
    c. Encourage and allow the child to express anger in acceptable ways (*e.g.*, loud talking or running outside around the house).

MATERNAL FOCUS INTERVENTIONS

1. Explore fears and concerns during each trimester (Reeder, 1997).
    a. First trimester
       • Ambivalence, new role expectations, uncertainty about adequacy
    b. Second trimester
       • Success as a new mother
    c. Third trimester
       • Feels unattractive; fears for own well-being, performance during labor, and well-being of fetus.
2. Help her and her partner identify unrealistic expectations.
3. Acknowledge her anxiety and the normalcy of it.
4. Discuss these concerns with the woman alone, her partner alone, and then together as indicated.

OLDER ADULT FOCUS INTERVENTIONS

1. Explore the person's worries (*e.g.*, financial, security, health, living arrangements, crime, violence).

Death Anxiety

DEFINITION

Death Anxiety: The state in which an individual experiences apprehension, worry, or fear related to death or dying.

Author's Note:

The inclusion of death anxiety in the NANDA Classification creates a diagnostic category with the etiology in the label. This opens the NANDA list to thousands and thousands of diagnostic labels with etiology, such as separation anxiety, divorce anxiety, infidelity anxiety, failure anxiety, and travel anxiety. Many diagnostic labels can take this same path: fear as claustrophobic fear, diarrhea as traveler's diarrhea, decisional conflict as end-of-life decisional conflict.

This author recommends that etiology be deleted in the diagnostic label except for syndrome diagnoses, which require the etiology in the label. Syndrome diagnoses have no "related to" factors.

DEFINING CHARACTERISTICS

Worrying about the impact of one's own death on significant others

Powerless over issues related to dying

Fear of loss of physical and/or mental abilities when dying

Anticipated pain related to dying

Deep sadness

Fear of the process of dying

Concerns of overworking the caregiver as terminal illness incapacitates self

Concern about meeting one's creator or feeling doubtful about the existence of a god or higher being

Total loss of control over any aspect of one's own death

Negative death images or unpleasant thoughts about any event related to death or dying

Fear of delayed demise

Fear of premature death because it prevents the accomplishment of important life goals

RELATED FACTORS

Impending death is the situation that causes this diagnosis. Additional factors can contribute to death anxiety.

Situational (Personal, Environmental)

Related to situational factors (anxiety)
Related to fear of being a burden
Related to fear of unmanageable pain
Related to fear of abandonment
Related to unresolved conflict (family, friends)
Related to fear that one's life lacked meaning
Related to social disengagement
Related to powerlessness and vulnerability

OUTCOME CRITERIA

The person will:

1. Share his or her feelings regarding dying.
2. Identify two methods or activities that diminish anxiety or fears

⬦ GENERIC INTERVENTIONS

1. Allow the person to share his or her perceptions of the situation (*e.g.*, Share with me what you are experiencing).
2. Encourage the person to share his or her conflicts and concerns (*e.g.*, If you could fix something before you die what would it be? What are you most concerned about?).
3. Explore the person's relationship between spirituality and approaching death:
   a. Afterlife beliefs
   b. Search for meaning
   c. Relationship with greater Other
4. Explore the person's interpretation of suffering (*e.g.*, punishment, testing bad luck, nature's course, will of greater Other, denial, redemption).
5. Encourage telling life stories and reminiscing.
6. Discuss leaving a legacy (*e.g.*, donation, personal articles, taped message for survivors).
7. Encourage reflective activities (*e.g.*, personal prayer, meditation, journal writing).

8. Encourage person to return the gift of love to others (*e.g.*, listening, praying for others, sharing personal wisdom gained from illness, creating legacy gifts)(Taylor, 1997).
9. Encourage friends and families to be emotionally and spiritually honest.
10. Explain advance directives and assist in process if desired.

Body Temperature, Risk for Altered

Hypothermia

Hyperthermia

Thermoregulation, Ineffective

Author's Note:

Risk for Altered Body Temperature includes those at risk for Hyperthermia, Hypothermia, or Ineffective Thermoregulation. If the person is at risk for only one of the diagnoses (*e.g.*, Hypothermia but not Hyperthermia), then it is more useful to label the problem with the more specific diagnosis (Risk for Hypothermia). If the person is at risk for two or more of the diagnoses, then Risk for Altered Body Temperature is more appropriate. The focus of nursing care for these diagnoses is that of preventing abnormal body temperatures by identifying and treating those with a normal temperature who demonstrate risk factors that can be controlled by nursing-prescribed interventions (*e.g.*, by removing or adding blankets or by controlling environmental temperature). If the alteration in body temperature is related to a pathophysiological complication that requires nursing and medical interventions, then the problem should be labeled as a collaborative problem (*e.g.*, Potential Complication: Fever related to atelectasis or Potential Complication: Severe Hypothermia related to hypothalamus injury). The focus of concern then becomes monitoring to detect and report significant temperature fluctuations and implementing
(Continued)

Author's Note (Continued)
collaborative interventions (*e.g.*, a warming or cooling blanket) as ordered. (See also diagnostic considerations for *Hyperthermia* and *Hypothermia*.)

Body Temperature, Risk for Altered

DEFINITION

Risk for Altered Body Temperature: The state in which an individual is at risk of failing to maintain body temperature within normal range (36°–37.5°C, or 98°–99.5°F).

RISK FACTORS

Major (Must Be Present, One or More)

Presence of risk factors (see Related Factors)

RELATED FACTORS

Pathophysiological

Related to impaired temperature control secondary to:
  Coma, increased intracranial pressure (ICP)
  Brain tumor, hypothalamic tumor, head trauma
  Cerebrovascular accident (CVA)
  Infection, inflammation
Related to decreased circulation secondary to:
  Anemia
  Neurovascular disease, peripheral vascular disease
Related to decreased ability to sweat secondary to (specify)

Treatment-Related

Related to cooling effects of:
  Parenteral fluid infusion, blood transfusion
  Dialysis
  Cooling blanket
  Operating suite

Situational (Personal, Environmental)

Related to:

Exposure to cold, rain, snow, wind; exposure to heat, sun, humidity extremes
Inappropriate clothing for climate
Inability to pay for shelter, heat, or air-conditioning
Extremes of weight
Consumption of alcohol
Dehydration/malnutrition

Maturational

Related to ineffective temperature regulation secondary to extremes of age (*e.g.*, newborn, older adult)

Hypothermia

DEFINITION

Hypothermia: The state in which an individual has or is at risk of having a sustained reduction of body temperature of below 35.5°C (96°F) rectally because of increased vulnerability to external factors.

DEFINING CHARACTERISTICS*

Major (80%–100%)

Reduction in body temperature below 35.5°C (96°F) rectally
Cool skin
Pallor (moderate)
Shivering (mild)

Minor (50%–79%)

Mental confusion, drowsiness, restlessness
Decreased pulse and respiration
Cachexia, malnutrition

*Adapted from Carroll, S. M. (1989). Nursing diagnosis: Hypothermia. In R. M. Carroll-Johnson (Ed.), *Classification of nursing diagnoses: Proceedings of the eighth conference.* Philadelphia: J.B. Lippincott.

RELATED FACTORS

Situational (Personal, Environmental)

Related to:
    Exposure to cold, rain, snow, wind
    Inappropriate clothing for climate
    Inability to pay for shelter or heat
Related to decreased circulation secondary to:
    Extremes of weight
    Consumption of alcohol
    Dehydration
    Inactivity

Maturational

Related to ineffective temperature regulation secondary to age

OUTCOME CRITERIA

The person will:

1. Identify risk factors for hypothermia
2. Relate methods of maintaining warmth/preventing heat loss
3. Maintain body temperature within normal limits

◆ GENERIC INTERVENTIONS
(for Risk for Hypothermia)

1. Teach client to reduce prolonged exposure to cold environment.
   a. Explain the importance of wearing a hat, gloves, and warm socks and shoes to prevent heat loss.
   b. Encourage the person to limit going outside when temperatures are very cold.
   c. Acquire an electric blanket, warm blankets, or down comforter for bed.
   d. Teach to wear close-knit undergarments to prevent heat loss.
2. Consult with social services to identify sources of financial assistance, warm clothing, blankets.
3. Teach the early signs of hypothermia: cool skin, pallor, blanching, redness.
4. Explain the need to drink 8 to 10 glasses of water daily.
5. Explain the need to avoid alcohol in very cold weather.

6. Teach to wear extra clothing in the morning when metabolism is at lowest point.

🔵 🏛 CHILD/OLDER ADULT FOCUS INTERVENTIONS

1. Explain to family members that newborns, infants, and the elderly are more susceptible to heat loss (see also *Ineffective Thermoregulation*).
2. For children and elderly during intraoperative experience, unless hypothermia is desired to reduce blood loss, consider the following interventions (Burkle, 1988):
   a. Increase ambient temperature of operating room (OR) before case.
   b. Use a portable radiant heating lamp to provide additional heat during surgery.
   c. Cover with warm blankets when arriving in OR.
   d. When possible, use a warming mattress.
   e. During prepping and surgery, keep as much of body surface covered as possible.
   f. Warm prep set, blood, fluids, anesthesia, irrigants.
   g. Replace wet gowns and drapes with dry ones.
   h. Keep head well covered.
   i. Continue heat-conserving interventions postoperatively.

Hyperthermia

DEFINITION

Hyperthermia: The state in which an individual has or is at risk of having a sustained elevation of body temperature greater than 37.8°C (100°F) orally or 38.8°C (101°F) rectally due to external factors.

DEFINING CHARACTERISTICS (Stacy, 1994)

Major (50%–100%)

Temperature greater than 37.8°C (100°F) orally or 38.8°C (101°F) rectally
Warm skin to touch
Tachycardia

Minor (50%–79%)

Flushed skin
Increased respiratory depth
Shivering/goose pimples
Feelings of warmth or
coolness

Specific or generalized aches
and pains (*e.g.*, headache)
Malaise, fatigue, weakness
Loss of appetite
Sweating

RELATED FACTORS

Treatment-Related

Related to reduced ability to sweat secondary to (specify medication)

Situational (Personal, Environmental)

Related to:
Exposure to heat, sun
Inappropriate clothing for
climate

No access to air conditioning

Related to decreased circulation secondary to:
Extremes of weight
Dehydration
Related to insufficient hydration for vigorous activity

Maturational

Related to ineffective temperature regulation secondary to age

OUTCOME CRITERIA

The person will:

1. Identify risk factors for hyperthermia
2. Relate methods of preventing hyperthermia
3. Maintain normal body temperature

◉ GENERIC INTERVENTIONS

(for Risk for Hyperthermia)

1. Teach the person the importance of maintaining an adequate fluid intake (at least 2,000 mL/d unless contraindicated by heart or kidney disease) to prevent dehydration.
2. Monitor intake and output.
3. See also *Fluid Volume Deficit*.

4. Assess whether clothing or bed covers are too warm for the environment or planned activity.

5. Teach the importance of increasing fluid intake during warm weather and exercise.

6. Explain the need to avoid alcohol, caffeine, and large, heavy meals during hot weather.

7. Explain the need to wear:
   a. Loose-fitting clothing
   b. A hat or use an umbrella

8. Avoid outdoor activity between 11 AM and 2 PM.

9. Take cool baths or showers several times a day during heat waves. Do not use soap.

10. Teach the early signs of hyperthermia or heat stroke:
    a. Flushed skin
    b. Headache
    c. Fatigue
    d. Loss of appetite

CHILD FOCUS INTERVENTIONS

1. Determine if fever is drug related (*e.g.*, anticholingergics, amphetamines, epinephrine, acetaminophen [large doses] antihistamines [large doses], phenothiazines).

2. Explain to parents that fever is a protection measure and not harmful unless high (*e.g.*, >41.1°C or 100°F).

3. Caution not to sponge, which causes extreme chilling.

OLDER ADULT FOCUS INTERVENTIONS

Refer to Ineffective Thermoregulation, Older Adult Focus Interventions.

Thermoregulation, Ineffective

DEFINITION

Ineffective Thermoregulation: The state in which an individual experiences or is at risk of experiencing an inability to maintain normal body temperature effectively in the presence of adverse or changing external factors.

Author's Note:

This diagnosis is indicated when the nurse can maintain or assist a client to maintain a body temperature within normal limits by manipulating external factors (*e.g.*, clothing) and environmental conditions. Persons who are at high risk for this diagnosis are the elderly and neonates. For those with temperature fluctuations due to disease, infections, or trauma, see *Altered Comfort*.

DEFINING CHARACTERISTICS

Major (Must Be Present)

Temperature fluctuations related to limited metabolic compensatory regulation in response to environmental factors

RELATED FACTORS

Situational (Personal, Environmental)

Related to:

Fluctuating environmental temperatures	Inadequate housing
	Wet body surface
Cold or wet articles (clothes, cribs, equipment)	Inadequate clothing for weather (excessive, insufficient)

Maturational

Related to limited metabolic compensatory regulation secondary to age (e.g., neonate, older adult)

OUTCOME CRITERIA

The infant will:

1. Have a temperature between 36.4° and 37°C

The parent will:

1. Explain techniques to avoid heat loss at home

🔈 CHILD FOCUS INTERVENTIONS

1. Reduce or eliminate the sources of heat loss in infants.
   a. Evaporation
      - When bathing, provide a warm environment.
      - Wash and dry in sections to reduce evaporation.
      - Limit time in contact with wet clothing or blankets.
   b. Convection
      - Avoid drafts (air conditioning, fans, windows, open portholes on isolette).
   c. Conduction
      - Warm all articles for care (stethoscopes, scales, hands of caregivers, clothes, bed linens).
   d. Radiation
      - Limit objects in the room that absorb heat (metal).
      - Place crib or bed as far away from walls (outside) or windows as possible.
2. Monitor temperature of infants.
   a. If temperature is below normal:
      - Wrap in two blankets.
      - Put on head cap.
      - Assess for environmental sources of heat loss.
      - If hypothermia persists for more than 1 hour, notify physician.
      - Assess for complications of cold stress: hypoxia, respiratory acidosis, hypoglycemia, fluid and electrolyte imbalances, weight loss.
   b. If temperature is above normal:
      - Loosen blanket.
      - Remove cap, if on.
      - Assess environment for thermal gain.
      - If hyperthermia persists for more than 1 hour, notify physician.
3. Assess for signs of sepsis (respiratory function, skin, poor feeding, irritability, signs of localized infections [skin, umbilicus, circumcision, eyes]).
4. Teach caregiver why infant is vulnerable to temperature fluctuations (cold and heat).
   a. Demonstrate how to conserve heat during bathing.

b. Instruct that it is not necessary to check temperature routinely at home.

c. Teach to check temperature if infant is hot, sick, or irritable.

🏛 OLDER ADULT FOCUS INTERVENTIONS

1. Explain age-related changes that interfere with thermoregulation (Miller, 1999).

   a. Cold (inefficient vasoconstriction, decreased cardiac output, decreased subcutaneous tissue, delayed and diminished shivering)

   b. Heat (delayed sweating response, diminished sweating response)

2. Explain that these changes will distort perception of environmental temperatures.

3. Investigate even a slight elevation of temperature. Use tympanic route for temperatures, not oral or axillary.

4. Teach how to prevent hypothermia and hyperthermia (refer to Hypothermia, Hyperthermia).

Bowel Incontinence

DEFINITION

Bowel Incontinence: The state in which an individual experiences a change in normal bowel habits characterized by involuntary passage of stool.

Author's Note:

This diagnosis represents a situation in which nurses have multiple responsibilities. Clients experiencing Bowel Incontinence have various responses that disrupt functioning, such as embarrassment and skin problems related to irritative nature of feces on skin.

For some spinal cord-injured persons, Bowel Incontinence related to lack of voluntary control over rectal sphincter would be descriptive.

DEFINING CHARACTERISTICS

Major (Must Be Present)

Involuntary passage of stool

RELATED FACTORS

Pathophysiological

Related to impaired rectal sphincter secondary to:
   Diabetes mellitus
   Anal or rectal surgery
   Anal or rectal injury
Related to cognitive impairment
Related to overdistension of rectum secondary to chronic constipation or fecal impaction
Related to lack of voluntary sphincter control secondary to:
   Progressive neuromuscular   Spinal cord compression
   disorder   Multiple sclerosis
   Spinal cord injury   CVA
Related to impaired reservoir capacity secondary to:
   Inflammatory bowel disease   Chronic rectal ischemia

Treatment-Related

Related to impaired reservoir capacity secondary to:
   Colectomy
   Radiation proctitis

Situational (Personal, Environmental)

Related to inability to recognize, interpret, or respond to rectal cues secondary to:
   Depression   Cognitive impairment

OUTCOME CRITERIA

The person will:

1. Evacuate a soft, formed stool every day, every other day, or every third day

◆ GENERIC INTERVENTIONS

1. Assess previous bowel elimination patterns, diet, and lifestyle.

2. Determine present neurological and physical status and functional level.
3. Plan a consistent, appropriate time for elimination.
    a. Daily bowel program for 5 days or until a pattern develops, then every-other-day bowel program; morning or evening
4. For persons with intact sacral reflex center:
    a. Position in an upright or sitting position if functionally able. If not functionally able (quadriplegic), position in left side-lying position; use digital stimulation: gloves, lubricant, index finger (adults).
    b. For the functionally able, use assistive devices: dil stick, digital stimulator, raised commode seat, and lubricant and gloves as appropriate.
5. For persons with upper extremity mobility and those with abdominal musculature innervation, teach bowel elimination facilitation techniques as appropriate:
    a. Valsalva's maneuver
    b. Forward bends
    c. Sitting push-ups
    d. Abdominal massage
6. For persons with absent sacral reflex center:
    a. Plan daily evacuation schedule, either morning or evening, with manual evacuation of rectal contents.
    b. Position in upright or sitting position if functionally able.
    c. Use assistive devices, raised commode seats, and lubricant as appropriate.
    d. Teach bowel facilitation techniques:
        • Valsalva's maneuver
        • Forward bends
        • Abdominal massage
        • Sitting push-ups if person is functionally able
7. For persons with decreased reservoir capacity, try to reduce stool volume by (Maas, 1990):
    a. Avoiding foods that provide a laxative effect
    b. Avoiding gas-producing foods
    c. Restricting fiber in diet
8. Maintain an elimination record of bowel schedule to include time, stool results, method(s) used, and number of involuntary stools if any.
9. Teach the importance of diet high in fiber and optimal fluid intake.

10. Cleanse skin after each bowel movement. Protect intact skin with an ointment (*e.g.*, aluminum paste). If skin is not intact, consult clinical nurse specialist or enterostomal therapist.
11. Provide physical activity and exercise appropriate to functional level (*e.g.*, abdominal exercises, walking).
12. Teach appropriate use of stool softeners and suppositories and hazards of enemas.
13. Teach signs and symptoms of fecal impaction and constipation.
14. Provide home care training for those who can be functionally independent with bowel program.

Breastfeeding, Effective

DEFINITION

Effective Breastfeeding: The state in which a mother–infant dyad exhibits adequate proficiency and satisfaction with the breastfeeding process.

Author's Note:

This diagnosis reportedly represents a wellness diagnosis. The newly proposed North American Nursing Diagnosis Association (NANDA) wellness diagnosis is defined as "a clinical judgment about an individual, family or community in transition from a specific level of wellness to a higher level of wellness" (NANDA Guidelines). This definition does not describe a mother–infant dyad seeking higher level breastfeeding. Instead, it describes "adequate proficiency and satisfaction with the breastfeeding process."

In the management of the breastfeeding experience, the nurse will find three situations:

Ineffective Breastfeeding
Risk for Ineffective Breastfeeding
Effective Breastfeeding or Potential for Enhanced Breastfeeding

(Continued)

Author's Note (Continued):

Effective Breastfeeding can be used to describe correct and satisfying breastfeeding of a mother and child in the early weeks. The interventions would focus on teaching basic breastfeeding.

If the nurse, most likely in a community or private practice, has a mother who reports proficiency and satisfaction with the breastfeeding process and desires additional teaching to achieve even greater proficiency and satisfaction, the nursing diagnosis of Potential for Enhanced Breastfeeding is appropriate. The focus of this teaching and continued support would not be to prevent Ineffective Breastfeeding or to maintain adequate proficiency and satisfaction, but rather to promote enhanced, higher quality breastfeeding.

DEFINING CHARACTERISTICS

Major (Must Be Present, One or More)

Mother is able to position infant at breast to promote a successful latch-on response.
Infant is content after feeding.
Regular and sustained suckling/swallowing occurs at the breast.
Infant weight patterns are appropriate for age.
Effective mother–infant communication patterns (infant cues, maternal interpretation and response).

Minor (May Be Present)

Signs and symptoms of oxytocin release (let-down or milk ejection reflex)
Adequate infant elimination patterns for age
Eagerness of infant to nurse
Maternal verbalization of satisfaction with the breastfeeding process

🖉 🍼 MATERNAL/CHILD FOCUS INTERVENTIONS

1. Assess knowledge and previous breastfeeding experiences; correct myths and misinformation.
2. Discuss advantages and disadvantages of breastfeeding.

3. Assist during first feedings (Reeder et al., 1997).
   a. Provide privacy and position comfortably.
   b. Demonstrate different positions.
   c. Assist in positioning infant, supporting head and body.
   d. Demonstrate how to support breast, with four fingers below and thumb above for first 2 weeks.
   e. Teach ways of waking baby (*e.g.*, gently tickling lips with breast).
   f. Teach how to break suction when removing infant from breast.
   g. Teach to rub infant's mouth with breast until infant's mouth is wide open.
4. Assess infant at breast for (Shrago & Bocar, 1990):
   a. Relaxed, flexed position
   b. Head aligned with trunk
   c. Wide-open mouth
   d. Visible lips, flanged outward
   e. Complete seal and strong vacuum
   f. One-half inch of areolar tissue beyond nipple in mouth
   g. Tongue curved under alveolar ridge
   h. Problems (*e.g.*, smacking sounds or dimpling of cheeks) during sucking
   i. Quiet sound of swallowing
5. Encourage to breastfeed long enough to remove sufficient milk to prevent engorgement. Instruct not to limit sucking time (Moon, 1989).
6. Instruct mother to offer both breasts at each feeding, alternating the beginning side each time.
7. Encourage feeding on demand and the convenience of infant sleeping in mother's room.
8. Teach mother to wear well-fitting support brassiere day and night; apply warm compresses for 15 to 20 minutes before nursing for engorgement.
   a. Share with father how breastfeeding may interfere with initial relationship with newborn (Gamble, 1993).

Breastfeeding, Ineffective

DEFINITION

Ineffective Breastfeeding: The state in which a mother, infant, or child experiences or is at risk of experiencing dissatisfaction or difficulty with the breastfeeding process.

DEFINING CHARACTERISTICS

Major (Must Be Present, One or More)

Actual or perceived inadequate milk supply
Infant's inability to attach correctly onto breast
No observable signs of oxytocin release
Observable signs of inadequate infant intake
Nonsustained suckling at the breast
Insufficient emptying of each breast at each feeding
Persistence of sore nipples beyond the first week of breast-feeding
Infant exhibiting fussiness and crying within the first hour after breastfeeding; unresponsive to other comfort measures
Infant arching and crying at the breast, resisting latching on

RELATED FACTORS

Physiological

Related to difficulty of neonate to attach or suck secondary to:
    Cleft lip/palate   Inverted nipples
    Prematurity   Inadequate let-down reflex
    Previous breast surgery

Situational (Personal, Environmental)

Related to maternal fatigue
Related to maternal anxiety
Related to maternal ambivalence
Related to multiple birth
Related to inadequate nutritional intake
Related to inadequate fluid intake
Related to history of unsuccessful breastfeeding
Related to nonsupportive partner/family

Related to lack of knowledge
Related to interruption in breastfeeding secondary to:
  Ill mother
  Ill infant

OUTCOME CRITERIA

The mother will:

1. Make an informed decision related to method of feeding infant (breast or bottle)
2. Identify activities that deter or promote successful breastfeeding

🔵 🟢 MATERNAL/CHILD FOCUS INTERVENTIONS

1. Assess for contributing factors to difficulty or dissatisfaction (refer to Related Factors).
2. If dissatisfied, explore specifics. Encourage mother to share her concerns openly. Evaluate her fatigue level, knowledge, anxiety, support system, and history of breastfeeding. (Refer to Effective Breastfeeding for basic teaching.)
3. Evaluate:
   a. Mother's state (comfort, anxiety, position)
   b. Infant's state (quiet, alert, crying, extremely hungry)
   c. Let-down reflex
   d. Baby at breast (Shrago & Bocar, 1990)
      • Alignment
      • Areolar grasp
      • Areolar compression
      • Audible swallowing
   e. Infant's intake and frequency of feedings
   f. Infant's output (six to eight diapers per day, bowel movement daily)
4. Teach management of sore nipples.
   a. Decrease nursing time to 5 to 10 minutes per side. Start baby on nontender side first. Allow for more frequent, short feedings. Suggest alternate positions to rotate infant's grasps. Allow breasts to dry after each feeding.

    b. Keep nursing pads dry.

    c. Use breast cream only after breasts are dry.

    d. Use breast shield as last measure, and remove after milk has let down.

    e. Be sure infant's mouth is positioned correctly on the breast.

5. If symptoms of mastitis or breast abscess develop (increased warmth, tenderness, redness), instruct to contact her advance practice nurse or physician.

6. If engorgement occurs:

    a. Massage breast before nursing by encircling breast with both hands and move hands downward toward nipple. Use lotion if desired.

    b. Use heat before nursing (hot shower, hot pack).

    c. If needed, massage breast again while infant is sucking in shorter sucks at end of feeding.

    d. Use ice packs between feedings.

    e. Wear a good support bra.

    f. Use mild analgesics as needed.

7. Respond to concerns regarding confidence and "not enough milk."

8. If supplementary feedings are used, consider the pouch and tubing device to continue breastfeeding and prevent nipple confusion.

9. Support mother's decision to continue with breastfeeding or to discontinue.

10. If breastfeeding is interrupted (*e.g.,* illness, maternal employment):

    a. Allow her to share her feelings.

    b. Determine if breastfeeding can be resumed if desired.

11. Teach how to express, handle, store, and transport breast milk safely.

12. Provide breast pump, or make mother aware of availability, if needed.

13. Encourage verbal expression of feelings.

14. Explore feelings and anticipation of problems. Older child may be jealous of contact with baby. Mother can use this time to read to older child.

15. Stress the need for rest.

    a. Encourage mother to make herself and infant a priority.

    b. Discuss temporary housekeeper.

      c. Encourage mother to limit visits from relatives for first 4 weeks.

16. Provide opportunities for significant others to ask questions.

17. Initiate referrals as indicated (lactation specialist, La Leche League).

Breastfeeding, Interrupted

DEFINITION

Interrupted Breastfeeding: A break in the continuity of the breast-feeding process as a result of inability or inadvisability to put baby to breast for feeding.

Author's Note:

This diagnosis represents a situation, not a response. If one examines the diagnosis *Ineffective Breastfeeding,* interrupted breastfeeding is listed as "related to." Nursing interventions do not treat the interruption but treat the effects of this interruption. The situation is interrupted breastfeeding; the responses can be varied. For example, if continued breastfeeding or use of a breast pump is contraindicated, the nurse will focus on the loss of this breastfeeding experience, using the nursing diagnosis of Grieving. If breastfeeding is continued with expression and storage of breast milk, teaching, and support, the diagnosis will be Risk for Ineffective Breastfeeding related to continuity problems secondary to, for example, maternal employment. If difficulty is experienced, the diagnosis would be Ineffective Breastfeeding related to interruption secondary to (specify) and lack of knowledge. Refer to Ineffective Breastfeeding for interventions.

DEFINING CHARACTERISTICS

Major (Must Be Present)

Infant does not receive nourishment at the breast for some or all of feedings.

Minor (May Be Present)

Maternal desire to maintain lactation and provide (or eventually provide) her breast milk for her infant's nutritional needs

Separation of mother and infant

Lack of knowledge about expression and storage of breast milk

RELATED FACTORS

Maternal or infant illness

Prematurity

Maternal employment

Contraindications to breastfeeding (*e.g.*, drugs, true breast milk jaundice)

Need to wean infant abruptly

Cardiac Output, Decreased

DEFINITION

Cardiac Output: Decreased: The state in which an individual experiences a reduction in the amount of blood pumped by the heart, resulting in compromised cardiac function.

> ### Author's Note:
> This diagnosis represents a situation in which nurses have multiple responsibilities. Individuals experiencing decreased cardiac output may present various responses that disrupt functioning, such as:
>
> Activity Intolerance
> Sleep Pattern Disturbance
>
> *(Continued)*

Author's Note (Continued):

Instead, they may be at risk for developing physiological complications, such as:

Dysrhythmias
Cardiogenic shock
Congestive heart failure

I recommend that the nurse not use Altered Cardiac Output: Decreased but instead select another diagnosis that better describes the situation (see *Activity Intolerance*).

By not using Altered Cardiac Output: Decreased, the nurse can more specifically describe the situations that nurses either treat as a nursing diagnosis or cotreat as a collaborative problem.

DEFINING CHARACTERISTICS

Low blood pressure
Rapid pulse
Restlessness
Cyanosis
Dyspnea
Angina
Dysrhythmia

Oliguria
Fatigability
Vertigo
Edema
   (peripheral, sacral)

Caregiver Role Strain

Risk for Caregiver Role Strain

Caregiver Role Strain

DEFINITION

Caregiver Role Strain: A state in which an individual is experiencing physical, emotional, social, and/or financial burden(s) in the process of giving care to another.

Author's Note:

There are 2.2 million unpaid home caregivers in the United States (Stone et al., 1987). These caregivers provide care for individuals of all ages, some across their entire life span (*e.g.*, children with permanent disabilities). The care receivers have physical or mental disabilities. These disabilities can be temporary or permanent Some disabilities are permanent but stable (*e.g.*, blind child), whereas others signal progressive deterioration (*e.g.*, Alzheimer's).

Caregiver Role Strain represents the burden of caregiving on the physical and emotional health of the caregiver and its effects on the family and social system of the caregiver and care receiver. Risk for Caregiver Role Strain can be a significant nursing diagnosis, because nurses can identify at-risk individuals and assist them to prevent this grave situation.

DEFINING CHARACTERISTICS

Reports insufficient time or physical energy
Difficulty performing caregiving activities required
Caregiving responsibilities interfering with other important roles (*e.g.*, work, spouse, friend, parent)
Apprehension about the future for the care receiver's health and ability to provide care
Apprehension about care receiver's care when caregiver is ill or deceased
Depressed feelings, anger

RELATED FACTORS

Pathophysiological

Related to unrelenting or complex care requirements secondary to:

Debilitating conditions (acute, progressive)
Progressive dementia
Addiction

Chronic mental illness
Unpredictable illness course
Disability

Treatment-Related

Related to 24-hour care responsibilities
Related to time (activities, *e.g.,* dialysis, transportation)

Situational (Personal, Environmental)

Related to unrealistic expectations of caregiver by care receiver

Related to pattern of ineffective coping

Related to compromised physical health

Related to unrealistic expectations of self

Related to history of poor relationship

Related to history of family dysfunction

Related to unrealistic expectations for caregiver by others (society, other family members)

Related to duration of caregiving required

Related to isolation

Related to insufficient respite

Related to insufficient recreation

Related to insufficient finances

Related to no or unavailable support

Maturational

Infant, child, adolescent related to unrelenting care requirements secondary to:

Mental disabilities (specify)

Physical disabilities (specify)

OUTCOME CRITERIA

The person will:

1. Share frustrations about caregiving responsibilities
2. Identify one source of support
3. Identify two changes that, if made, would improve daily life

The family will:

1. Relate an intent to listen without giving advice
2. Convey empathy to caregiver regarding daily responsibilities
3. Establish a plan for weekly support or help

⬙ **GENERIC INTERVENTIONS**

1. Assess for causative or contributing factors:
   a. Poor insight of situation
   b. Unrealistic expectations (caregiver, family)

    c. Reluctance or inability to access help
    d. Unsatisfactory caregiver–care receiver relationship
    e. Insufficient resources (*e.g.*, help, financial)
    f. Social isolation
    g. Insufficient leisure
    h. Competing roles (spouse, parenting, work)

2. Evaluate caregiver's and others' interpretation of the situation (Rolland, 1994).
    a. What information have they been told?
    b. Do they expect the situation to continue as is, improve, or worsen?
    c. Are they realistic?

3. Provide empathy, and promote a sense of competency.

4. Discuss the effects of present schedule and responsibilities on:
    a. Physical health
    b. Emotional status
    c. Relationships

5. Assist to identify for which activities assistance is desired:
    a. Care receiver's needs (hygiene, food, treatments, mobility)
    b. Laundry
    c. House cleaning
    d. Meals
    e. Shopping, errands
    f. Transportation
    g. Appointments (doctor, hairdresser)
    h. Yard work
    i. House repairs
    j. Respite (number of hours a week)
    k. Money management

6. Discuss with the family (Shields, 1992; Winslow, 1998):
    a. The importance of regularly acknowledging the burden of the situation for the caregiver
    b. The benefits of listening without giving advice
    c. The importance of emotional and appraisal support
       • Regular phone calls
       • Cards, letters
       • Visits
    d. The need to give caregiver "permission" to enjoy self (*e.g.*, vacations, day trips)
    e. The need to provide caregiver with opportunities to respond to "How can I help you?"

7. Identify all possible sources of volunteer help: family (siblings, cousins), friends, neighbors, church, community groups.
8. Role play how to ask for help with activities identified in item 4.
9. Identify community resources available:
    a. Support groups
    b. Counseling
    c. Social service
    d. Transportation
    e. Home-delivered meals
    f. Day care
10. Engage others to work actively to increase state, federal, and private agencies' financial support for resources to enhance caregiving in the home.

🏛 OLDER ADULT FOCUS INTERVENTIONS

1. If appropriate, discuss if and when an alternative source of care (*e.g.*, nursing home, senior housing) may be indicated.
2. If elder abuse is suspected, refer to Ineffective Family Coping: Disabling.

Risk for Caregiver Role Strain

DEFINITION

Risk for Caregiver Role Strain: The state in which an individual is at high risk to experience physical, emotional, social, and/or financial burden(s) in the process of giving care to another.

Author's Note:
Refer to Caregiver Role Strain.

RISK FACTORS

Presence of risk factors (refer to Related Factors)

RELATED FACTORS

Primary caregiver responsibilities for a recipient who requires regular assistance with self-care or supervision because of physical or mental disabilities

In addition to one or more of the following:

Related to unrelenting or complex care requirements secondary to:
  (Care receiver characteristics)
    Unable to perform self-care activities
    Not motivated to perform self-care activities
    Cognitive problems
    Psychological problems
    Unrealistic expectations of caregiver
  (Caregiver/spouse characteristics)
    Pattern of ineffective coping
    Compromised physical health
    Unrealistic expectations of self
Related to history of poor relationship
Related to history of family dysfunction
Related to unrealistic expectations for caregiver by others (society, other family members)
Related to duration of caregiving required
Related to isolation
Related to insufficient respite
Related to insufficient recreation
Related to insufficient finances
Related to no or unavailable support

OUTCOME CRITERIA

The person will:

1. Identify activities that are important for self
2. Relate a plan on how these activities can continue despite caregiving responsibilities
3. Relate an intent to enlist the help of at least two persons

⊞ GENERIC INTERVENTIONS

1. Explain the causes of caregiver role strain. Refer to intervention 1 of *Caregiver Role Strain*. Assist with anticipating the effects of the caregiving role.
2. Stress the importance of daily health-promotion activities:
    a. Rest–exercise balance

      b. Effective stress management
      c. Low-fat, high-complex carbohydrate diet
      d. Supportive social networks
      e. Appropriate screening practices for age
      f. See *Health Seeking Behaviors* for specific interventions.

3. Discuss the need for respite and short-term relief.
4. Maintain a good sense of humor. Associate with others who laugh.
5. Caution about spending too much time complaining, which is depressing for all involved and may lead to avoidance.
6. Advise to initiate phone contacts or visits with friends or relatives rather than "waiting for others to do it."
7. Emphasize the importance of respites to prevent isolating behaviors that foster depression.
8. Discuss the implications of caring for ill family member with all family members. Include:
      a. Available resources (finances, environmental)
      b. 24-hour responsibility
      c. Effects on other household members
      d. Likelihood of progressive deterioration
      e. Sharing of responsibilities (with other household members, siblings, neighbors)
      f. Likelihood of exacerbating long-standing conflicts
      g. Impact on lifestyle
      h. Alternative or assistive options (*e.g.*, community-based health care providers, life care centers, group living, nursing home)
9. Assist to identify for which activities assistance is desired:
      a. Care receiver's needs (hygiene, food, treatments, mobility)
      b. Laundry
      c. House cleaning
      d. Meals
      e. Shopping, errands
      f. Transportation
      g. Appointments (doctor, hairdresser)
      h. Yard work
      i. House repairs
      j. Respite (number of hours a week)
      k. Money management
10. Identify community resources available:
      a. Support group
      b. Counseling

c. Social service
d. Transportation
e. Home-delivered meals
f. Day care

Comfort, Altered*

Acute Pain

Chronic Pain

Nausea

Comfort, Altered

DEFINITION

Altered Comfort: The state in which an individual experiences an uncomfortable sensation in response to a noxious stimulus.

> **Author's Note:**
> This diagnosis, Altered Comfort, can represent a variety of uncomfortable sensations, such as pruritus, immobility, or nothing by mouth (NPO) status. When an individual experiences nausea and vomiting, the nurse should assess whether Nausea or Risk for Altered Nutrition is the appropriate category. Short-lived episodes of nausea or vomiting (*e.g.*, postoperatively) can be best described with Nausea related to nausea/vomiting secondary to effects of anesthesia or analgesics. When the nausea/ vomiting is at risk of compromising nutritional intake, use Risk for Altered Nutrition: Less than body requirements related to nausea and vomiting secondary to (specify).

*This diagnosis is not currently on the NANDA list but has been included for clarity and usefulness.

DEFINING CHARACTERISTICS

Major (Must Be Present)

The person reports or demonstrates a discomfort (*e.g.*, pain, nausea, vomiting, pruritus).

Minor (May Be Present)

Autonomic response to acute pain
  Blood pressure increased
  Pulse increased
  Respirations increased
  Diaphoresis
  Dilated pupils
Guarded position
Facial mask of pain
Crying, moaning
Abdominal heaviness

RELATED FACTORS

Any factor can contribute to altered comfort. The most common are listed below.

Biopathophysiological

(Pregnancy)
  Related to uterine contractions during labor
  Related to trauma to perineum during labor and delivery
  Related to involution of uterus and engorged breasts
Related to tissue trauma and reflex muscle spasms secondary to:
  (Musculoskeletal disorders)

Fractures	Arthritis
Contractures	Spinal cord disorders
Spasms	

  (Visceral disorders)

Cardiac	Intestinal
Renal	Pulmonary
Hepatic	

  (Vascular disorders)

Vasospasm	Phlebitis
Occlusion	Vasodilation (headache)

Cancer
Related to inflammation of:

Nerve	Joint

Tendon	Muscle
Bursa	Juxtoarticular structures

Related to fatigue, malaise, and/or pruritus secondary to contagious disease

Rubella	Mononucleosis
Chickenpox	Pancreatitis
Hepatitis	

Related to effects of cancer on (specify)

Related to abdominal cramps, diarrhea, and vomiting secondary to gastroenteritis, influenza, or gastric ulcers

Related to inflammation and smooth-muscle spasms secondary to renal calculi or gastrointestinal infections

Treatment-Related

Related to tissue trauma and reflex muscle spasms secondary to:

Surgery

Accidents

Burns

Diagnostic tests

Venipuncture

Invasive scanning

Biopsy

Related to nausea and vomiting secondary to chemotherapy, anesthesia, or side effects of (specify)

Situational (Personal, Environmental)

Related to fever

Related to immobility/improper positioning

Related to overactivity

Related to pressure points (tight cast, elastic bandage)

Related to allergic response

Related to chemical irritants

Related to unmet dependency needs

Related to severe repressed anxiety

Maturational

Infancy: Colic

Infancy and early childhood: Teething, ear pain

Middle childhood: Recurrent abdominal pain, growing pains

Adolescence: Headaches, chest pain, dysmenorrhea

Acute Pain

DEFINITION

Acute Pain: The state in which an individual experiences and reports the presence of severe discomfort or an uncomfortable sensation lasting from 1 second to less than 6 months.

Author's Note:

The NANDA list contains Pain and Chronic Pain. For clarity and usefulness, the author has organized diagnoses associated with pain and discomfort under two levels:

Altered Comfort
   Acute Pain
   Chronic Pain

DEFINING CHARACTERISTICS
(Simon, Nolan, & Baumann, 1995)

Major (80%–100%)

Communication of pain descriptors

Minor (60%–79%)

Clenched jaws or fists
Altered ability to continue previous activities
Agitation
Anxiety
Irritability
Rubs painful part
Grunts
Unusual posture (knees to abdomen)
Physical inactivity or immobility
Problems with concentration
Changes in sleep patterns
Fear of reinjury
Withdraws when touched
Widely opened or tightly shut eyes
Pinched features
Nausea and vomiting

RELATED FACTORS

Refer to *Altered Comfort*.

OUTCOME CRITERIA

The person will:

1. Convey that others validate that the pain exists
2. Relate relief after a satisfactory relief measure as evidenced by (specify)

The child will, according to age and ability:

1. Identify the source of the pain
2. Identify activities that increase and decrease pain
3. Describe comfort from others during the pain experience

⬛ GENERIC INTERVENTIONS

1. Reduce lack of knowledge.
   a. Explain causes of the pain to the person, if known.
   b. Relate how long the pain will last, if known.
   c. Explain diagnostic tests and procedures in detail by relating the discomforts and sensations that will be felt, and approximate the length of time involved (*e.g.*, "During the intravenous pyelogram, you might feel a momentary hot flash through your entire body.").
2. Provide accurate information to reduce fear of addiction.
3. Relate your acceptance of person's response to pain.
   a. Acknowledge the presence of the pain.
   b. Listen attentively concerning pain.
   c. Convey that you are assessing the pain because you want to understand it better (not determine if it is really present).
4. Assess the family for the presence of misconceptions about pain or its treatment.
5. Discuss the reasons why an individual may experience increased or decreased pain (*e.g.*, fatigue [increased] or presence of distractions [decreased]).
   a. Encourage family members to share their concerns privately (*e.g.*, fear that the person will use pain for secondary gains if they give the person too much attention).

     b. Assess whether the family doubts the pain, and discuss the effects of this on the person's pain and on the relationship.

     c. Encourage the family to give attention also when pain is not exhibited.

6. Provide person with opportunities to rest during the day and with periods of uninterrupted sleep at night (must rest when pain is ↓).

7. Discuss with the person and family the therapeutic uses of distraction, along with other methods of pain relief.

8. Teach a method of distraction during acute pain (*e.g.*, painful procedure) that is not a burden (*e.g.*, count items in a picture; count anything in the room, such as patterns on wallpaper; count silently to self; breathe rhythmically; listen to music and increase the volume as the pain increases).

9. Teach noninvasive pain-relief measures.

    a. Relaxation

      • Instruct on techniques to reduce skeletal muscle tension, which will reduce the intensity of the pain.

      • Promote relaxation with a back rub, massage, or warm bath.

      • Teach a specific relaxation strategy (*e.g.*, slow, rhythmic breathing or deep breath—clench fists—yawn).

    b. Cutaneous stimulation

      • Discuss with the person the various methods of skin stimulation and their effects on pain.

      • Discuss each of the following methods and the precautions:

        ◦ Hot water bottle, warm tub

        ◦ Electric heating pad, moist heat pack

        ◦ Hot summer sun

        ◦ Thin plastic wrap over painful area to retain body heat (*e.g.*, knee, elbow)

      • Discuss each of the following methods and the precautions:

        ◦ Cold towels (wrung out)

        ◦ Cold-water immersion for small body parts

        ◦ Ice bag, cold gel pack, ice massage

      • Explain the therapeutic uses of menthol preparations and massage/back rub.

10. Provide the person with optimal pain relief with prescribed analgesics.
11. After administering a pain-relief medication, return in 30 minutes to assess effectiveness.
12. Give accurate information to correct family misconceptions (*e.g.*, addiction, doubts about pain).
13. Provide individuals with opportunities to discuss their fears, anger, and frustrations in private; acknowledge the difficulty of the situation.

✌ CHILD FOCUS INTERVENTIONS

1. Assess the child's pain experience.
    a. Determine the child's concept of the cause of pain, if feasible.
    b. Ask child to point to the area that hurts.
    c. For children younger than 4 or 5 years, use Oucher Scale of five faces from very happy (1) to crying (5).
    d. For children older than 4 years, ask to rate the pain using a scale of 0–5 (0 = no pain, and 5 = worst pain).
    e. Ask the child what makes the pain better and what makes it worse.
    f. Assess if fear or loneliness is contributing to pain.
2. Promote security with honest explanations and opportunities for choice.
    a. Tell the truth. Explain:
        • How much it will hurt
        • How long it will last
        • What will help the pain.
    b. Do not threaten (*e.g.*, *do not* tell the child, "If you don't hold still, you won't go home.").
    c. Explicitly explain and reinforce to the child that pain is not a means of punishment.
    d. Explain to the parents that the child may cry more openly when they are present but that their presence is important for promoting trust.
    e. Explain to the child that the procedure is necessary so he or she can get better, and it is important to hold still so it can be done quickly.
    f. Discuss with the parents the importance of truth-telling. Instruct parents to:
        • Tell child when they are leaving and when they will return

- Relate to the child that they cannot take away the pain but that they will be there (except in circumstances when parents are not permitted to remain)

  g. Allow the parents opportunities to share their feelings about witnessing their child's pain and their helplessness.

3. Prepare the child for a painful procedure.
   a. Discuss the procedure with the parents; determine what they have told the child.
   b. Explain the procedure in words suited to the child's age and developmental level.
   c. Relate the discomforts that will be felt (*e.g.*, what the child will feel, taste, see, or smell).
   d. Encourage the child to ask questions before and during the procedure; ask the child to share with you what he or she thinks is going to happen and why.
   e. Share with the child (who is old enough—older than 3½ years):
      - You expect that the child will hold still and that such behavior will be pleasing to you.
      - It is all right to cry or squeeze your hand if it hurts.
   f. Arrange to have parents present for procedures (especially for children 18 months to 5 years).

4. Explain to the child that he or she can be distracted from the procedure if that is the child's wish. (The use of distraction without the child's knowledge of the impending discomfort is not advocated because the child will learn to mistrust.)
   a. Tell a story with a puppet.
   b. Ask the child to name or count objects in a picture.
   c. Ask the child to look at the picture and to locate certain objects ("Where is the dog?").
   d. Ask child to tell you about a pet.
   e. Ask child to count your blinks.

5. Provide the child with privacy during the painful procedure; use a treatment room rather than the child's bed.

6. Assist the child with the aftermath of pain.
   a. Tell the child when the painful procedure is over.
   b. Pick up the small child to indicate that it is over.

    c. Encourage the child to discuss the pain experience (draw or act out with dolls).

    d. Encourage the child to perform the painful procedure using the same equipment on a doll under supervision.

    e. Praise the child for endurance, and convey that the pain was handled well, regardless of the child's behavior (unless the child was violent to others).

    f. Give the child a souvenir of the pain (Band-Aid, badge for bravery).

    g. Teach the child to keep a record of painful experiences and to place a star next to those for which he or she held still (*e.g.*, gold stars on a paper for each injection or venipuncture).

◗ MATERNAL FOCUS INTERVENTIONS
(Reeder et al., 1997)

1. Assess contractions and discomfort (onset, frequency, duration, intensity, description of discomfort).
2. Determine the presence of other discomforts not related to labor (*e.g.*, chronic or recent illness).
3. Assess goals and expectations:
   a. Regarding labor
   b. Pain-relief methods
   c. Persons to be present
   d. Medications
4. Explain pain-relief methods available:
   a. Relaxation techniques
   b. Breathing patterns
   c. Acupressure
   d. Massage
   e. Cold/heat applications
   f. Positioning
   g. Physical activities
   h. Distraction
   i. Medications
5. Determine what types of methods are desired. Encourage the patient to try several methods.
6. Coach her with the method, and include her labor support person.
7. Stand and walk as much as possible during first stage.
8. Change positions at least every hour.

9. For backaches, try squatting, kneeling, or an all-fours position (hands and knees).
10. Encourage use of heat (bath, showers, heating pad) to lower abdomen, groin, back, perineum, or thigh pain.
11. For back pain, apply could pack to back or neck (20–30 minutes).
12. If mother panics during transition, be firm and direct:
    a. "I'm here, and I'm in charge."
    b. "I'm here for you."
    c. Make her look at you.
    d. Hold her wrist.
    e. Exaggerate your coaching breathing.
13. Assist her with the aftermath of labor.
    a. Praise her for her hard work.
    b. Allow her to relive difficult moments.
    c. Explain why pain increased.
    d. Acknowledge support person's help.

Chronic Pain

DEFINITION

Chronic Pain: The state in which an individual experiences pain that is persistent or intermittent and lasts for more than 6 months.

DEFINING CHARACTERISTICS

Major (Must Be Present)

The person reports that pain has existed for more than 6 months (may be the only assessment data present).

Minor (60%–79%) (Simon, Nolan, & Baumann, 1995)

Disruption of social and family relationships
Irritability
Physical inactivity or immobility
Depression
Rubbing of painful part
Anxiety
"Beaten look"

Self-focusing
Skeletal muscle tension
Somatic preoccupation
Agitation
Fatigue
Decreased libido
Restlessness

RELATED FACTORS

Refer to *Altered Comfort*.

OUTCOME CRITERIA

The person will:

1. Relate that others validate that the pain exists
2. Practice selected noninvasive pain-relief measures to manage the pain
3. Relate improvement of pain and increase in daily activities as evidenced by (specify)

✥ GENERIC INTERVENTIONS

1. Refer to Acute Pain.
2. Assess the effects of chronic pain on the individual's life, using the person and family.
   a. Performance (job, role responsibilities)
   b. Social interactions
   c. Finances
   d. Activities of daily living (sleep, eating, mobility, sexual)
   e. Cognition/mood (concentration, depression)
   f. Family unit (response of members)
3. Explore expectations of course of pain, treatment, and side effects; clarify if unrealistic.
4. Discuss the effectiveness of combining physical and psychological techniques and pharmacotherapy.
5. Discuss with the individual and family the various treatment modalities available (family therapy, group therapy, behavior modification, biofeedback, hypnosis, acupuncture, exercise program, cognitive strategies).
6. Discuss the suffering caused by the pain experience: decreased endurance, poor appetite, interrupted sleep,

diminished enjoyment, anxiety, fear, difficulty concentrating, and diminished social and sexual relationships (Kongable, 1998).

🕿 CHILD FOCUS INTERVENTIONS

1. Assess pain experiences by using developmentally appropriate assessment scales and by assessing behavior.
2. Set goals for pain management with child and family (short and long term), and evaluate regularly.
3. Promote the "normal" aspects of the child's life: play, school, relationships with family, physical activity.
4. Promote a trusting environment for child and family.
   a. Believe the child's pain.
   b. Encourage child's perception that interventions are attempts to help.
   c. Have child, family, and nurse participate in controlling pain.
5. Use interdisciplinary team for pain management as necessary (*e.g.*, nurse, physician, child life therapist, mental health therapist, occupational therapist, physical therapist, nutritionist).

Nausea

DEFINITION

Nausea: The state in which an individual experiences an unpleasant, wave like sensation in the back of the throat, epigastrium, or throughout the abdomen that may or may not lead to vomiting.

DEFINING CHARACTERISTICS

Usually precedes vomiting, but may be experienced after vomiting or when vomiting does not occur

Accompanied by pallor, cold and clammy skin, increased salivation, tachycardia, gastric stasis, and diarrhea

Accompanied by swallowing movements affected by skeleted muscles

Reports "nausea" or "sick to stomach"

RELATED FACTORS

Biopathophysiological
Gastrointestinal
    Acute gastroenteritis
    Peptic ulcer disease
    Irritable bowel syndrome
    Pancreatitis
Migraine headaches
Pregnancy
Infections (*e.g.*, food poisoning)
Drug overdose
Renal calculi

Treatment-Related

Related to effects of chemotherapy, theophylline, digitalis, or antibiotics
Related to effects of anesthesia

Situational

Motion sickness

OUTCOME CRITERIA

The individual will

1. Report decreased nausea.
2. Name foods or beverages that do not increase nausea.

INTERVENTIONS

1. Explain the cause of the nausea and the duration if known.
2. Encourage the client to eat small, frequent meals and to eat slowly. Cool, bland foods and liquids are usually well tolerated.
3. Eliminate unpleasant sights and odors from the eating area.
4. Instruct the client to avoid the following:
   a. Hot or cold liquids
   b. Foods containing fat and fiber
   c. Spicy foods
   d. Caffeine

5. Encourage the client to rest in a semi-Fowler's position after eating and to change position slowly.
6. Teach techniques to reduce nausea:
    a. Avoid the smell of food preparation and other noxious stimuli.
    b. Loosen clothing before eating.
    c. Sit in fresh air.
    d. Avoid lying flat for at least 2 hours after eating.
7. Consult with a nurse practitioner or physician if there is a high risk for dehydration or malnutrition.

Communication, Impaired*

Communication, Impaired Verbal

Communication, Impaired

DEFINITION

Impaired Communication: The state in which an individual experiences, or is at high risk to experience, a decreased ability to send or receive messages (*i.e.*, has difficulty exchanging thoughts, ideas, or desires).

Author's Note:

Impaired Communication and Impaired Verbal Communication are diagnoses to describe individuals who desire to communicate but are encountering problems. Impaired Communication may not be useful to describe an individual in whom communication problems are a manifestation of a psychiatric illness or a coping problem. If nursing interventions are focusing on reducing hallucinations, fear, or anxiety, the diagnosis of Fear or Anxiety is more appropriate.

---

*This diagnosis was developed by Rosalinda Alfaro-LeFevre and is not currently on the NANDA list; it has been included for clarity or usefulness.

DEFINING CHARACTERISTICS

Major (Must Be Present, One or More)

Impaired ability to speak
Inappropriate or absent speech or response

Minor (May Be Present)

Incongruence between verbal
and nonverbal messages
Stuttering
Dysarthria
Aphasia
Slurring

Problem finding the correct
word when speaking
Weak or absent voice
Statements of not understanding or being misunderstood

RELATED FACTORS

Pathophysiological

Related to disordered, unrealistic thinking secondary to schiz-
ophrenic disorder, delusional disorder, psychotic or paranoid
disorders
Related to impaired motor function of muscles of speech sec-
ondary to: *or*
Related to ischemia of temporal or frontal lobe secondary to:
Expressive or receptive aphasia
CVA
Oral trauma
Facial trauma
Brain damage (*e.g.*, birth/head trauma)
CNS depression/increased ICP
Tumor (head, neck, or spinal cord)
Chronic hypoxia/decreased cerebral blood flow
Quadriplegia
Nervous system diseases (*e.g.*, myasthenia gravis, multiple
sclerosis, muscular dystrophy)
Vocal cord paralysis
Related to impaired ability to produce speech secondary to:
Respiratory impairment (*e.g.*, shortness of breath)
Laryngeal edema/infection
Oral deformities
Cleft lip or palate
Malocclusion or fractured jaw
Missing teeth
Dysarthria
Related to auditory impairment

Treatment-Related

Related to impaired ability to produce speech secondary to:
Endotracheal intubation
Tracheostomy/tracheotomy/laryngectomy
Surgery of the head, face, neck, or mouth
Pain (especially of the mouth or throat)
Lethargy secondary to CNS depressants, anesthesia

Situational (Personal, Environmental)

Related to decreased attention secondary to fatigue, anger, anxiety, or pain
Related to no access to hearing aid or malfunction of hearing aid
Related to psychological barrier (*e.g.*, fear, shyness)
Related to lack of privacy
Related to loss of recent memory recall
Related to unavailable interpreter

Maturational

Infant/child
Related to inadequate sensory stimulation
Older adult (auditory losses)
Related to hearing impairment
Related to cognitive impairments secondary to (specify)

OUTCOME CRITERIA

The person will:

1. Wear a hearing aid (if appropriate)
2. Receive messages through alternative methods (*e.g.*, written communication, sign language, speaking distinctly into "good" ear)
3. Relate/demonstrate an improved ability to communicate
4. Demonstrate increased ability to understand
5. Relate decreased frustration with communication

⬛ GENERIC INTERVENTIONS

1. Use factors that promote hearing and understanding.
   a. Talk distinctly and clearly, facing the person.
   b. Minimize unnecessary sounds in the room.
      • Have only one person talk.

- Be aware of background noises (*e.g.*, close the door, turn off the television or radio).
  c. Repeat, then rephrase, a thought if the person does not seem to understand the whole meaning.
  d. Use touch and gestures to enhance communication.
  e. If person can understand only sign language, have an interpreter present as often as possible.
  f. If the person is in a group (*e.g.*, diabetes class), place the individual in the front of the room near the teacher.
  g. Approach the person from the side on which hearing is best (*i.e.*, if hearing is better with left ear, approach the person from the left).
  h. If the person can lip read, look directly at the person, and talk slowly and clearly.
  i. Assess functioning of hearing aids (*e.g.*, batteries).

2. Provide alternative methods of communication.
   a. Use pad and pencil, alphabet letters, hand signals, eye blinks, head nods, bell signals.
   b. Make flash cards with pictures or words depicting frequently used phrases (*e.g.*, "Wet my lips," "Move my foot," glass of water, bedpan).
   c. Encourage person to point, use gestures, and pantomime.
   d. Consult with speech pathologist for assistance in acquiring flash cards.

3. Provide a nonrushed environment.
   a. Use normal loudness level, and speak unhurriedly in short phrases.
   b. Encourage person to take plenty of time talking and to enunciate words carefully with good lip movements.
   c. Decrease external distractions.
   d. Delay conversation when the person is tired.

4. Use techniques to increase understanding.
   a. Use uncomplicated one-step commands and directives.
   b. Encourage the use of gestures and pantomime.
   c. Match words with actions; use pictures.
   d. Terminate conversation on a note of success (*e.g.*, move back to an easier item).
   e. Use same words with same task.

5. Make a concerted effort to understand when the person is speaking.
   a. Allow enough time to listen if the person speaks slowly.
   b. Rephrase the person's message aloud to validate it.
   c. Respond to all attempts at speech even if they are unintelligible (*e.g.*, "I do not know what you are saying. Can you try to say it again?").
   d. Ignore mistakes and profanity.
   e. Do not pretend you understand if you do not.
   f. Allow the person time to respond; do not interrupt. Supply words only occasionally.
6. Teach techniques to improve speech.
   a. Ask the person to slow down speech and say each word clearly, while providing an example.
   b. Encourage the person to speak in short phrases.
   c. Suggest a slower rate of talking or taking a breath before beginning to speak.
   d. Encourage the person to take time and concentrate on forming the words.
   e. Ask the person to write down the message or to draw a picture if verbal communication is difficult.
   f. Encourage the person to speak in short phrases.
   g. Ask questions that can be answered with a yes or no.
   h. Focus on the present; avoid topics that are controversial, emotional, abstract, or lengthy.
7. Verbally address the problem of frustration about inability to communicate, and explain that patience is needed for the nurse and the person who is trying to talk.
8. Give the person opportunities to make decisions about care (*e.g.*, "Do you want a drink?" "Would you rather have orange juice or prune juice?").
9. Teach techniques to significant others and repetitive approaches to improve communications.
10. If a translator is needed, refer to Impaired Verbal Communication.
11. If person is hearing impaired, refer to Older Adult Focus Interventions.

OLDER ADULT FOCUS INTERVENTIONS

1. If person can hear with a hearing aid, make sure that it is on and functioning.

2. If person can hear with one ear, speak slowly and clearly into the good ear. (It is more important to speak distinctly than to speak loudly.)
3. If person can read and write, provide pad and pencil at all times (even when going to another department).
4. If person can understand only sign language, have an interpreter with him or her as much as possible.
5. Write and speak all important messages.
6. Validate the person's understanding by asking questions that require more than "yes" or "no" answers. Avoid asking "Do you understand?"
7. Assess if cerumen impaction is impairing hearing.

Communication, Impaired Verbal

DEFINITION

Impaired Verbal Communication: The state in which an individual experiences, or is at high risk to experience, a decreased ability to speak but can understand others.

DEFINING CHARACTERISTICS

Major (Must Be Present)

Inability to speak words but can understand others *or*
Articulation or motor planning deficits

Minor (May Be Present)

Shortness of breath

RELATED FACTORS

See *Impaired Communication.*

OUTCOME CRITERIA

The person will:

1. Demonstrate improved ability to express self
2. Relate decreased frustration with communication

⊕ GENERIC INTERVENTIONS

1. Identify a method by which person can communicate basic needs.
2. Provide alternative methods of communication.
   a. Use pad and pencil, alphabet letters, hand signals, eye blinks, head nods, bell signals.
   b. Make flash cards with pictures or words depicting frequently used phrases (*e.g.*, "Wet my lips," "Move my foot," glass of water, bedpan).
   c. Encourage person to point, use gestures, and pantomime.
   d. Consult with speech pathologist for assistance in acquiring flash cards.
3. For individuals with dysarthria:
   a. Reduce environmental noise.
   b. Encourage the person to make a conscious effort to slow down speech and to speak louder (*e.g.*, "Take a deep breath between sentences.").
   c. Ask person to repeat words that are unclear.
   d. If person is tired, ask questions that require only short answers.
   e. If speech is unintelligible, teach the person to use gestures, written messages, and communication cards.
4. Do not alter your speech, tone, or type of message, because the person's ability to understand is not affected; speak on an adult level.
5. Verbally address the problem of frustration about inability to communicate, and explain that patience is needed for the nurse and the person who is trying to talk.
6. Write the method of communication that is used on person's care plan.
7. Teach significant others techniques and repetitive approaches to improve communication.
8. Encourage the family to share feelings concerning communication problems.
9. Seek consultation with a speech pathologist early in treatment regimen.
10. For individuals with language barriers (Giger & Davidhazar, 1995):
    a. Communicate in an unhurried, caring manner. Be polite and formal.
    b. Speak in a low, moderate voice. Listen carefully; validate mutual understanding.

    c. Use gestures and pictures.

    d. Keep the message simple; do not use medical or technical terms.

    e. If an interpreter is needed:
- Clarify what language is spoken at home.
- Attempt to use same gender and similar age as client.
- Avoid interpreters from rival tribe, nation.
- Ask to translate verbatim.

11. Use AT&T telephone translating system when necessary.

Confusion

Acute Confusion

Chronic Confusion

Author's Note:

I have added Confusion to the diagnostic list to provide the nurse with an option when the origins, onset, or duration of the confusion is unknown. By providing this diagnostic option, the nurse can refrain from too quickly labeling the confusion as acute or chronic. Careful assessment is indicated. Until data collection is complete, the diagnosis can be written as Confusion related to unknown etiology as evidenced by (specify supporting data).

Confusion*

DEFINITION

Confusion: The state in which the individual experiences or is at risk of experiencing a disturbance in cognition, attention, memory, and orientation of an undetermined origin or onset.

   *This diagnosis is not currently on the NANDA list but has been included for clarity and usefulness.

DEFINING CHARACTERISTICS

Major (Must Be Present, One or More)

Disturbances of:

Consciousness	Memory
Attention	Orientation
Perception	Thinking

Minor (May Be Present)

Misperceptions
Hypervigilance
Agitation

Acute Confusion

DEFINITION

Acute Confusion: The state in which there is an abrupt onset of a cluster of global, fluctuating disturbances in consciousness, attention, perception, memory, orientation, thinking, sleep–wake cycle, and psychomotor behavior (American Psychological Association, 1994).

DEFINING CHARACTERISTICS

Major (Must Be Present, One or More)

Abrupt onset of a cluster of fluctuating disturbances of:

Consciousness	Orientation
Attention	Thinking
Perception	Sleep–wake cycle
Memory	

Psychomotor behavior (reaction time, speed of movement, flow of speech, involuntary movements, handwriting)

Minor (May Be Present)

Hypervigilance
Hallucinations
Illusions

RISK FACTORS

Presence of risk factors (see Related Factors)

RELATED FACTORS

Pathophysiological

Related to cerebral hypoxia or disturbance in cerebral metabolism secondary to (Miller, 1999):

Fluid and electrolyte disturbances
    Dehydration
    Volume depletion
    Acidosis/alkalosis
    Hypercalcemia
    Hypokalemia
    Hyponatremia/hypernatremia
    Hypoglycemia/hyperglycemia

Nutritional deficiencies
    Folate or vitamin B_{12} deficiency
    Anemia
    Niacin deficiency
    Magnesium deficiency

Cardiovascular disturbances
    Myocardial infarction
    Congestive heart failure
    Dysrhythmias
    Heart block
    Temporal arteritis

Respiratory disorders
    Chronic obstructive pulmonary disease
    Pulmonary embolism
    Tuberculosis
    Pneumonia

Infections
    Sepsis
    Meningitis, encephalitis
    Urinary tract infection

Metabolic and endocrine disorders
    Hypothyroidism
    Hypopituitarism
    Parathyroid disorders
    Hypoadrenocorticism
    Postural hypotension
    Hypothermia/hyperthermia
    Hepatic or renal failure

CNS disorders
    Multiple infarctions
    Parkinson's disease
    Neurosyphilis
    Alzheimer's disease
    Head trauma
    Tumors
    Seizures and postconvulsive states
    Normal pressure hydrocephalus

Collagen and rheumatoid disease
    Polymyalgia rheumatica
    Temporal arteritis
    Periarteritis nodosa
    Lupus erythematosus

Treatment-Related

Related to a disturbance in cerebral metabolism secondary to:
Surgery
Therapeutic drug intoxication (*e.g.*, neuroleptics, narcotics)
General anesthesia
Side effects of medication

Diuretics	Barbiturates
Digitalis	Methyldopa
Propanolol	Disulfiram
Atropine	Lithium
Oral hypoglycemics	Phenytoin
Anti-inflammatory agents	Antianxiety agents
Anticholinergics	Over-the-counter cold, cough, and sleeping
Phenothiazines	preparations

Situational (Personal, Environmental)

Related to disturbance in cerebral metabolism secondary to:
Withdrawal from alcohol
Withdrawal from sedatives, hypnotics
Heavy metal or carbon monoxide intoxication
Related to pain, bowel impaction, immobility, or depression
Related to chemical intoxications (specify):

Alcohol	Opiates
Cocaine	Barbiturates
Amphetamines	Hallucinogenics

OUTCOME CRITERIA

The person will:

1. Have diminished episodes of confusion

⊞ GENERIC INTERVENTIONS

1. Assess for causative and contributing factors.
   a. Ensure that a thorough diagnostic workup has been completed.
      • Laboratory
         ○ Complete blood count, electrolytes, chemistry
         ○ B_{12} and folate, thiamine
         ○ RPR

- ○ TSH, T$_4$
- ○ Drug levels—ETOH, barbiturates
- ○ Serum thyroxine and serum-free thyroxine
- ○ Serum glucose and fasting blood sugar (FBS)
- ○ Urinalysis
- Diagnostic
  - ○ Electroencephalogram
  - ○ Computed tomography scan
  - ○ Electrocardiogram
  - ○ Chest x-ray, skull x-ray
  - ○ Spinal tap
  - ○ Psychiatric evaluation

2. Promote communication that contributes to the person's sense of integrity.
   a. Examine attitudes about confusion (in self, caregivers, significant others).
      - Provide education to family, significant other(s), and caregivers regarding the situation and methods of coping.
   b. Maintain standards of empathic, respectful care.
   c. Attempt to obtain information that will provide useful and meaningful topics for conversations (likes, dislikes; interests, hobbies; work history). Interview early in the day.
   d. Encourage significant others and caregivers to speak slowly with low voice pitch and at an average volume (unless hearing deficits are present), as one adult to another, with eye contact, and as if expecting person to understand.
   e. Provide respect and promote sharing.
      - Pay attention to what person is saying.
      - Pick out meaningful comments, and continue talking.
      - Call person by name, and introduce yourself each time a contact is made; use touch if welcomed.
      - Use name the person prefers; avoid "Pops" or "Mom."
      - Convey to person that you are concerned and friendly (through smiles, an unhurried pace).
   f. Use memory aids, if appropriate.

3. Provide sufficient and meaningful sensory input.
   a. Keep person oriented to time and place.
   b. Encourage family to bring in familiar objects from home (*e.g.*, photographs with nonglare glass, blanket).
   c. Discuss current events, seasonal events (snow, water activities); share your interests (travel, crafts).
   d. Assess if person can perform an activity with hands (*e.g.*, latch rugs, wood crafts).
   e. When teaching a task or activity (*e.g.*, eating), break it into small, brief steps by giving only one instruction at a time.
4. Promote a well role.
   a. Discourage the use of nightclothes during the day.
   b. Encourage self-care and grooming activities.
   c. Promote socialization during meals.
   d. Plan an activity each day.
   e. Encourage participation in decision making.
5. Do not endorse confusion.
   a. Do not argue with person.
   b. Never agree with confused statements.
   c. Direct person back to reality; do not allow him or her to ramble.
   d. Adhere to the schedule; if changes are necessary, advise person of them.
   e. Avoid talking to coworkers about other topics in person's presence.
   f. Provide simple explanations that cannot be misinterpreted.
   g. Remember to acknowledge your entrance with a greeting and your exit with a closure. ("I will be back in 10 minutes.")
   h. Avoid open-ended questions.
   i. Replace five- to six-step tasks with two- to three-step tasks.
6. Promote the client's safety.
   a. Ensure that person carries identification.
   b. Adapt the environment so person can pace or walk if desired.
   c. Keep the environment uncluttered.
   d. Keep medications, cleaning solutions, and other toxic chemicals in inaccessible places.
   e. If person cannot manipulate call button, use another method (*e.g.*, bell, an extension from bed call system).

7. Discourage use of restraints; explore other alternatives (Quinn, 1994).
    a. If person's behavior disrupts treatment (*e.g.*, nasogastric tube, urinary catheter, intravenous line), reevaluate whether treatment is appropriate.
    b. Evaluate if restlessness is associated with pain. If analgesics are used, adjust dosage to reduce side effects.
    c. Put person in a room with others who can help watch him or her.
    d. Enlist aid of family or friends to watch person during confused periods.
    e. Give person something to hold (*e.g.*, a stuffed animal).

Chronic Confusion

DEFINITION

Chronic Confusion: A state in which the individual experiences an irreversible, long-standing, and/or progressive deterioration of intellect and personality.

DEFINING CHARACTERISTICS

Major (Must Be Present, One or More)

Cognitive or intellectual losses
  Loss of memory
  Loss of time sense
  Inability to make choices, decisions
Inability to problem solve, reason
  Altered perceptions
  Loss of language abilities
  Poor judgment
Affective or personality losses
  Loss of affect
  Diminished inhibition
  Increasing self-preoccupations
  Loss of tact, control of temper
  Psychotic features
  Antisocial behavior
  Loss of recognition (others, environment, self)
  Loss of energy reserve
Conative or planning losses
  Loss of general ability to plan

Impaired ability to set goals, plan
Progressive lowered stress threshold
Purposeful wandering
Violent, agitated, or anxious behavior
Purposeless behavior
Withdrawal or avoidance behavior
Compulsive repetitive behavior

RELATED FACTORS

Pathophysiological (Hall, 1991)

Related to progressive degeneration of the cerebral cortex secondary to:
Alzheimer's disease
Multi-infarct disease (MID)
Combination of senile dementia of Alzheimer's type and MID
Related to disturbance in cerebral metabolism, structure, or integrity secondary to:
Pick's disease
Creutzfeldt-Jakob disease
Toxic substance injection
Degenerative neurological disease
Brain tumors
Huntington's chorea
End-stage diseases
Acquired immunodeficiency disease (AIDS)
Cancer
Cardiac failure
Cirrhosis
Renal failure
Chronic obstructive pulmonary disease
Psychiatric disorders

OUTCOME CRITERIA

The person will:

1. Participate to maximum level of independence in a therapeutic milieu
2. Have decreased frustration when environmental stressors are reduced
3. Have diminished episodes of combativeness

4. Eliminate episodes of combative behavior
5. Increase hours of sleep at night
6. Stabilize or increase weight

⊜ GENERIC INTERVENTIONS

1. Refer to interventions 2 through 7 under *Acute Confusion*.
2. Promote communication that contributes to the person's sense of integrity (Miller, 1999).
   a. Adapt communication to the ability level.
   b. Avoid "baby talk" and a condescending tone.
   c. It may be necessary to use simple sentences and to present one idea at a time.
   d. If person does not understand, repeat sentence.
   e. Use positive statements; avoid "don'ts."
3. Attempt to determine source of the fear and frustration that is associated with the person's combative episodes (Hall, 1991):
   a. Negative, restrictive feedback from others
   b. Restraints
   c. Misinterpretation of environmental stimuli (*e.g.*, television)
   d. Misinterpretation of possessions and ownership
   e. Mistaking others for spouses, family members
   f. Fear of water (*e.g.*, bathing)
4. Eliminate misleading stimuli (*e.g.*, mirrors, TV, radio).
5. Ensure physical comfort and maintenance of basic health needs (e.g., elimination, nutrition, bathing, toileting, hygiene, grooming, safety). Refer to individual nursing diagnoses for individuals to assist a cognitively impaired person with self-care.
6. Use various modalities to promote stimulation for the individual.
   a. Music therapy
      • Provide soft, familiar music during meals.
      • Play music to individuals that they preferred in their younger years.
   b. Recreation therapy
      • Encourage arts and crafts (knitting and crocheting).
      • Suggest creative writing.
      • Provide puzzles.
      • Organize group games.

    c. Remotivation therapy
- Topics for remotivation sessions are based on suggestions from group leaders and the interest of the group. Examples are pets, bodies of water, canning fruits and vegetables, transportation, holidays (Janssen & Giberson, 1988).
- Use associations and analogies.
  - "If ice is cold, then fire is . . . ?"
  - "If day is light, then night is . . . ?"

    d. Sensory training
- Stimulate vision (with brightly colored items of different shapes, pictures, color decorations, kaleidoscopes).
- Stimulate smell (with flowers, coffee, cologne).
- Stimulate hearing (ring a bell, play records).
- Stimulate touch (sandpaper, velvet, steel wool pads, silk, stuffed animals).
- Stimulate taste (spices, salt, sugar, sour substances)

    e. Reminiscence therapy (Smith, 1990; Burnside & Haight, 1994)
- Consider instituting reminiscence therapy on a one-to-one or group basis. Discuss purpose and goals with client care team. Prepare yourself well before initiating. Refer to Burnside and Haight (1994) for specific protocols for one-to-one and group reminiscence.

7. Implement techniques to lower the stress threshold in individuals in middle or later stages of dementia (Hall & Buckwalter, 1987; Miller, 1999).
   a. Reduce competing or excessive stimuli.
   b. Plan and maintain a consistent routine.
   c. Focus on the person's ability level.
   d. Reduce fatigue and anxiety.
   e. Allow for wandering.
   f. Be alert to individual's expressions of fatigue or increasing anxiety, and immediately reduce stimuli.

8. Discuss the proposed benefits of selected nutrients: zinc, choline, lecithin, selenium, magnesium, beta carotene, folic acid, and vitamins C and E (Miller, 1999).

Constipation

Perceived Constipation

Risk for Constipation

Constipation

DEFINITION

Constipation: The state in which an individual experiences stasis of the large intestine, resulting in infrequent elimination and/or hard, dry feces.

DEFINING CHARACTERISTICS

Major (Must Be Present, One or More)

Hard, formed stool *and/or*
Defecation fewer than three times a week

Minor (May Be Present)

Decreased bowel sounds
Reported feeling of rectal fullness
Reported feeling of pressure in rectum
Straining and pain on defecation
Palpable impaction
Feeling of inadequate emptying

RELATED FACTORS

Pathophysiological

Related to defective nerve stimulation, weak pelvic floor muscles, and immobility secondary to:
Spinal cord lesions
Spinal cord injury
Spina bifida
Dementia
CVA, stroke

Neurological diseases (multiple sclerosis [MS], Parkinson's)

Related to decreased metabolic rate secondary to:

Obesity

Pheochromocytoma

Diabetic neuropathy

Hypopituitarism

Uremia

Hypothyroidism

Hyperparathyroidism

Related to decreased response to urge to defecate secondary to:

Affective disorders

Related to pain upon defecation (*e.g.*, hemorrhoids, back injury)

Related to decreased peristalsis secondary to hypoxia (cardiac, pulmonary)

Treatment-Related

Related to side effects of (specify):

Antacids (calcium, aluminum)

Iron

Barium

Aluminum

Aspirin

Phenothiazines

Calcium

Anticholinergics

Anesthetics

Narcotics (codeine, morphine)

Diuretics

Antiparkinsonian agents

Related to effects of anesthesia and surgical manipulation on peristalsis

Related to habitual laxative use

Related to mucositis secondary to radiation

Situational (Personal, Environmental)

Related to decreased peristalsis secondary to: for example, immobility, pregnancy, stress, lack of exercise

Related to irregular evacuation patterns

Related to cultural or health beliefs

Related to lack of privacy

Related to inadequate fiber in diet

Related to fear of rectal or cardiac pain

Related to faulty appraisal
Related to inadequate fluid intake
Related to inability to perceive bowel cues

OUTCOME CRITERIA

The person will:

1. Describe therapeutic bowel regimen
2. Report or demonstrate improved bowel elimination
3. Explain rationale for interventions

GENERIC INTERVENTIONS

1. Teach the importance of a balanced diet.
   a. Review list of foods high in bulk:
      - Fresh fruits with skins
      - Bran
      - Nuts and seeds
      - Whole-grain breads and cereals
      - Cooked fruits and vegetables
      - Fruit juices
   b. Include approximately 800 g of fruits and vegetables (about four pieces of fresh fruit and large salad) for normal daily bowel movement.
   c. Gradually increase amount of bran as tolerated (may add to cereals, baked goods, etc.). Explain the need for fluid intake with bran.
2. Encourage daily intake of at least 2 L of fluids—8 to 10 glasses—unless contraindicated. Limit coffee to two to three cups per day.
3. Recommend a glass of warm water to be taken 30 minutes before breakfast; this may act as stimulus to bowel evacuation.
4. Establish a regular time for elimination. Use a commode chair or toilet instead of bedpan, if possible.
5. Assist person to normal semisquatting position to allow optimum usage of abdominal muscles and effect of force of gravity.
6. Teach how to massage along lower abdomen gently while on toilet.
7. Teach the importance of responding to urge to defecate.

8. If fecal impaction is present, instill warm mineral oil and retain it for 20 to 30 minutes. Using a well-lubricated glove, break up hard stool and remove pieces. Monitor for vagal stimulation (dizziness, slow pulse).

9. Explain the hazards of enema and non–bulk-producing laxative use (refer to Perceived Constipation).

10. Explain how to use bulk-producing laxatives (*e.g.*, psyllium hydrophilic mucilloid [Metamucil, Effersyllium Citrucel, Fiber-con]).

11. Emphasize the need for regular exercise.
    a. Suggest walking
    b. If walking is prohibited:
       - Teach client to lie in bed or sit on chair and bend one knee at a time to chest (10–20 times each knee) three to four times a day.
       - Teach client to sit in chair or lie in bed and turn torso from side to side (10–20 times) 6 to 10 times a day.

12. Reduce rectal pain, if possible, by instructing person in corrective measures:
    a. Gently apply a lubricant to anus to reduce pain on defecation.
    b. Apply cool compresses to area to reduce itching.
    c. Take sitz bath or soak in tub of warm water (43°–46°C) for 15-minute intervals if soothing.
    d. Take stool softeners or mineral oil as an adjunct to other approaches.
    e. Consult with physician concerning use of local anesthetics and antiseptic agents.

13. Protect the skin from contamination:
    a. Evaluate the surrounding skin area.
    b. Cleanse properly with nonirritating agent (*e.g.*, use gentle motion; use soft tissues following defecation).
    c. Suggest a sitz bath following defecation.
    d. Gently apply protective emollient or lubricant.

14. Initiate health teaching if indicated:
    a. Teach the methods to prevent rectal pressure, which contributes to hemorrhoids.
    b. Avoid prolonged sitting and straining at defecation.
    c. Soften stools (*e.g.*, low-roughage diet, high fluid intake).

🌀 CHILD FOCUS INTERVENTIONS

1. Discuss some causes of constipation in infants and children (underfeeding; high protein, low carbohydrate diet; lack of roughage; dehydration).
2. If bowel movements are infrequent with hard stools:
   a. With infants, add corn syrup to feeding or fruit to diet. Avoid apple juice or sauce.
   b. With children, add bran cereal, prune juice, fruits, and vegetables.
3. Persistent constipation should be evaluated medically.

🌀 MATERNAL FOCUS INTERVENTIONS

1. Explain the risks of constipation in pregnancy and postpartum (Reeder, 1997).
   a. Decreased gastric motility
   b. Prolonged intestinal time
   c. Pressure of enlarging uterus
   d. Distended abdominal muscles (postpartum)
   e. Relaxation of intestines (postpartum)
2. Explain aggravating factors for hemorrhoid development (straining at defecation, constipation, prolonged standing, wearing constrictive clothing).
3. If the woman has a history of constipation, discuss how to use bulk-producing laxatives to keep stool soft. Advise patient to avoid other types of laxatives (*e.g.*, stimulants, mineral oil).
4. Postdelivery, assess bowel sounds, presence of abdominal distention, hemorrhoids, and perineal swelling and if passing flatus.
5. Postdelivery, provide relief from pain of hemorrhoids, episiotomy, or perineal lacerations.
6. Consider the need for stool softeners, laxative, or rectal suppository. Promote defecation 2 to 3 days postdelivery.

🏛 OLDER ADULT FOCUS INTERVENTIONS

1. Discuss that individual bowel patterns vary (*e.g.*, three times a day to three times a week).
2. Discuss medication that can contribute to constipation (anticholinergics, narcotics, iron sulfate, psychotropic medications, aluminum and calcium antacids, tricyclic antidepressants, overuse of antidiarrheals).

MATERNAL FOCUS INTERVENTIONS

Refer to *Constipation.*

Perceived Constipation

DEFINITION

Perceived Constipation: The state in which an individual self-prescribes the daily use of laxatives, enemas, or suppositories to ensure a daily bowel movement.

DEFINING CHARACTERISTICS
(McLane & McShane, 1986)

Major (80%–100%)

Expectation of a daily bowel movement with the resulting overuse of laxatives, enemas, and/or suppositories
Expected passage of stool at the same time every day

RELATED FACTORS

Pathophysiological

Related to faulty appraisal secondary to: for example, obsessive-compulsive disorders, central nervous system (CNS) deterioration, depression

Situational (Personal, Environmental)

Related to inaccurate information secondary to: for example, cultural beliefs, family beliefs

OUTCOME CRITERIA

The person will:

1. Verbalize acceptance with bowel movement every 2 to 3 days
2. Not use non–bulk-producing laxatives
3. Relate the causes of constipation
4. Describe the hazards of enema or laxative use
5. Relate an intent to increase fiber, fluid, and exercise in daily life as discussed

⊞ GENERIC INTERVENTIONS

1. Explore with person their bowel patterns and expectations.
2. Gently explain that bowel movements are needed every 2 to 3 days, not daily.
3. Explain the hazards of regular laxative, enema, or suppository use:
   a. Temporary relief
   b. Impaired nutrient metabolism, riboflavin, calcium, magnesium, zinc, potassium
   c. Water deficiency
   d. Malabsorption of fat-soluble vitamins A, D, E, and K
   e. Diarrhea–constipation cycle
   f. Possible interactions with other medications (*e.g.*, diuretics, digoxin [Lanoxin])
4. Teach the importance of a balanced diet (refer to Colonic Constipation).
5. Encourage intake of at least 6 to 10 glasses of water (unless contraindicated).
6. Recommend a glass of warm water to be taken 30 minutes before breakfast; this may act as stimulus to bowel evacuation.
7. Establish a regular time for elimination.
8. Emphasize the need for regular exercise.
   a. Suggest walking:
   b. If walking is prohibited:
      • Teach client to lie in bed or sit on chair and bend one knee at a time to chest (10–20 times each knee) three to four times a day.
      • Teach client to sit in chair or lie in bed and turn torso from side to side (20–30 times) 6 to 10 times a day.
9. Emphasize that normal bowel function is possible without laxatives, enemas, or suppositories.

Risk for Constipation

DEFINITION

Constipation: The state in which an individual is at high risk of experiencing stasis of the large intestine, resulting in infrequent elimination and/or hard, dry feces.

RISK FACTORS

Refer to *Related Factors—Constipation*.

OUTCOME CRITERIA

The person will:

1. Report a pattern of soft, formed feces every 1–3 days.
2. Identify the effects of fluid, fiber, and activity on bowel elimination.

GENERIC INTERVENTIONS

Refer to *Constipation*.

Coping, Ineffective Individual

Defensive Coping

Ineffective Denial

Coping, Ineffective Individual

DEFINITION

Ineffective Individual Coping: The state in which the individual experiences or is at risk of experiencing an inability to manage internal or environmental stressors adequately because of inadequate resources (physical, psychological, behavioral, or cognitive).

> **Author's Note:**
> This diagnosis can be used to describe a variety of situations in which an individual does not adapt effectively to stressors.
> *(Continued)*

Author's Note (Continued):
Examples can be isolating behaviors, aggression, and destructive behavior. If the response is inappropriate use of the defense mechanisms of denial or defensiveness, the diagnosis Ineffective Denial or Defensive Coping can be used instead of Ineffective Individual Coping.

DEFINING CHARACTERISTICS (Vincent, 1985)

Major (Must Be Present, One or More)

Verbalization of inability to cope or ask for help *or*
Inappropriate use of defense mechanisms *or*
Inability to meet role expectations

Minor (May Be Present)

Chronic worry, anxiety
Reported difficulty with life stressors
Alteration in social participation
Destructive behavior toward self or others
High incidence of accidents
Frequent illnesses
Verbal manipulation
Inability to meet basic needs
Nonassertive response patterns
Change in usual communication pattern
Substance abuse

RELATED FACTORS

Pathophysiological

Related to chronicity of condition or complex self-care regimens
Related to changes in body integrity secondary to:
   Loss of body part
   Disfigurement secondary to trauma
Related to altered affect caused by changes secondary to:
   Body chemistry
   Tumor (brain)
   Intake of mood-altering substance
   Mental retardation

Treatment-Related

Related to separation from family and home (*e.g.*, hospitalization, confinement to a nursing home)

Related to disfigurement caused by surgery

Related to altered appearance owing to drugs, radiation, or other treatment

Situational (Personal, Environmental)

Related to increased food consumption in response to stressors

Related to changes in physical environment secondary to:

War	Poverty
Natural disaster	Homelessness
Relocation	Inadequate finances
Seasonal work (migrant worker)	

Related to disruption of emotional bonds secondary to:

Death	Foster home
Separation or divorce	Orphanage
Desertion	Educational institution
Relocation	Institutionalization
Jail	

Related to sensory overload secondary to:

Factory environment

Urbanization: crowding, noise pollution, excessive activity

Related to inadequate psychological resources secondary to:

Poor self-esteem

Excessive negative beliefs about self

Negative role modeling

Helplessness

Lack of motivation to respond

Related to culturally related conflicts with (specify):

Premarital sex

Abortion

Maturational

Child or adolescent

Related to:

Inconsistent methods of discipline

Fear of failure

Childhood trauma

Parental substance abuse

Parental rejection

Repressed anxiety
Panic level of anxiety
Poor impulse control
Poor social skills
Peer rejection

Adolescent

Related to inadequate psychological resources to adapt to:
Physical and emotional changes

Independence from family	Sexual awareness
	Educational demands
Relationships	Career choices

Young adult

Related to inadequate psychological resources to adapt to:

Career choices	Marriage
Educational demands	Parenthood
Leaving home	

Middle adult

Related to inadequate psychological resources to adapt to:

Physical signs of aging	Problems with relatives
Career pressures	Social status needs
Childrearing problems	Aging parents

Older adult

Related to inadequate psychological resources to adapt to:

Physical changes	Retirement
Changes in financial status	Response of others to older persons
Changes in residence	

OUTCOME CRITERIA

The person will:

1. Verbalize feelings related to emotional state
2. Identify personal coping patterns and the consequences of the behavior that results
3. Identify personal strengths and accept support through the nursing relationship
4. Make decisions and follow through with appropriate actions to change provocative situations in personal environment

✥ GENERIC INTERVENTIONS

1. Assess individual's present coping status.
   a. Determine onset of feelings and symptoms and their correlation with events and life changes.

       b. Assess ability to relate facts.

       c. Listen carefully, and observe facial expressions, gestures, eye contact, body positioning, tone, and intensity of voice.

       d. Determine risk of client inflicting self-harm, and intervene appropriately (see *Risk for Self-Harm*).

2. Offer support as person talks.

       a. Reassure that the feelings he or she has must be difficult.

       b. When person is pessimistic, attempt to provide a more hopeful, realistic perspective.

3. If person is angry (Thomas, 1998):

       a. Maintain an environment with low levels of stimuli.

       b. Explore why the person is angry.

       c. Do not argue or become defensive.

       d. Focus on what can be done rather than what has not been done.

       e. Offer options to increase sense of control.

       f. Acknowledge that everyone gets angry, but certain actions are not acceptable.

       g. If violence is a risk, refer to *Risk for Violence*.

4. Encourage a self-evaluation of his or her own behavior.

       a. "Did that work for you?"

       b. "How did it help?"

       c. "What did you learn from that experience?"

5. Assist the person to problem solve in a constructive manner.

       a. What is the problem?

       b. Who or what is responsible for the problem?

       c. What are the options? (Make a list.)

       d. What are the advantages and disadvantages of each option?

6. Discuss possible alternatives (*i.e.*, talk about the problem with those involved, try to change the situation, or do nothing and accept the consequences).

7. Assist the individual to identify problems that cannot be controlled directly and help him or her to practice stress-reducing activities for control (*e.g.*, exercise program, yoga).

8. Instruct person in relaxation techniques; emphasize the importance of setting 15 to 20 minutes aside each day to practice relaxation.

9. Mobilize the person into a gradual increase in activity.

10. Find outlets that foster feelings of personal achievement and self-esteem.
11. Provide opportunities to learn and use stress management techniques (*e.g.*, jogging, yoga).
12. Establish a network of persons who understand the situation.
13. For depression-related problems beyond the scope of nurse generalists, refer to appropriate professionals (marriage counselor, psychiatric nurse therapist, psychologist, psychiatrist).

🌀 CHILD FOCUS INTERVENTIONS
(Johnson & Saunders, 1995)

1. Establish eye contact before giving instructions.
2. Set firm, responsible limits.
3. State rules simply; do not lecture.
4. Maintain regular routine.
5. Advise parents to avoid disagreeing with each other in child's presence.
6. Maintain a calm, simple environment.
7. If hyperactive, provide for periods of activity using large muscles.
8. Provide immediate and constant feedback.
9. Advise parents to consult with educational professionals for educational programming.

Defensive Coping

DEFINITION

Defensive Coping: The state in which an individual repeatedly presents falsely positive self-evaluation as a defense against underlying perceived threats to positive self-regard.

DEFINING CHARACTERISTICS
(Norris & Kunes-Connell, 1987)

Major (80%–100%)

Denial of obvious problems/weaknesses
Projection of blame/responsibility
Rationalization of failures

Hypersensitivity to slight criticism
Grandiosity

Minor (50%–79%)

Superior attitude toward others
Difficulty in establishing or maintaining relationships
Hostile laughter or ridicule of others
Difficulty in testing perceptions against reality
Lack of follow through or participation in treatment or therapy

RELATED FACTORS

See *Chronic Low Self-Esteem, Powerlessness,* and *Impaired Social Interaction.*

OUTCOME CRITERIA

The person will:

1. Establish realistic goals in concert with caregivers
2. Work effectively toward the achievement of these goals without progress being compromised by defensive dynamics

◆ GENERIC INTERVENTIONS

1. Reduce demands on the individual as stress level or signs of defensive coping increase.
2. Establish a therapeutic stance that will reduce defensive binds and increase effective actions.
   a. Maintain a neutral, matter-of-fact tone with a consistent positive regard. Ensure that all staff relate in a consistent fashion with consistent expectations.
   b. Focus on simple here-and-now, goal-directed topics when encountering the client's defenses.
   c. Encourage client to express goals, and establish agreement with the client in at least one or two areas.
   d. Do not defend or dwell on the client's negative projections or displacements.
   e. Disengage from disagreement.
   f. Do not challenge distortions or unrealistic/grandiose self-expressions. Try instead to redirect the conversation toward more neutral topics or more

      realistic topics about which some agreement has already been established.

   g. Encourage the person to evaluate his or her own progress.

   h. Identify for the person actions that have interfered with achieving established goals.

   i. Practice role-playing less defensive responses with difficult situations.

   j. Evaluate interactions, progress, and approach with other team members to ensure overall consistency within the treatment milieu.

3. Work to establish a therapeutic relationship with the client to decrease the need to defend and permit a more direct addressing of underlying, related factors (see *Chronic Low Self-Esteem*).

   a. Validate the client's reluctance to trust in the beginning.

   b. Engage the client in diversional, non–goal-directed, noncompetitive activities (*e.g.*, relaxation therapy, games, outing).

   c. Encourage self-expression of neutral themes, positive reminiscences, and so forth.

   d. Encourage other means for self-expression (*e.g.*, writing or art) if verbal interaction is difficult or if this is an area of personal strength.

   e. Listen passively to some grandiose or negative self-expression to reinforce your "positive regard."

Ineffective Denial

DEFINITION

Ineffective Denial: The state in which individuals minimize or disavow symptoms or a situation to the detriment of their health.

Author's Note:
This type of denial differs from the denial in response to a loss. The denial in response to an illness or loss is necessary to maintain psychological equilibrium and is beneficial. Ineffective Denial is
(Continued)

Author's Note (Continued):
not beneficial when the individual will not participate in regimens to improve health or the situation (*e.g.*, denial of substance abuse). If the cause of the Ineffective Denial is not known, Ineffective Denial related to unknown etiology can be used, for example, Ineffective Denial related to unknown etiology as manifested by repetitive refusal to admit that barbiturate use is a problem.

DEFINING CHARACTERISTICS
(Lynch & Phillips, 1989)

Major (Must Be Present, One or More)

Delays seeking or refuses health care attention to the detriment of health
Does not perceive personal relevance of symptoms or danger

Minor (May Be Present)

Does not admit fear of death or invalidism
Minimizes symptoms
Displaces source of symptoms to other areas of the body
Unable to admit impact of disease on life pattern
Makes dismissive gestures or comments when speaking of distressing events
Displaces fear of impact of the condition
Displays inappropriate affect

RELATED FACTORS

Pathophysiological

Related to inability to consciously tolerate the consequences of any chronic or terminal illness

Treatment-Related

Related to prolonged treatment with no positive results

Situational/Psychological

Related to inability to tolerate consciously the consequences of:
Drug use   Financial crisis

Alcohol use
Smoking
Obesity
Loss of job
Loss of spouse/significant
other

Feelings of negative self-
concept, inadequacy,
guilt, loneliness,
despair, failure

Related to feelings of increased anxiety/stress, need to escape
personal problems, anger, and frustration

Related to feelings of omnipotence

Related to culturally permissive attitudes toward alcohol/
drug use

Biological/Genetic

Related to family history of alcoholism

OUTCOME CRITERIA

The person will:

1. Identify fears or anxieties
2. Express a sense of hope
3. Use alternative coping mechanisms

✥ GENERIC INTERVENTIONS

1. Provide opportunities to share fears and anxieties.
2. Focus on present response.
3. Assist in lowering anxiety level (see *Anxiety* for additional interventions).
4. Avoid confronting person on use of denial.
5. Carefully explore with person his or her interpretation of
the situation.
   a. Reflect self-reported cues used to minimize the
   situation (*e.g.,* "a little," "only").
   b. Identify recent detrimental behavior, and discuss
   the effects of this behavior on health.
6. Emphasize strengths and past successful coping.
7. Provide positive reinforcement for any expressions of
insight.
8. Do not accept rationalization or projection. Be polite,
caring, but firm.

9. If substance abuse is present (Heatter, 1995):
   a. Review observations and findings with client and family.
   b. Present evidence of damage (physical, social, financial, spiritual, familial).
   c. Establish goals.
   d. Provide self-help manuals or other pamphlets.
   e. Acquire commitment to keep daily log of alcohol/drug use.
   f. At next visit:
      • Review log.
      • Review progress.
      • Refer those who are dependent and desire to continue abstinence.

Coping, Ineffective Community

DEFINITION

Ineffective Community Coping: The state in which a community's pattern of activities for adaptation and problem solving are unsatisfactory for meeting the demands or needs of the community.

Author's Note

This diagnosis is useful for nurses who practice with aggregates. An aggregate is a group of persons "who have in common one or more personal or environmental characteristics" (Williams, 1977). Therefore, an aggregate can be the population of a small town, high school girls, or Hispanic men with hypertension.

This diagnosis may be more frequently used as a risk diagnosis than an actual one. Nurses practicing with community aggregates would identify risk factors that could cause Ineffective Community Coping. The focus would be on assisting the community to prevent the diagnosis.

DEFINING CHARACTERISTICS

Major (Must Be Present, One or More)

Failure of community to meet its own expectations
Unresolved community conflicts
Expressed difficulty in meeting demands for change
Expressed vulnerability

Minor (May Be Present)

Angry
Indifferent
Helpless
Overwhelmed

Bitter
Apathetic
Hopeless

RISK FACTORS

Presence of risk factors (see Related Factors)

RELATED FACTORS

Situational (Personal, Environmental)

Related to lack of knowledge of resources
Related to inadequate communication patterns
Related to inadequate community cohesiveness
Related to inadequate problem solving
Related to inadequate community resources
Related to inadequate law enforcement services
Related to overwhelming community destruction secondary to:

Flood
Earthquake
Avalanche

Hurricane
Epidemic

Related to traumatic effects of airplane crash, large fire,
 industrial disaster, or environmental accident
Related to threat to community safety (*e.g.*, murder, rape,
 kidnapping, robberies)
Related to sudden rise in community unemployment

Maturational

Related to inadequate resources for children, adolescents,
 working parents, or older adults

OUTCOME CRITERIA

The community will:

1. Access information to improve coping
2. Use communication channels to access assistance

INTERVENTIONS

1. Assess for causative or contributing factors.
   a. Lack of knowledge of available resources
   b. Inadequate problem solving
   c. Inadequate communication links
   d. Overwhelming, multiple stressors
   e. Threat to community safety
2. Provide opportunities for community members to face and discuss the situation (*e.g.*, schools, churches, synagogues, town hall) and demonstrate acceptance of their anger, withdrawal, or denial.
3. Do not offer false reassurance. Emphasize their ability to cope effectively.
4. Explore techniques that may improve coping. Elicit suggestions from group.
5. Discuss resources that can be accessed. Prepare the group to accept outside help.
   a. Emergency shelter, funds, food, clothes
   b. Counseling
   c. Transportation
   d. Health care
6. Plan how to access isolated persons in the community.
7. Establish a method to access information and support (*e.g.*, local health department, hospital, churches, synagogues, community center).
8. Initiate referrals as indicated.
   a. Counseling
   b. Public assistance

⬛ Coping, Potential for Enhanced Community

DEFINITION

Potential for Enhanced Community Coping: A state in which a community's pattern for adaptation and problem solving is satisfactory for meeting the demands or needs of the community, but it desires to improve management of current and future problems or stressors.

> **Author's Note:**
> This diagnosis can be used to describe a community that desires to improve an already effective pattern of coping. For a community to be able to be assisted to a higher level of functioning, its basic needs for food, shelter, safety, a clean environment, and a supportive network must first be addressed. When these needs are met, programs can focus on higher functioning, such as wellness and self-actualization. Community programs can be designed after a community assessment and because of community requests. Community programs can focus on enhancing health promotion with topics related to optimal nutrition, weight control, regular exercise programs, constructive stress management, social support, role responsibilities, and preparing for and coping with life cycle events, such as retirement, parenting, or pregnancy.

DEFINING CHARACTERISTICS

Major (Must Be Present)

Successful coping with a previous crisis

Minor (May Be Present)

Active planning by community for predicted stressors
Active problem solving by community when faced with issues
Agreement that community is responsible for stress management
Positive communication among community members
Positive communication between community/aggregates and larger community

Programs available for recreation and relaxation
Resources sufficient for managing stressors

RISK FACTORS

Presence of risk factors (see Related Factors)

RELATED FACTORS

Situational (Personal, Environmental)

Related to availability of community programs to augment (specify):
Nutritional status
Weight control
Stress management
Exercise program
Self-actualization
Social support

Maturational

Related to availability of community programs to augment coping with life cycle events, for example:

Aging	Parenting
Adolescence	Retirement
Pregnancy	"Empty nest"

OUTCOME CRITERIA

The community will:

1. Access programs designed to improve overall community well-being

INTERVENTIONS

1. Meet with influential members of the target population to determine health-promotion needs (Archer, 1983).
   a. For what needs could the nursing agency develop services?
   b. How can the agency promote or market the services to motivate people to use them?
   c. Will enough members of the targeted population use the service?

      d. Based on past programming, what improvements can be made for the future?

      e. Are similar services provided by another agency or organization (hospital, religious)?

2. Plan the development of programs targeted for a specific population.

3. Delineate the geographical area to be served and the site of the program.

4. Develop detailed program objectives and the evaluation framework to be used: content, time needed, ideal teaching method for targeted group, teaching aids (*e.g.*, large-print materials).

5. Establish resources needed and sources.
   a. Space
   b. Transportation facilities
   c. Optimal day of week, time of year
   d. Supplies, audiovideo equipment
   e. Financial (budgeted, donations)

6. Market the program.
   a. Media (*e.g.*, newspaper, television, radio)
   b. Posters (food market, train station)
   c. Flyers (distribute in school to home)
   d. Word of mouth (religious organizations, community clubs, schools)
   e. Guest speakers (community clubs, schools)

7. Provide program, and evaluate whether the desired results (objectives) were achieved.
   a. Number of participants
   b. Actual expenditures versus budgeted
   c. Participant evaluations
   d. Revisions for future programs

Family Coping: Potential for Growth

DEFINITION

Family Coping: Potential for Growth: Effective management of adaptive tasks by a family member involved with the individual's health challenge who now is exhibiting the desire and readiness for enhanced health and growth in regard to self and in relation to the client.

Author's Note:

This diagnosis describes a family that seeks the opportunity to adapt together to changes and to have a sense of control over outcomes.

DEFINING CHARACTERISTICS

Family member attempts to describe the growth impact of a crisis on his or her own values, priorities, goals, or relationships.

Family member moves in the direction of a health-promoting and enriching lifestyle that supports and monitors maturational processes, audits and negotiates treatment programs, and generally chooses experiences that optimize wellness.

Individual expresses interest in making contact on a one-to-one basis or in a mutual-aid group with another person who has experienced a similar situation.

RELATED FACTORS

See *Health Seeking Behaviors* and *Altered Family Processes*.

🔁 GENERIC INTERVENTIONS

1. Help to establish goals.
2. Assist with mutual problem solving.
3. Encourage sharing of thoughts, perceptions, and feelings (Stolte, 1996).
4. Explore if family members can change roles as needed.
5. Assist members to communicate with each other. If indicated, suggest letter-writing, role-playing.
6. Help to anticipate challenges to family functioning (Duvail & Miller, 1985).
   a. Beginning families
   b. Childbearing families
   c. Preschool children
   d. School age

e. Teenage
f. Launching young adult
g. Middle-age family
h. Aging family
7. See also *Altered Family Processes*.

Ineffective Family Coping: Compromised

DEFINITION

Ineffective Family Coping: Compromised: The state in which a usually supportive primary person (family member or close friend) is providing insufficient, ineffective, or compromised support, comfort, assistance, or encouragement that may be needed by the client to manage or master adaptive tasks related to his or her health challenge.

> **Author's Note:**
> This nursing diagnosis describes situations that are similar to the diagnosis Altered Family Processes. Until clinical research differentiates this category from the preceding ones, use Altered Family Processes.

DEFINING CHARACTERISTICS

Subjective

Client expresses or confirms a concern or complaint about a significant other's response to his or her health problem.

Significant person describes preoccupation with personal reactions (*e.g.*, fear, anticipatory grief, guilt, anxiety) to client's illness, disability, or other situational or developmental crises.

Significant person describes or confirms an inadequate understanding or knowledge base that interferes with effective assistive or supportive behaviors.

Objective

Significant person attempts assistive or supportive behaviors with less than satisfactory results.

Significant person withdraws or enters into limited or temporary personal communication with the client in times of need.

Significant person displays protective behavior disproportionate (too little or too much) to the client's abilities or need for autonomy.

RELATED FACTORS

See *Altered Family Processes.*

Ineffective Family Coping: Disabling

DEFINITION

Ineffective Family Coping: Disabling: The state in which a family demonstrates, or is at risk to demonstrate, destructive behavior in response to an inability to manage internal or external stressors due to inadequate resources (physical, psychological, or cognitive).

Author's Note:

The diagnosis Ineffective Family Coping: Disabling describes a family that has a history of demonstrating destructive overt or covert behavior or has adapted detrimentally to a stressor. This diagnosis differs from Altered Family Processes, which describes a family that usually functions constructively but is challenged by a stressor that has altered or may alter its functioning. Sustained Altered Family Processes may progress to Ineffective Family Coping.

DEFINING CHARACTERISTICS

Major (Must Be Present, One or More)

Abusive or neglectful care of individual(s)
Decisions/actions that are detrimental to family well-being
Neglectful relationships with other family members

Minor (May Be Present)

Distortion of reality regarding the client's health problem
Intolerance
Rejection
Abandonment
Desertion
Psychosomaticism
Taking on illness signs of client
Agitation
Depression
Aggression
Hostility
Impaired restructuring of a meaningful life for self
Prolonged preoccupation with client
Client's development of helpless, inactive dependence

RELATED FACTORS

Related to impaired ability to fulfill role responsibilities
  secondary to any acute or chronic illness

Situational (Personal, Environmental)

Related to impaired ability to manage stressors constructively
  secondary to:
    Addiction
    Alcoholism
    Negative role modeling
    Low self-esteem
    History of ineffective relationship with own parents
    History of abusive relationships with parents
Related to unrealistic expectations of child by parent
Related to unrealistic expectations of self by parent
Related to unrealistic expectations of parent by child
Related to unmet psychosocial needs of child by parent
Related to unmet psychosocial needs of parent by child

OUTCOME CRITERIA

The person will:

1. Identify responses that are neglectful or harmful
2. Verbalize the need for assistance with situation
3. Relate community resources available

◤ GENERIC INTERVENTIONS

1. Assist family to evaluate past and present family functioning.
2. Provide all family members an opportunity to discuss their appraisal of the situation.
3. Discourage blaming but allow ventilation of anger.
4. Clarify feelings of members.
5. Assist family with appraisal of the situation.
   a. What is wrong?
   b. What are the causes?
   c. Who has contributed to the problem?
   d. What are the options?
   e. What are the advantages/disadvantages of each option?
6. If indicated, ask members to consider the problem from the perspective of another family member.
7. If a member is ill, assist family to have more realistic expectations.
8. If domestic abuse is suspected:
   a. Know your state's laws regarding domestic abuse (*e.g.*, mandatory reporting).
   b. Provide an opportunity to validate abuse and talk about feelings.
   c. Be direct and nonjudgmental (Blair, 1986).
      • How do you handle stress?
      • How does your partner or caregiver handle stress?
      • How do you and your partner argue?
      • Are you afraid of your partner?
      • Have you ever been hit, pushed, or injured by your partner?
   d. Encourage a realistic appraisal of the situation; dispel guilt and myths.
      • Violence is not normal for most families.
      • Violence may stop, but it usually becomes increasingly worse.

- Alcohol and drugs do not cause violence.
- The victim is not responsible for the violence.
- You do not deserve this.
- You have a right to be protected.

  e. Provide options, but allow them to make a decision at their own pace.
  f. Discuss the importance of a "safety plan." For specifics of a safety plan, refer to a hotline or programs specific for domestic violence.
  g. Provide a list of community agencies available to victim and abuser (emergency and long term):
    - Hotlines
    - Legal services
    - Shelters
    - Counseling agencies
  h. Discuss the availability of the social service department for assistance.
  i. Consult with the legal resources in the community, and familiarize the victim with the state laws regarding:
    - Eviction of abuser
    - Counseling
    - Temporary support
    - Protection orders
    - Criminal law
    - Types of police interventions
  j. Document findings and dialogue for possible future court use.

🕸 CHILD FOCUS INTERVENTIONS

1. Report suspected cases of child abuse.
    a. Know your state's child abuse laws and procedures for reporting child abuse (*e.g.*, Bureau of Child Welfare, Department of Social Services, Child Protective Services).
    b. Maintain an objective record:
      - Description of injuries
      - Conversations with parents and child in quotes
      - Description of behaviors, not interpretation (*e.g.*, avoid "angry father"; instead, write "Father screamed at child, 'If you weren't so bad, this wouldn't have happened.' ")

- Description of parent–child interactions (*e.g.*, shies away from mother's touch)
- Nutritional status
- Growth and development compared with age-related norms

2. Provide the child with acceptance and affection.
3. Assist child with grieving if foster home placement is necessary.
4. Allow opportunities for child to ventilate feelings.
5. Provide interventions that promote parents' self-esteem and sense of trust.
   a. Tell them it was good that they brought the child to the hospital.
   b. Promote their confidence by presenting a warm, helpful attitude and acknowledging any competent parenting activities.
   c. Provide opportunities for parents to participate in their child's care (*e.g.*, feeding, bathing).
6. Refer abusive parents to community agencies and professionals for counseling.
7. Disseminate information to the community about the problem of child abuse (*e.g.*, parent-school organizations, radio, television, newspaper).

OLDER ADULT FOCUS INTERVENTIONS

1. Identify suspected cases of elder abuse; observe for these signs:
   a. Failure to adhere to therapeutic regimens
   b. Evidence of malnutrition, dehydration
   c. Bruises, swelling, lacerations, burns, bites
   d. Pressure ulcers
   e. Caregiver not allowing nurse to be alone with elder
2. If suspected: (Anetzberger, 1987)
   a. Know your state's laws regarding elder abuse.
   b. Consult with supervisor for procedures.
   c. Maintain an objective record, including:
      - Description of injuries
      - Conversations with elder and caregivers
      - Description of behaviors
      - Nutritional, hydration status
   d. Consider the elder's right to choose to live at risk of harm providing he or she is capable of making that choice.

e. Do not initiate an action that could increase the elder's risk of harm or antagonize the abuser.

f. Respect the elder's right to secrecy and the right for self-determination.

3. Disseminate information to community regarding prevention.

Decisional Conflict

DEFINITION

Decisional Conflict: The state in which an individual or group experiences uncertainty about a course of action when the choice involves risk, loss, or challenge.

DEFINING CHARACTERISTICS (Hiltunen, 1987)

Major (80%–100%)

Verbalization of uncertainty about choices
Verbalization of undesired consequences of alternative actions being considered
Vacillation between alternative choices
Delayed decision making

Minor (50%–79%)

Verbalized feeling of distress while attempting a decision
Self-focusing
Physical signs of distress or tension (*e.g.*, increased heart rate, increased muscle tension, restlessness, etc.) whenever the decision comes within focus of attention
Questioning personal values and beliefs while attempting to make a decision

RELATED FACTORS

Many situations can contribute to Decisional Conflict, particularly those that involve complex medical interventions of great risk. Any decisional situation can precipitate conflict for an individual; thus, the examples listed below are not exhaustive but reflect situations that may be problematic and possess factors that increase the difficulty.

Treatment-Related

Related to risks versus benefits of (specify test, treatment):
   (Surgery)

Tumor removal	Joint replacement
Cataract	Hysterectomy
Laminectomy	Transplant
Orchiectomy	Cesarean section
Cosmetic	

(Diagnostics)

Amniocentesis	X-rays
Ultrasound	

   Chemotherapy
   Radiation
   Dialysis
   Mechanical ventilation
   Enteral feedings
   Intravenous hydration
   Use of medications during labor
   HIV antiviral therapy

Situational (Personal, Environmental)

Related to risks versus benefits of:
   Personal

Marriage	Institutionalization
Separation	(child, parent)
Divorce	Breastfeeding versus
Parenthood	bottle feeding
Birth control	Abortion
Artificial insemination	Sterilization
Adoption	Nursing home placement
Circumcision	Transport from rural
Foster home placement	facilities

   Work/task

Career change	Business investments
Relocation	Professional ethics

Related to lack of relevant information
Related to confusing information

Related to:
    Disagreement within support systems
    Inexperience with decision making
    Unclear personal values/beliefs
    Conflict with personal values/beliefs
    Resignation
    Family history of poor prognosis
    Hospital environment—loss of control
    Ethical dilemmas of:
        Quality of life
        Cessation of life-support systems
        "Do not resuscitate" orders
        Termination of pregnancy
        Organ transplant

Maturational

Related to risks versus benefits of:
    (Adolescent)

Peer pressure	Use of birth control
Sexual activity	Whether to continue a
Alcohol/drug use	relationship
Illegal/dangerous	College
situations	Career choice

    (Adult)

Career change	Relocation
Retirement	

    (Older adult)

Retirement	Nursing home placement

OUTCOME CRITERIA

The individual or group will:

1. Relate the advantages and disadvantages of choices
2. Share fears and concerns regarding choices and responses of others
3. Make an informed choice

⊞ GENERIC INTERVENTIONS

1. Establish a trusting and meaningful relationship that promotes mutual understanding and caring.

2. Facilitate a logical decision-making process.
   a. Assist the person in recognizing what the problem is, and clearly identify that a decision needs to be made.
   b. Explore what the outcomes of not deciding would be.
   c. Have person make a list of all the possible alternatives or options.
   d. Help identify the probable outcomes of the various alternatives.
   e. Help person to face fears.
   f. Correct misinformation.
   g. Aid in evaluating the alternatives based on actual or potential threats to beliefs/values.
   h. Encourage the person to make a decision.
3. Encourage the person's significant others to be involved in the entire decision-making process.
4. Assist the individual in exploring personal values and relationships that may have an impact on the decision.
5. Support individual making informed decision, even if decision conflicts with own values.
   a. Consult own spiritual leader.
6. Actively reassure the person that the decision is his or hers to make and that he or she has the right to do so.
7. Do not allow others to undermine the person's confidence in making own decision.
8. Collaborate with family members to clarify the process.

🐚 CHILD FOCUS INTERVENTIONS

1. Include children and adolescents in decision-making process.

🏛 OLDER ADULT FOCUS INTERVENTIONS

1. Ensure that older adult is involved in decisions.
2. Facilitate communication among the elder, family, and professionals.
3. If needed, use simple explanations, and provide the pros and cons of the decision.

Diarrhea

DEFINITION

Diarrhea: The state in which an individual experiences or is at risk of experiencing frequent passage of liquid stool or unformed stool.

DEFINING CHARACTERISTICS

Major (Must Be Present, One or More)

Loose, liquid stools *and/or*
Increased frequency of stools (more than three times a day)

Minor (May Be Present)

Urgency
Cramping/abdominal pain
Increased frequency of bowel sounds
Increased fluidity or volume of stools

RELATED FACTORS

Pathophysiological

Related to malabsorption or inflammation secondary to:

Kwashiorkor	Crohn's disease
Gastritis	Colon cancer
Peptic ulcer	Spastic colon
Diverticulitis	Celiac disease (sprue)
Ulcerative colitis	Irritable bowel

Related to lactase deficiency
Related to increased peristalsis secondary to increased metabolic rate (hyperthyroidism)
Related to dumping syndrome
Related to infectious process secondary to:

Trichinosis	Shigellosis
Dysentery	Typhoid fever
Cholera	Infectious hepatitis
Malaria	Microsporidia
Cryptosporida	

Related to excessive secretion of fats in stool secondary to liver dysfunction

Related to inflammation and ulceration of gastrointestinal mucosa secondary to high levels of nitrogenous wastes (renal failure)

Treatment-Related

Related to malabsorption or inflammation secondary to surgical intervention of the bowel

Related to side effects of (specify):

Thyroid agents	Cancer chemotherapeutic
Antacids (magnesium	agents
hydroxide)	Analgesics
Laxatives	Cimetidine
Stool softeners	Iron sulfate
Antibiotics	Antivirals (HIV)

Related to high-solute tube feedings

Situational (Personal, Environmental)

Related to stress or anxiety
Related to irritating foods (fruits, bran cereals)
Related to change in water or food secondary to travel
Related to change in bacteria in water
Related to bacteria, virus, or parasite to which no immunity is present
Related to hot weather
Related to increased caffeine consumption

Maturational

Infant: Related to breast milk

OUTCOME CRITERIA

The person will:

1. Describe contributing factors when known
2. Explain rationale for interventions
3. Report less diarrhea

🔁 GENERIC INTERVENTIONS

1. Assess for causative or contributing factors: tube feedings, dietary indiscretions/contaminated foods, food allergies, foreign travel, fecal impaction.

2. Reduce diarrhea.
   a. Discontinue solids.
   b. Ingest clear liquids (fruit juices, Gatorade, broth).
   c. Avoid milk products, fat, high fiber, (whole-grain products, fresh fruits, and vegetables).
   d. Gradually add semisolids and solids (crackers, yogurt, rice, bananas, applesauce).
3. Increase oral intake to maintain a normal urine-specific gravity (pale yellow urine).
4. Encourage fluids high in potassium and sodium (water, apple juice, flat ginger ale).
5. Caution against use of very hot or very cold liquids.
6. Explain to client and significant others the interventions required to prevent future episodes.
7. If related to tube feedings:
   a. Change to continuous-drip tube feedings.
   b. Administer more slowly if signs of gastrointestinal intolerance occur.
   c. If refrigerated, warm in hot water to room temperature.
   d. Dilute strength of feeding temporarily.
   e. Follow tube feeding with specified amount of water to ensure hydration.
8. Teach precautions to take when traveling to foreign lands (Maresca, 1986; Bennett, 1995).
   a. Avoid foods served cold, salads, milk, fresh cheese, cold cuts, and salsa.
   b. Drink carbonated or bottled beverages; avoid ice.
   c. Peel fresh fruits and vegetables.
   d. Consult with primary health care provider for prophylactic use of bismuth subsalicylate (*e.g.*, Pepto-Bismol), 30 to 60 mL q.i.d. during travel and 2 days after return, or antimicrobials for treatment of traveler's diarrhea. Avoid opiate-containing antidiarrheals (*e.g.*, Lomotil, Imodium)
9. Explain how to prevent transmission of infection (handwashing, proper storing, cooking, and handling of food).

❷ CHILD FOCUS INTERVENTIONS

1. For breastfed infants:
   a. Discontinue solids.

  b. Offer clear liquid supplements.

  c. Continue breastfeeding.

2. For formula-fed infant or milk-fed child:

  a. Discontinue formula, milk products, and solid foods.

  b. Avoid high carbohydrate fluids (*e.g.*, soft drinks, gelatin, fruit juices, caffeinated drinks, chicken or beef broth).

  c. Use oral rehydration solutions (*e.g.*, Pedialyte, Lytran, Ricelyte, Resol).

   • Provide 60–80 mL/kg over a 2-hour period for mild to moderate diarrhea.

  d. Gradually add plain solids (Jell-O, bananas, rice, cereal, crackers).

  e. Gradually return to regular diet (except milk products) after 36 to 48 hours; after 3 to 5 days, gradually add milk products (half-strength skim milk to full-strength skim milk to half-strength whole milk to full-strength whole milk).

  f. Gradually introduce formula (half-strength formula to full-strength formula).

3. Explain the BRAT diet (bananas, rice, applesauce, tea, and toast) to counter the effects of diarrhea.

🏛 OLDER ADULT FOCUS INTERVENTIONS

1. Determine if impaction is present; if so, remove it (refer to Constipation for specific interventions).

2. Monitor closely for hypovolemia and electrolyte imbalance (potassium, sodium).

Disuse Syndrome

DEFINITION

Disuse Syndrome: The state in which an individual is experiencing or at risk for deterioration of body systems or altered functioning as a result of prescribed or unavoidable musculoskeletal inactivity.

Author's Note:
Disuse Syndrome represents an individual experiencing or at risk for the adverse effects of immobility. Syndrome nursing diagnoses should not be written as Risk, because clustered under them are risk and actual diagnoses. Disuse Syndrome identifies an individual as vulnerable to certain complications and experiencing altered functioning in a health pattern. In most situations, syndrome diagnoses do not require causative or contributing factors (*i.e.*, Disuse Syndrome related to spinal cord injury). When the causative or contributing factors to Disuse Syndrome are personal, environmental, or maturational, it may be useful to specify the related factors.
　　If an individual who is immobile manifests the signs and symptoms of Impaired Skin Integrity or another diagnosis, the specific diagnosis should be used. The nurse should continue to use Disuse Syndrome so that deterioration of the other body systems does not occur.

DEFINING CHARACTERISTICS

Presence of a cluster of actual or risk nursing diagnoses related to inactivity:

- *Risk for Impaired Skin Integrity*
- *Risk for Constipation*
- *Risk for Altered Respiratory Function*
- *Risk for Altered Peripheral Tissue Perfusion*
- *Risk for Infection*
- *Risk for Activity Intolerance*
- *Risk for Impaired Physical Mobility*
- *Risk for Injury*
- *Risk for Sensory/Perceptual Alterations*
- *Powerlessness*
- *Body Image Disturbance*

RELATED FACTORS (Optional)

Pathophysiological

Related to:
　　Decreased sensorium
　　Unconsciousness
　　Neuromuscular impairment
　　　　Multiple sclerosis　　　　　　Muscular dystrophy

Parkinsonism	Partial or total paralysis
Guillain-Barré syndrome	Spinal cord injury

Musculoskeletal conditions

Fractures	Rheumatic diseases

End-stage disease

AIDS	Cardiac disease
Renal disease	Cancer

Psychiatric/mental health disorders

Major depression	Severe phobias
Catatonic state	

Treatment-Related

Related to:

Surgery (amputation, skeletal)	Prescribed immobility
	Mechanical ventilation
Traction/casts/splints	Invasive vascular lines

Situational (Personal, Environmental)

Related to depression, fatigue, debilitated state, or pain

Maturational

Related to:

Newborn, infant, child, or adolescent

Down syndrome	Osteogenesis imperfecta
Legg-Calvé-Perthes disease	Cerebral palsy
	Spina bifida
Risser turnbuckle jacket	Autism
Juvenile arthritis	Mental/physical disability

Older adult

Decreased motor agility	Presenile dementia
Muscle weakness	

OUTCOME CRITERIA

The person will demonstrate continued:

1. Intact skin/tissue integrity
2. Maximum pulmonary function
3. Maximum peripheral blood flow
4. Full ROM
5. Bowel, bladder, and renal functioning
6. Use of social contacts and activities when possible

The person will:

1. Explain rationale for treatments
2. Make decisions regarding care when possible
3. Share feelings regarding immobile state

⬢ GENERIC INTERVENTIONS

1. Assist to reposition, turning frequently from side to side (hourly if possible).
2. Encourage deep breathing and controlled coughing exercises five times every hour.
3. Auscultate lung fields every 8 hours.
4. Maintain usual pattern of bowel elimination. Refer to *Constipation* for specific interventions.
5. Prevent pressure ulcers (Maklebust & Sieggreen, 1996).
   a. Use repositioning schedule that relieves vulnerable area most often.
   b. Turn person or instruct person to turn or shift weight every 30 minutes to 2 hours.
   c. Keep bed as flat as possible to reduce shearing forces; limit Fowler's position to 30 minutes at a time.
   d. Use foam blocks or pillows to provide a bridging effect.
   e. Use enough personnel to lift person up in bed or chair.
6. Observe for erythema and blanching, and palpate for warmth and tissue sponginess with each position change.
7. Do not massage reddened areas.
8. Refer to *Impaired Skin Integrity* for additional interventions.
9. Elevate extremity above the level of the heart (may be contraindicated if severe cardiac or respiratory disease is present).
10. Perform ROM exercises (frequency to be determined by condition of the individual).
11. Position the person in alignment to prevent complications.
12. Provide a daily intake of fluid of 2,000 mL or greater (unless contraindicated); refer to *Fluid Volume Deficit* for specific interventions.
13. Provide weight bearing when possible (*e.g.*, Tilt table).

14. Encourage the person to share feelings and fears regarding restricted movement.
15. Encourage the person to wear own clothes rather than pajamas.
16. Include the individual in planning schedule for daily routine.
17. Be creative; vary the physical environment and daily routine when possible.
18. Provide opportunities for individual to control decisions.

🍥 CHILD FOCUS INTERVENTIONS

1. Provide child with play appropriate for condition.
2. Encourage child to share feelings regarding immobilization.
3. Encourage child to keep a diary of experiences.
4. If possible, provide child with lunchmates (*e.g.*, staff, other children).

Diversional Activity Deficit

DEFINITION

Diversional Activity Deficit: The state in which an individual or group experiences or is at risk of experiencing decreased stimulation from or interest in leisure activities.

DEFINING CHARACTERISTICS

Major (Must Be Present)

Observed or statements of boredom/depression from inactivity

Minor (May Be Present)

Constant expression of unpleasant thoughts or feelings
Yawning or inattentiveness
Flat facial expression
Body language (shifting of body away from speaker)
Restlessness/fidgeting
Weight loss or gain
Hostility

RELATED FACTORS

Pathophysiological

Related to difficulty accessing or participating in usual activities secondary to communicable disease or pain

Treatment-Related

Related to difficulty accessing or participating in usual activities secondary to isolation or immobility

Situational (Personal, Environmental)

Related to unsatisfactory social behaviors
Related to no peers or friends
Related to monotonous environment
Related to long-term hospitalization or confinement
Related to lack of motivation
Related to difficulty accessing or participating in usual activities secondary to:
  Excessive long hours of stressful work
  No time for leisure activities
  Career changes (*e.g.*, teacher to homemaker, retirement)
  Children leaving home ("empty nest")
  Immobility
  Decreased sensory perception (*e.g.*, blindness, hearing loss)
  Multiple role responsibilities

Maturational

Infant/child
  Related to lack of appropriate stimulation, toys, peers
Older adult
  Related to difficulty accessing or participating in usual activities secondary to:

Sensory motor deficits	Lack of peer group
Lack of transportation	Limited finances
Fear of crime	Confusion

OUTCOME CRITERIA

The person will:

1. Relate feelings of boredom and discuss methods of finding diversional activities
2. Relate methods of coping with feelings of anger or depression caused by boredom

3. Report an increase in enjoyable activities
4. Engage in an enjoyable activity by (date)

⊞ GENERIC INTERVENTIONS

1. Stimulate motivation by showing interest and encouraging sharing of feelings and experiences.
2. Help the person to work through feelings of anger and grief.
3. Vary daily routine when possible (*e.g.*, give bath in the afternoon so that the person can watch a special show or talk with a visitor who drops in).
4. Include the individual in planning daily schedule.
5. Plan time for visitors.
6. Be creative; vary the physical environment when possible.
7. Place the person near a window, if possible.
8. Discuss previously enjoyed hobbies. Consult with recreational or occupational therapist.
9. Provide reading material, radio, television "books on tape" (if person is visually impaired).
10. Plan an activity daily to give person something to look forward to, and always keep your promises.
11. Discourage the use of television as the primary source of recreation unless it is highly desired.
12. Consider using a volunteer to spend time reading to the person or helping with an activity.
13. If appropriate, enlist person to help others with an activity.
14. In an institutional setting (Rantz, 1991):
    a. Encourage participation in recreational therapy.
    b. Praise involvement.
    c. Allow person to choose which recreational activities are of interest.
    d. Focus on capabilities not the deficits.
    e. Consider using reminiscence, music, or pet therapy.
    f. Organize book discussions.

⊕ CHILD FOCUS INTERVENTIONS

1. Provide an environment with accessible playthings that suit the child's developmental age, and ensure that they are well within reach.

2. Encourage family to bring in child's favorite playthings, including items from nature that will help to keep the real world alive (*e.g.*, goldfish, leaves in fall).

Dysreflexia

Risk for Dysreflexia

Dysreflexia

DEFINITION

Dysreflexia: The state in which an individual with a spinal cord injury at T7 or above experiences or is at risk of experiencing a potential life-threatening uninhibited sympathetic response of the nervous system to a noxious stimulus.

Author's Note:

This is a situation that the nurse or client can prevent or treat. If the nurse's initial treatment does not abate the symptoms, medical treatment is imperative. An individual does not experience dysreflexia as a continued state but rather is at risk for it, so if it is experienced, it must be abated. Thus, Risk for Dysreflexia better describes the clinical situation than does Dysreflexia.

DEFINING CHARACTERISTICS

Major (Must Be Present, One or More)

Individual with spinal cord injury at T7 or above with:
Paroxysmal hypertension (sudden periodic elevated blood pressure in which systolic pressure is over 140 mm Hg and diastolic is above 90 mm Hg)
Bradycardia or tachycardia (pulse rate of fewer than 60 or more than 100 beats/min)
Diaphoresis (above the injury)
Red splotches on the skin (above the injury)

Pallor (below the injury)
Headache (a diffuse pain in different portions of the head and not confined to any nerve distribution area)
Apprehension

Minor (May Be Present)

Chilling
Conjunctival congestion
Horner's syndrome (contraction of the pupil, partial ptosis of the eyelid, enophthalmos, and sometimes loss of sweating over the affected side of the face)
Paresthesia
Pilomotor reflex
Blurred vision
Nasal congestion
Chest pain
Metallic taste in the mouth

RELATED FACTORS

Pathophysiological

Related to visceral stretching and irritation secondary to:
(Bowel)

Constipation	Fecal impaction
Acute abdominal condition	

(Bladder)

Distended bladder	Infection
Urinary calculi	

Related to stimulation of skin (abdominal, thigh)
Related to spastic sphincter

Treatment-Related

Related to removal of fecal impaction
Related to clogged or nonpatent catheter
Related to visceral stretching and irritation secondary to surgical incision

Situational (Personal, Environmental)

Related to lack of knowledge of prevention or treatment
Related to sexual activity
Related to menstruation

OUTCOME CRITERIA

The individual/family will:

1. State factors that cause dysreflexia
2. Describe the treatment for dysreflexia
3. Relate when emergency treatment is indicated

✦ GENERIC INTERVENTIONS

1. If signs of dysreflexia occur, *raise the head of the bed*, and remove the noxious stimuli.
2. Check for distended bladder.
3. If catheterized:
   a. Check catheter for kinks or compression.
   b. Irrigate with only 30 mL saline very slowly.
   c. Replace catheter if it will not drain.
4. If not catheterized, insert catheter using an anesthetic ointment and remove 500 mL, then clamp for 15 minutes; repeat cycle until bladder is drained.
5. For fecal impaction:
   a. First apply dibucaine hydrochloride ointment (Nupercaine) to the anus and 1 in (2.54 cm) into the rectum.
   b. Gently check rectum with a well-lubricated glove.
   c. Insert rectal suppository, or gently remove impaction.
6. Assess for other causes:
   a. Skin stimulation: spray lesion with a topical anesthetic agent.
   b. Other stimuli: these include cold draft, objects that pressure skin.
   c. Bladder infection: send urine for culture.
7. Continue to monitor blood pressure every 3 to 5 minutes.
8. Immediately consult physician for pharmacological treatment if hypertension or noxious stimuli are not eliminated.
9. Teach signs and symptoms and treatment of dysreflexia to person and family.
10. Teach when immediate medical intervention is warranted.
11. Explain what situations can trigger dysreflexia (menstrual cycle, sexual activity, bladder or bowel routines).
12. Advise consultation with physician for long-term pharmacological management if individual is very vulnerable.

Risk for Dysreflexia

DEFINITION

Risk for Dysreflexia: The state in which an individual with a spinal cord injury at T7 or above is at risk of experiencing a potential for life-threatening uninhibited sympathetic response of the nervous system to a noxious stimulus.

RELATED FACTORS

Refer to Related Factors in *Dysreflexia*.

OUTCOME CRITERIA

Refer to *Dysreflexia*.

INTERVENTIONS

1. Teach signs and symptoms and treatment of dysreflexia to person and family.
2. Teach when immediate medical intervention is warranted.
3. Explain what situations can trigger dysreflexia (menstrual cycle, sexual activity, bladder or bowel routines).
4. Teach to observe for early signs of bladder infections and skin lesions (pressure ulcers, ingrown toenails).
5. Advise consultation with physician for long-term pharmacologic management if individual is very vulnerable.

Energy Field Disturbance

DEFINITION

Energy Field Disturbance: The state in which a disruption of the flow of energy surrounding a person's being results in a disharmony of the body, mind, and/or spirit.

Author's Note:

This new addition to the NANDA list is unique for two reasons. It represents a specific theory—human energy field theory—and the interventions used require specialized instruction and supervised practice. Meehan (1991) recommends:

- At least 6 months' experience in professional practice in an acute care setting
- Guided learning by a nurse with at least 2 years' experience
- Conformance with practice guidelines
- Thirty hours of instruction in the theory and practice
- Thirty hours of supervised practice with relatively healthy individuals
- Successful completion of written and practice evaluations

This diagnosis may be considered unconventional by some. Perhaps each nurse needs to be reminded that there are many theories, philosophies, and frameworks of nursing practice, just as there are many definitions of clients and practice settings; some nurses practice on street corners with homeless persons, whereas others practice in an office attached to their home. Nursing diagnoses should not represent only the practices of nurses in the mainstream practice setting (acute care, long-term care, and home health). Rather than criticize a diagnosis as having little applicability to one's own practice, perhaps we should celebrate the diversity among us. Fundamentally, nurses are all connected as each of us and all of us seek to improve the condition of clients, families, groups, and communities.

DEFINING CHARACTERISTICS

Perception of changes in patterns of the energy flow, such as:

Temperature change	
Warmth	Coolness
Visual changes	
Image	Color
Disruption of the field	
Vacant	Hole
Spike	Bulge
Movement	
Wave	Spike
Tingling	Dense
Flowing	
Sounds	
Tone	Words

RELATED FACTORS

Pathophysiological

Related to slowing or blocking of energy flows secondary to: illness (specify), injury, or pregnancy

Treatment-Related

Related to slowing or blocking of energy flows secondary to: immobility, labor and delivery, or perioperative experience

Situational (Personal, Environmental)

Related to the slowing or blocking of energy flows secondary to pain, anxiety, fear, or grieving

Maturational

Related to age-related developmental difficulties or crises (specify)

OUTCOME CRITERIA

The person will:

1. Report relief of symptoms after therapeutic touch
2. Report increased sense of relaxation
3. Report a decrease in pain using a scale of 0 to 10 before and after therapies

⊕ GENERIC INTERVENTIONS

The following phases of therapeutic touch are learned separately but are rendered concurrently. The presentation of these interventions is for the purpose of describing the process for nurses who do not practice therapeutic touch. This discussion may help nurses support colleagues who practice therapeutic touch and initiate referrals. As discussed previously, preparing for therapeutic touch requires specialized instruction that is beyond the scope of this book.

1. Explain therapeutic touch, and obtain verbal permission.
2. Prepare the client and environment for therapeutic touch.
   a. Provide as much privacy as possible.

      b. Give person permission to stop the therapy at any time.

      c. Allow person to assume a comfortable position (*e.g.*, lying or sitting on a bed or couch).

3. Shift from a direct focus on the environment to an inner focus, which is perceived as the center of life within the nurse (centering).

4. Assess by scanning the person's energy field for openness and symmetry (Krieger, 1979).

      a. Move hands, palms toward person, at a distance of 2 to 4 in over the person's body from head to feet in a smooth, light movement.

      b. Sense the cues to energy imbalance (*e.g.*, warmth, coolness, tightness, heaviness, tingling, emptiess).

5. Facilitate a rhythmic flow of energy by moving hands more vigorously from head to toe (unruffling/clearing).

6. Focus intent on the specific repatterning of areas of imbalance and impeded flow. Using your hands as focal points, move the hands in gentle, sweeping movements from head to feet one time.

7. Encourage the person to provide feedback.

8. Document the procedure and the feedback.

Environmental Interpretation Syndrome, Impaired

DEFINITION

Impaired Environmental Interpretation Syndrome: Consistent lack of orientation to person, place, time, or circumstances for more than 3 to 6 months, necessitating a protective environment.

Author's Note:

Impaired Environmental Interpretation Syndrome describes an individual who needs a protective environment because of consistent
(Continued)

DEFINING CHARACTERISTICS

Major (Must Be Present, One or More)

Consistent disorientation in known and unknown environments

Chronic confusional states

Minor (May Be Present)

Loss of occupation or social functioning from memory decline

Inability to follow simple directions, instructions

Inability to reason

Inability to concentrate

Slow in responding to questions

RELATED FACTORS

Dementia (Alzheimer's disease, multi-infarct dementia, Pick's disease, AIDS dementia)

Parkinson's disease

Huntington's disease

Depression

Alcoholism

Family Processes, Altered

Family Processes, Altered: Alcoholism

Family Processes, Altered

DEFINITION

Altered Family Processes: The state in which a normally supportive family experiences, or is at risk to experience, a stressor that challenges its previously effective functioning ability.

Author's Note:

The nursing diagnosis Altered Family Processes describes a family that usually functions optimally but is challenged by a stressor that has altered or may alter the family's function. This diagnosis differs from Ineffective Family Coping: Disabling, which describes a family that has a pattern of destructive behavioral responses. Unsuccessful resolution of a problem can change Altered Family Processes to Ineffective Family Coping: Disabling.

DEFINING CHARACTERISTICS

Major (Must Be Present, One or More)

Family system cannot or does not:
   Adapt constructively to crisis
   Communicate openly and effectively among family members

Minor (May Be Present)

Family system cannot or does not:
   Meet physical needs of all its members
   Meet emotional needs of all its members
   Meet spiritual needs of all its members
   Express or accept a wide range of feelings
   Seek or accept help appropriately

RELATED FACTORS

Any factor can contribute to *Altered Family Processes*. Some common factors are listed below.

Pathophysiological

Related to impact of illness (specify)
Related to change in the family member's ability to function

Treatment-Related

Related to:
    Disruption of family routines due to time-consuming treatments (e.g., home dialysis)
    Physical changes due to treatments of ill family member
    Emotional changes in all family members due to treatments of ill family member
    Financial burden of treatments for ill family member
    Hospitalization of ill family member

Situational (Personal, Environmental)

Related to loss of family member
    Death
    Going away to school
    Separation
    Divorce
    Incarceration
    Desertion
    Hospitalization
Related to gain of family member (*e.g.*, birth, adoption, marriage, elderly relative)
Related to losses associated with:
    Poverty
    Disaster
    Relocation
    Economic crisis
    Change in family roles
        Working mother
        Retirement
        Birth of child with defect
Related to conflict (moral, goal, cultural)
Related to breach of trust among members
Related to social deviance by family member (*e.g.*, crime)

OUTCOME CRITERIA

The person (family members) will:

1. Frequently verbalize feelings to professional nurse and each other
2. Participate in care of ill family member
3. Facilitate return of ill family member from sick role to well role
4. Maintain functional system of mutual support for each member
5. Seek appropriate external resources when needed

⊞ GENERIC INTERVENTIONS

1. Assist family with appraisal of the situation.
   a. What is at stake? Encourage family to have a realistic perspective by providing accurate information and answers to questions.
   b. What are the choices? Assist family to reorganize roles at home and set priorities to maintain family integrity and reduce stress.
   c. Where is help available? Direct family to community agencies, home health care organizations, and sources of financial assistance as needed (see *Impaired Home Maintenance Management* for additional interventions).
2. Create a private and supportive hospital environment for family.
3. Acknowledge strengths to family when appropriate.
   a. "I can tell you are a very close family."
   b. "You know just how to get your mother to eat."
   c. "Your brother means a great deal to you."
4. Involve family members in care of ill member when possible (feeding, bathing, dressing, ambulating).
5. Involve family members in patient care conferences when appropriate.
6. Encourage family to acquire substitutes to care for the ill person to provide the family with time away.
7. Encourage verbalization of guilt, anger, blame, hostility, and subsequent recognition of own feelings in family members.
8. Aid family members to change their expectations of the ill member in a realistic manner.

9. Provide the family with anticipatory guidance as illness continues.
   a. Inform parents of the effects of prolonged hospitalization on children (appropriate to developmental age).
   b. Prepare family members for signs of depression, anxiety, and dependency, which are a natural part of the illness experience.
10. Enlist help of other professionals when problems extend beyond realm of nursing (*e.g.*, social worker, clinical psychologist, nurse therapist, clinical specialist, psychiatrist, child care specialist).

Family Processes, Altered: Alcoholism

DEFINITION

Altered Family Processes: Alcoholism: The state in which the psychosocial, spiritual, economic, and physiological functions of the family members and system are chronically disorganized because of the effects of alcohol abuse.

Author's Note:

Alcoholism is a family disease. This nursing diagnosis represents the consequences of the disturbed family dynamics related to alcohol abuse by a family member. The NANDA definition of Altered Family Processes is "the state in which a family that normally functions effectively experiences a dysfunction" (NANDA, 1992, p. 41). The alcoholic family does not have a history of effective functioning. The diagnosis Ineffective Family Coping: Disabling would be more descriptive of the alcoholic family. The diagnosis could be stated as Ineffective Family Coping: Alcoholism. Further assessments will determine the effects of alcoholism on physical, psychological, spiritual, financial, and developmental aspects of the family unit. If clinical research validates that alcoholism affects all of these dimensions in all or most families, the diagnosis Alcoholic Family Process Syndrome may prove very useful.

DEFINING CHARACTERISTICS
(Lindeman et al., 1994)

Major (80%–100%)

Behaviors:
    Loss of control of drinking
    Denial of problems
    Alcohol abuse
    Impaired communication
    Rationalization
    Broken promises
    Inability to meet emotional needs of members
    Manipulation
    Inappropriate expression of anger
    Dependency
    Refusal to get help
    Blaming
    Enabling behaviors
    Ineffective problem-solving skills
    Inadequate understanding or knowledge of alcoholism
    Criticizing

Roles and relationships:
    Deterioration in family relationships
    Disturbed family dynamics
    Marital problems
    Ineffective spouse communication
    Disruption of family roles
    Inconsistent parenting
    Family denial
    Intimacy dysfunction
    Closed communication systems

Feelings:

Decreased self-esteem	Hurt
Anger	Unhappiness
Frustration	Guilt
Powerlessness	Distress
Tension	Emotional isolation
Insecurity	Vulnerability
Suppressed rage	Worthlessness
Anxiety	Shame
Repressed emotions	Loneliness
Responsibility for alcoholic's behavior	Mistrust
	Hopelessness
Lingering resentment	Rejection
Embarrassment	

Minor (70%–79%)

Behaviors
   Inability to express or accept wide range of feelings
   Orientation toward tension relief rather than achievement
      of goals
   Family's special occasions are alcohol-centered
   Escalating conflict
   Lying
   Failure to send clear messages
   Inability to get help or receive help appropriately
   Ineffective decision making
   Contradictory, paradoxical communication
   Failure to deal with conflict
   Harsh self-judgment
   Isolation
   Nicotine addiction
   Difficulty having fun
   Control of communication
   Inability to adapt to change
   Immaturity
   Power struggles
   Stress-related physical illnesses
   Inability to deal with traumatic experiences constructively
   Seeking approval and affirmation
   Lack of reliability
   Disturbances in academic performance in children
   Disturbances in concentration
   Chaos
   Substance abuse other than alcohol
   Difficulty with life cycle transitions
   Verbal abuse of spouse or parent
   Failure to accomplish current or past developmental tasks
   Agitation
Feelings:

Being different from other persons	Unresolved grief
	Loss
Depression	Feeling misunderstood
Hostility	Abandonment
Fear	Confused love and pity
Emotional control by others	Moodiness
Confusion	Failure
Dissatisfaction	Being unloved
Self-blaming	Lack of identity

Roles and relationships:
   Triangulating family relationship
   Inability to meet spiritual needs of its members
   Reduced ability of family members to relate to each other
     for mutual growth and maturation
   Lack of skills necessary for relationships
   Lack of cohesiveness
   Disrupted family rituals
   Family unable to meet security needs of members
   Family does not demonstrate respect for autonomy and in-
     dividuality of its members
   Decreased sexual communication
   Low perception of parental support
   Pattern of rejection
   Economic problems
   Neglected obligations

RELATED FACTORS

Because the cause of this diagnosis is alcohol abuse by a family member, no related factors are needed.

OUTCOME CRITERIA

The family will:

1. Acknowledge the alcoholism in the family
2. Relate the effects of alcoholism on the family unit
3. Identify destructive response patterns
4. Set short- and long-term goals
5. Describe resources available for individual and family therapy

⬢ GENERIC INTERVENTIONS

1. Establish a trusting relationship.
    a. Be consistent; keep promises.
    b. Be accepting and noncritical.
    c. Do not pass judgment on what is revealed.
    d. Focus on family member responses.
2. Allow the family as individuals and as a group to share their pent-up feelings.
3. Emphasize that family members are not responsible for the person's drinking.

4. Explore the family's beliefs about their situation and their goals.
   a. Discuss characteristics of alcoholism
      • Review a screening test, which outlines characteristics of alcoholism (*e.g.*, the Michigan Alcoholism Screening Test)
   b. Discuss causes, and correct misinformation.
   c. Assist to establish short- and long-term goals.
5. Discuss methods families use to control the person's alcoholic behaviors (*e.g.*, hiding alcohol or car keys, anger, silence, threats, crying) or to cover up or minimize the negative effects of drinking on the person (*e.g.*, making excuses for work, family, or friends; putting the person to bed; bailing the person out of jail).
6. Assist family members to gain insight into the effects of their attempts to control the drinking:
   a. Does not stop drinking
   b. Increases family anger
   c. Removes the responsibility for drinking from the person
   d. Prevents the person from suffering the consequences of his or her drinking behavior
7. Emphasize that helping the alcoholic means first helping themselves.
   a. Focus on changing their response.
   b. Allow the person to be responsible for his or her drinking behavior.
   c. Describe activities that will improve their life as individuals and as a family.
   d. Initiate one stress-management technique (*e.g.*, aerobic exercises, assertiveness course, walking, meditation, relaxation breathing).
   e. Plan time as a family together outside the home (*e.g.*, museum, zoos, picnics). If the alcoholic person is included, the person must contract not to drink during the activity and agree on a consequence if he or she does.
8. Discuss with the family that during recovery, their usual family dynamics will be dramatically changed.
9. Discuss the possibility of relapse and the contributing factors.
10. If additional family or individual nursing diagnoses exist, refer to *Child Abuse* or *Domestic Violence* under *Ineffective Family Coping: Disabling*.

11. Initiate health teaching regarding community resources and referrals as indicated:
    a. AL-ANON
    b. Alcoholics Anonymous
    c. Family therapy
    d. Individual therapy
    e. Self-help groups (*e.g.*, Adult Children of Alcoholics)

Fatigue

DEFINITION

Fatigue: The self-recognized state in which an individual experiences an overwhelming sustained sense of exhaustion and decreased capacity for physical and mental work that is not relieved by rest.

> **Author's Note:**
> Fatigue is different from tiredness. Tiredness is a transient, temporary state from lack of sleep, improper nutrition, sedentary lifestyle, or a temporary increase in work or social responsibilities. Fatigue is a pervasive, subjective, drained feeling that cannot be eliminated. Persons with fatigue are taught energy conservation techniques. Activity Intolerance is different from Fatigue in that the person with Activity Intolerance will be assisted to increase endurance to progress and increase activity. The person with chronic Fatigue will not return to the previous level of functioning.

DEFINING CHARACTERISTICS
(Voith et al., 1987)

Major (80%–100%)

Verbalization of an unremitting and overwhelming lack of energy
Inability to maintain usual routines

Minor (50%–79%)

Perceived need for additional energy to accomplish routine tasks
Increase in physical complaints
Emotionally labile or irritable
Impaired ability to concentrate
Decreased performance
Lethargic or listless
Lack of interest in surroundings/introspection
Decreased libido
Accident prone

RELATED FACTORS

Many factors can cause fatigue. It may be useful to combine related factors, such as related to muscle weakness, build-up of waste products, inflammatory process, and infections secondary to AIDS.

Pathophysiological

Related to:
    Acute infections (*e.g.*, mononucleosis, hepatitis, viruses)
    Chronic infections
Related to inadequate tissue oxygenation secondary to:
    Congestive heart failure
    Chronic obstructive lung disease
    Anemia
    Peripheral vascular disease
Related to biochemical changes secondary to:
    Endocrine/metabolic disorders

Diabetes mellitus	Pituitary disorders
Hypothyroidism	Addison's disease

    Chronic diseases (*e.g.*, renal failure, cirrhosis, Lyme disease)
Related to muscle wasting secondary to:

Myasthenia gravis	Parkinson's disease
Multiple sclerosis	AIDS
Amyotrophic lateral sclerosis	

Related to hypermetabolic state, competition between body and tumor for nutrients, anemia, and stressors associated with cancer
Related to nutritional deficits or changes in nutrient metabolism secondary to:

Nausea	Side effects of medications
Vomiting	Gastric surgery
Diarrhea	Diabetes mellitus

Related to chronic inflammatory process secondary to:

AIDS	Cirrhosis
Arthritis	Inflammatory bowel disease
Lupus erythematosus	Renal failure
Hepatitis	

Treatment-Related

Related to chemotherapy

Related to radiation therapy

Related to side effects of (specify)

Related to surgical damage to tissue and anesthesia

Related to increased energy expenditure secondary to, for example, amputation, gait disorder, use of walker, crutches

Situational (Personal, Environmental)

Related to prolonged decreased activity and deconditioning secondary to:

Anxiety	Social isolation
Fever	Nausea/vomiting
Diarrhea	Depression
Pain	

Related to excessive role demands

Related to overwhelming emotional demands

Related to extreme stress

Related to sleep disturbance

Maturational

Child/adolescent

Related to hypermetabolic state secondary to:

Mononucleosis	Fever

Related to insufficient nutrients secondary to:

Obesity	Excessive dieting
Eating disorders	

Adult/adolescent

(Pregnancy, postpartum)

Related to effects of newborn care on sleep patterns and need for continuous attention

Related to changes in metabolic, respiratory, circulatory, gastrointestinal, renal, and endocrine function during first trimester

OUTCOME CRITERIA

The person will:

1. Discuss the causes of fatigue
2. Share feelings regarding the effects of fatigue on his or her life
3. Establish priorities for daily and weekly activities
4. Participate in activities that stimulate and balance physical, cognitive, affective, and social domains

⬛ GENERIC INTERVENTIONS

1. Explain the causes of the person's fatigue.
2. Allow expression of feelings regarding the effects of fatigue on person's life.
3. Assist the individual to identify strengths, abilities, interests.
4. Instruct individual to record fatigue levels each hour during a 24-hour period (select a usual day).
   a. Ask to rate fatigue 0 to 10 using the Rhoten (1982) fatigue scale (0 = not tired, peppy; 10 = total exhaustion).
   b. Record the activities at the time of each rating.
5. Analyze together the 24-hour fatigue levels.
   a. Times of peak energy
   b. Times of exhaustion
   c. Activities associated with increasing fatigue
6. Assist individual to identify what tasks can be delegated.
7. Plan the important tasks during periods of high energy.
8. Assist individual to identify priorities and eliminate nonessential activities.
9. Teach energy-conservation techniques.
   a. Place work items within easy reach.
   b. Reduce trips up and down stairs.
   c. Distribute difficult tasks throughout the week.
   d. Rest before difficult tasks, and stop before fatigue ensues.
   e. Install grab rails.
   f. Eat small meals (five times daily).

g. Request drivers instead of driving.

h. Delegate or barter for household chores.

10. Teach energy-conservation techniques.

11. Explain the psychological and physiological benefits of exercise, and discuss what is realistic.

12. Provide significant others with opportunities to discuss their feelings in private.

13. Explain the effects of conflict and stress on energy levels.

14. Assist to learn effective coping skills (*e.g.*, sharing, assertiveness, relaxation techniques).

15. Refer to community services (Meals on Wheels, housekeeper).

MATERNAL FOCUS INTERVENTIONS

1. Explain the reason for fatigue in first and third trimesters.
   a. Increased basal metabolic rate
   b. Changes in hormonal levels
   c. Anemia
   d. Increased cardiac output (third trimester)

2. Emphasize the need for naps and 8 hours of sleep.

3. Discuss the importance of exercise (*e.g.*, walking).

4. Advise to avoid overexertion.

5. For postpartum women, discuss factors that increase fatigue (Gardner & Campbell, 1991):
   a. Labor more than 30 hours, difficult labor or reports of high labor pain.
   b. Hemoglobin <10 g/dL or postpartum hemorrhage
   c. Preexisting chronic disease
   d. Episiotomy, tear, or cesarean section
   e. Sleeping difficulties
   f. Ill neonate or a congenital anomaly
   g. Nonsupportive partner
   h. Dependent children at home
   i. Child care problems
   j. Unrealistic expectations

OLDER ADULT FOCUS INTERVENTIONS

1. Consider if chronic fatigue is the consequence of late life depression.

2. Refer individual suspected of depression for evaluation.

Fear

DEFINITION

Fear: The state in which an individual or group experiences a feeling of physiological or emotional disruption related to an identifiable source that is perceived as dangerous.

Author's Note:
See Anxiety.

DEFINING CHARACTERISTICS

Major (Must Be Present, One or More)

Feelings of dread, fright, apprehension, alarm
Behaviors of avoidance, narrowing of focus on danger, and deficits in attention, performance, control, and self-assurance

Minor (May Be Present)

Verbal reports of panic, obsessions
Behavioral acts of:

Crying	Dysfunctional immobility
Aggression	Compulsive mannerisms
Escape	Increased questioning/
Hypervigilance	verbalization

Visceral-somatic activity
  Musculoskeletal

Trembling	Fatigue/weakness
Muscle tightness	of the limbs

  Cardiovascular

Palpitations	Increased blood pressure
Rapid pulse	

  Respiratory

Shortness of breath	Increased rate

  Gastrointestinal

Anorexia	Diarrhea/urge to defecate
Nausea/vomiting	Dry mouth/throat

Genitourinary
    Urinary frequency/urgency
Skin
    Flush/pallor   Paresthesia
    Sweating
CNS/perceptual
    Syncope   Absentmindedness
    Insomnia   Nightmares
    Lack of concentration   Dilated pupils
    Irritability

RELATED FACTORS

Fear can occur as a response to a variety of health problems, situations, or conflicts. Some common sources are indicated below.

Pathophysiological

Related to perceived immediate and long-term effects of:
    Loss of body part   Cognitive impairment
    Loss of body function   Long-term disability
    Disabling illness   Terminal disease
    Sensory impairment

Treatment-Related

Related to loss of control and unpredictable outcome
  secondary to:
    Hospitalization
    Surgery and its outcome
    Anesthesia
    Invasive procedures
    Radiation

Situational (Personal, Environmental)

Related to loss of control and unpredictable outcome
  secondary to:
    Pain   Divorce
    New environment   Success
    New persons   Failure
    Lack of knowledge   Language barrier
    Change or loss of significant
      other
Related to potential loss of income

Maturational

Preschool, school-age
  Related to:

Separation from parents, peers	Animals
Not being liked	Bodily harm
Being alone	Age-related fears (dark,
Strangers	strangers, ghosts,
	monsters)

Adolescent
  Related to uncertainty of:

Appearance	Scholastic success
Peer support	

  Related to vulnerability to violence
  Related to separation from support system
Adult
  Related to uncertainty of:

Marriage	Job security
Pregnancy	Effects of aging
Parenthood	

Older adult
  Related to:
    Anticipated dependence
    Prolonged suffering
    Vulnerability to crime
    Financial insecurity
    Abandonment

OUTCOME CRITERIA

The adult will:

1. Relate increase in psychological and physiological comfort
2. Differentiate real from imagined situations
3. Describe effective and ineffective coping patterns
4. Identify own coping responses

The child will:

1. Discuss fears
2. Relate an increase in psychological comfort

◆ GENERIC INTERVENTIONS

1. Orient to environment using simple explanations.
2. Speak slowly and calmly.

3. Allow personal space.
4. Use simple direct statements (avoid detail).
5. Encourage expression of feelings (helplessness, anger).
6. Encourage responses that reflect reality. Discuss which aspects can be changed and which cannot.
7. Provide an emotionally nonthreatening atmosphere. Set up a consistent daily schedule.
8. When intensity of feelings has decreased, bring behavioral cues into the person's awareness.
9. Teach relaxation techniques.
   a. Slow, rhythmic breathing
   b. Progressive relaxation of muscle groups
   c. Self-coaching
   d. Thought stopping
   e. Guided imagery

🌀 CHILD FOCUS INTERVENTIONS

1. Accept the child's fear and provide an explanation, if possible, or some form of control; share with child that these fears are okay.
   a. Fear of imaginary animals, intruders ("I don't see a lion in your room, but I will leave the light on for you, and if you need me again, please call.")
   b. Fear of parent being late (Establish a contingency plan, *e.g.*, "If you come home from school and Mommy is not here, go to Mrs. S. next door.")
   c. Fear of vanishing down a toilet or bathtub drain. Wait until child is out of tub before releasing drain. Wait until child is off the toilet before flushing. Leave toys in bathtub, and demonstrate how they do not go down the drain.
   d. Fear of dark. Give child a night light.
   e. Fear of dogs, cats:
      • Allow child to watch a child and a dog playing from a distance.
      • Do not force child to touch the animal.
2. Discuss with parents the normalcy of fears in children; explain the necessity of acceptance and the negative outcomes of punishment or of forcing the child to overcome the fear.
3. Provide the child with opportunity to observe how other children cope successfully with feared object.

◎ MATERNAL FOCUS INTERVENTIONS

1. Explore fears and emotional responses to pregnancy (Reeder, Martin, & Koniak-Griffin, 1997).
   a. First trimester
      - Uncertainty about future role as mother
      - Uncertainty about timing of pregnancy
   b. Third trimester
      - Fears about own well-being and "performance" during labor
      - Fears about well-being of the fetus

Fluid Volume Deficit

DEFINITION

Fluid Volume Deficit: The state in which an individual who is not NPO experiences or is at risk of experiencing vascular, interstitial, or intracellular dehydration.

Author's Note:

This diagnosis represents situations in which nurses can prescribe definitive treatment to prevent fluid depletion or to reduce or eliminate related factors, such as insufficient oral intake. Situations that represent hypovolemia caused by hemorrhage or NPO status should be considered collaborative problems, not nursing diagnoses. Nurses monitor to detect these situations and collaborate with doctors for treatment. These situations can be labeled Potential Complication: Hemorrhage or Potential Complication: Hypovolemia.

DEFINING CHARACTERISTICS

Major (Must Be Present, One or More)

Insufficient oral fluid intake
Negative balance of intake and output
Weight loss
Dry skin/mucous membranes

Minor (May Be Present)

Increased serum sodium
Decreased urine output or excessive urine output
Concentrated urine or urinary frequency
Decreased skin turgor
Thirst, nausea, or anorexia

RELATED FACTORS

Pathophysiological

Related to excessive urinary output
    Uncontrolled diabetes
    Diabetes insipidus (inadequate antidiuretic hormone)
Related to increased capillary permeability and evaporative loss from burn wound
Related to losses secondary to:
    Fever or increased metabolic rate
    Abnormal drainage (*e.g.*, wound, excessive menses, etc.)
    Peritonitis
    Diarrhea

Situational (Personal, Environmental)

Related to vomiting/nausea
Related to decreased motivation to drink liquids secondary to: depression or fatigue
Related to fad diets/fasting
Related to high-solute tube feedings
Related to difficulty swallowing or feeding self secondary to: oral pain or fatigue
Related to extreme heat/sun, dryness
Related to excessive loss through indwelling catheters or drains
Related to insufficient fluids for exercise effort or weather conditions
Related to excessive use of laxatives, enemas, diuretics, or alcohol

Maturational

Infant/child
    Related to increased vulnerability secondary to decreased fluid reserve and decreased ability to concentrate urine

Older adult
  Related to increased vulnerability secondary to decreased
  fluid reserve and decreased sensation of thirst

OUTCOME CRITERIA

The person will:

1. Increase intake of fluids to a minimum of 2,000 mL (unless contraindicated)
2. Relate the need for increased fluid intake during stress or heat
3. Maintain a urine-specific gravity within a normal range
4. Demonstrate no signs and symptoms of dehydration

◤ GENERIC INTERVENTIONS

1. Assess likes and dislikes; provide favorite fluids within dietary restrictions.
2. Plan an intake goal for every 8 hours (*e.g.*, 1,000 mL during day; 800 mL during evening; 300 mL at night).
3. Assess the person's understanding of the reasons for maintaining adequate hydration and methods for reaching goal of fluid intake.
4. Have person maintain a written record (log) of fluid intake and urinary output (if necessary).
5. Monitor intake; ensure at least 1,500 mL of oral fluids is taken every 24 hours.
6. Monitor output; ensure an output of at least 1,000 to 1,500 mL/24 h. Monitor for a decrease in urine-specific gravity.
7. Weigh daily in same type of clothing at same time. A 2% to 4% weight loss indicates mild dehydration; 5% to 9% weight loss indicates moderate dehydration.
8. Monitor levels of serum electrolytes, blood urea nitrogen, urine and serum osmolality, creatinine, hematocrit, and hemoglobin.
9. Teach that coffee, tea, and grapefruit juice are diuretics and can contribute to fluid loss.
10. Consider the additional fluid losses associated with vomiting, diarrhea, fever, tubes, drains.
11. For wound drainage:
    a. Keep careful records of the amount and type of drainage.

   b. Weigh dressings, if necessary, to estimate fluid loss.
   c. Cover wounds to minimize fluid loss.

🌀 CHILD FOCUS INTERVENTIONS

1. Monitor weight, body temperature, moisture in oral cavity, urine volume and concentration.
2. Offer:
   a. Appealing forms of fluids (popsicles, frozen juice bars, snow cones, water, milk, Jell-O with vegetable coloring added; let child help make it)
   b. Unusual containers (colorful cups, straws)
   c. A game or activity (have child take a drink when it is child's turn in a game)

🏛 OLDER ADULT FOCUS INTERVENTIONS

1. Teach to drink 8 to 10 glasses of fluid daily, not including caffeine drinks unless contraindicated (*e.g.*, renal or cardiac insufficiency).
2. Advise at least 4 glasses of water: caution on caffeine and sugar drinks.
3. Explain not to rely on thirst as an indicator of a need for fluids.
4. Teach to monitor hydration by color of urine.
5. Evaluate if person is restricting intake to avoid incontinence.

Fluid Volume Excess

DEFINITION

Fluid Volume Excess: The state in which an individual experiences or is at risk of experiencing intracellular or interstitial fluid overload.

> **Author's Note:**
> This diagnosis represents situations in which nursing can pre-
> scribe definitive treatment to reduce or eliminate factors that con-
> tribute to edema or can teach preventive actions. Situations that
> represent vascular fluid overload should be considered collabora-
> tive problems, not nursing diagnoses. They can be labeled Poten-
> tial Complication: Congestive Heart Failure or Potential Compli-
> cation: Hypervolemia.

DEFINING CHARACTERISTICS

Major (Must Be Present, One or More)

Edema (peripheral, sacral)
Taut, shiny skin

Minor (May Be Present)

Intake greater than output
Shortness of breath
Weight gain

RELATED FACTORS

Pathophysiological

Related to compromised regulatory mechanisms secondary to
acute or chronic renal failure
Related to increased preload, decreased contractility, and
decreased cardiac output secondary to:
Myocardial infarction
Congestive heart failure
Left ventricular failure
Valvular disease
Tachycardia/arrhythmias
Related to portal hypertension, lower plasma colloidal
osmotic pressure, and sodium retention secondary to liver
disease, cirrhosis, cancer, or ascites
Related to impaired venous return secondary to:
Varicose veins
Peripheral vascular disease

Thrombus
Chronic phlebitis
Immobility

Treatment-Related

Related to sodium and water retention secondary to corticosteroid therapy

Situational (Personal, Environmental)

Related to excessive sodium intake/fluid intake
Related to low protein intake (*e.g.*, fad diets, malnutrition)
Related to dependent venous pooling/venostasis secondary to
immobility, tight cast or bandage, or standing or sitting for
long periods
Related to venous compression by pregnant uterus
Related to inadequate lymphatic drainage secondary to
mastectomy

Maturational

Older adult
Related to impaired venous return secondary to increased
peripheral resistance and decreased efficiency of the
valves

OUTCOME CRITERIA

The person will:

1. Relate causative factors and methods of preventing edema
2. Exhibit decreased peripheral and sacral edema

⬍ GENERIC INTERVENTIONS

1. For edema:
   a. Monitor skin for signs of pressure ulcers.
   b. Gently wash between skin folds and dry carefully.
   c. Avoid tape when possible.
   d. Change position at least every 2 hours.
2. Assess for evidence of dependent venous pooling or
   venostasis.
3. Keep edematous extremity elevated above the level of the
   heart whenever possible (unless contraindicated by heart
   failure).

4. Assess dietary intake and habits that may contribute to fluid retention (*e.g.*, salt intake).
5. Teach the person to:
   a. Read labels for sodium content
   b. Avoid convenience foods, canned foods, and frozen foods
   c. Cook without salt, and use spices to add flavor (lemon, basil, tarragon, mint)
   d. Use vinegar in place of salt for flavor (*e.g.*, 2–3 teaspoons of vinegar to 4–6 quarts, according to taste)
6. Instruct person to avoid panty girdles/garters, knee-highs, and leg crossing and to practice keeping legs elevated when possible.
7. For inadequate lymphatic drainage in arm:
   a. Keep extremity elevated on pillows.
   b. Take blood pressures in unaffected arm.
   c. Do not give injections or start intravenous fluids in affected arm.
   d. Protect the affected arm from injury.
   e. Teach the person to avoid using strong detergents, carrying heavy bags, holding a cigarette, injuring cuticles or hangnails, reaching into a hot oven, wearing jewelry or a wristwatch, or using Ace bandages.
   f. Caution the person to see a physician if the arm becomes red, swollen, or unusually hard.
8. Protect edematous skin from injury.

🜨 MATERNAL FOCUS INTERVENTIONS

1. Explain the cause of fluid retention (*e.g.*, increased estrogen production, posture that affects blood flow and renal function).
2. Explain the importance of lying on side at night and during the day (several times).
3. Teach woman to:
   a. Elevate feet often
   b. Drink at least 2,000 mL of fluids (three to four servings)
   c. Eat enough protein and avoid highly salted foods
4. Assess for early signs of pregnancy-induced hypertension:
   a. Weight gain of over 2 lb in 1 week
   b. Finger edema

Fluid Volume Imbalance, Risk for

DEFINITION

Risk for Fluid Volume Imbalance: A state in which an individual is at risk to experience a decrease, increase, or rapid shift from one to the other of intravascular, interstitial, and/or intracellular fluid.

> **Author's Note:**
> This diagnosis can represent a multitude of clinical conditions, such as edema, hemorrhage, dehydration, and compartmental syndrome. If the nurse is monitoring an individual for fluid volume imbalance, labeling the specific imbalance as a collaborative problem, such as hypovolemia, compartmental syndrome, increased intracranial pressure, GI bleeding, or postpartum hemorrhage, would be more useful clinically. For example, most intraoperative clients are monitored for hypovolemia; if the procedure is neurosurgery, cranial pressure would also be monitored. If the procedure is orthopedic, compartmental syndrome would be addressed. Refer to Section III for specific collaborative problems and interventions.

RISK FACTORS

Need to be developed (NANDA, 1999)

OUTCOME CRITERIA

Refer to *Fluid Volume Deficit.*

INTERVENTIONS

Refer to *Fluid Volume Deficit.*

Grieving*

Grieving, Anticipatory

Grieving, Dysfunctional

Grieving

DEFINITION

Grieving: A state in which an individual or family experiences a natural human response involving psychosocial and physiological reactions to an actual or perceived loss (person, object, function, status, relationship).

> **Author's Note:**
> Grieving, Anticipatory Grieving, and Dysfunctional Grieving represent three types of responses of individuals or families experiencing a loss. Grieving describes normal grieving after a loss and participation in grief work.
> Anticipatory Grieving describes someone engaged in grief work before an expected loss. Dysfunctional Grieving is a maladaptive process that occurs when grief work is suppressed or absent or when there is a prolonged exaggerated response. For all three diagnoses, the nursing goal is to promote grief work. In addition, for Dysfunctional Grieving, the nurse will direct interventions to reduce excessive, prolonged problematic responses.

DEFINING CHARACTERISTICS

Major (Must Be Present)

The person reports an actual or perceived loss (person, object, function, status, relationship)

*This diagnosis is not currently on the NANDA list but has been included for clarity or usefulness.

Minor (May Be Present)

Denial
Guilt
Anger
Despair
Feelings of worthlessness
Suicidal thoughts
Crying
Sorrow

Delusions
Phobias
Anergia
Inability to concentrate
Visual, auditory, and tactile
  hallucinations about
  the object or person
Longing/searching behaviors

RELATED FACTORS

Many situations can contribute to feelings of loss. Some common situations are listed below.

Pathophysiological

Related to loss of function or independence secondary to:
Neurological
Cardiovascular
Sensory
Musculoskeletal

Digestive
Renal
Trauma

Treatment-Related

Related to losses associated with, for example, long-term dialysis, surgery (mastectomy, colostomy, hysterectomy)

Situational (Personal, Environmental)

Related to the negative effects and losses (*e.g.*, chronic pain, terminal illness, death)
Related to losses in lifestyle associated with:
Childbirth
Marriage
Separation
Divorce

Child leaving home
  (*e.g.*, college or marriage)
Retirement

Related to loss of normalcy secondary to, for example, handicap, scars, illness

Maturational

Related to losses attributed to aging, friends, occupation, function, home
Related to loss of hopes, dreams

OUTCOME CRITERIA

The individual will:

1. Express grief
2. Describe the meaning of the death or loss
3. Share grief with significant others (children, spouses)

⬡ GENERIC INTERVENTIONS

1. Promote a trust relationship.
2. Support the person and the family's grief reactions.
3. Explain grief reactions:
   a. Shock and disbelief
   b. Developing awareness
   c. Restitution
   d. Somatic manifestations
4. Assess for experiences with loss.
5. Recognize and reinforce the strengths of each family member.
6. Encourage the family members to evaluate their feelings and support one another. Allow each member privacy to share grief.
7. Promote grief work with each response.
   a. Denial
      - Explain the use of denial by one family member to the other members.
      - Do not push client to move past denial without emotional readiness.
   b. Isolation
      - Reinforce the person's self-worth by allowing privacy.
      - Encourage client/family to increase social activities gradually (*e.g.*, support groups, church groups).
   c. Depression
      - Identify the level of depression, and develop the approach accordingly.
      - Use empathic sharing; acknowledge grief ("It must be very difficult.").
   d. Anger
      - Explain to family that anger serves to try to control one's environment more closely because of inability to control loss.
      - Encourage verbalization of the anger.

  e. Guilt
  - Encourage client to identify positive contributions/aspects of the relationship.
  - Avoid arguing and participating in the person's system of "should's" and "should not's."
  f. Fear
  - Focus on the present, and maintain a safe and secure environment.
  g. Rejection
  - Explain this response to family members.
  h. Hysteria
  - Reduce environmental stresses (*e.g.*, limit personnel).
  - Provide person with a safe, private area to display grief.
8. Identify factors that can impede successful completion of the mourning process (Varcorolis, 1998):
  a. High dependence on deceased
  b. Unresolved conflicts
  c. Age of deceased
  d. Inadequate support system
  e. Number of previous losses
  f. Physical and psychological health of person grieving
9. Teach the person and the family signs of resolution. Refer to *Dysfunctional Grieving.*
10. Identify agencies that may be helpful.

🌀 CHILD FOCUS INTERVENTIONS

1. Encourage parents and staff to be truthful, and offer explanations that can be understood.
2. Encourage parents or significant others to nurture children during the grieving process.
3. Explore with child his or her concept of death in the context of maturational level.
4. Correct misconceptions about death, illness, and rituals (funerals).
5. Prepare the child for grief responses of others.
6. If the child plans to attend the funeral or visit the funeral home, a thorough explanation of the setting, rituals, and expected behaviors of mourners is necessary beforehand. (The family can plan the visit of the child to be short and to occur before the other mourners arrive.)
7. Allow child to share fears.

8. Allow child to remain with significant others while they grieve at home.

9. Provide accurate explanations for sibling illness or death.

🔵 MATERNAL FOCUS INTERVENTIONS

1. Assist parents of a deceased infant (newborn, stillbirth, miscarriage) with grief work (Mina, 1985):

   a. Use baby's name when discussing loss.
   b. Allow parents to share the hopes and dreams.
   c. Provide access to hospital chaplain or own religious leader.
   d. Encourage parents to see and hold their infant to validate the reality of the loss.
   e. Prepare a memory packet (wrapped in clean baby blanket) (photograph [Polaroid], identification bracelet, footprints with birth certificate, lock of hair, crib card, fetal monitor strip, infant's blanket).
   f. Encourage parents to share the experience with siblings at home (refer to pertinent literature for consumers).
   g. Provide for follow-up support and referral services after discharge (*e.g.*, social service, support group).

2. Assist others to comfort grieving parents.

   a. Stress the importance of openly acknowledging the death.
   b. If the baby or fetus was named, use the name in discussions.
   c. Send sympathy cards.

Grieving, Anticipatory

DEFINITION

Anticipatory Grieving: The state in which an individual/group experiences reactions in response to an expected significant loss.

DEFINING CHARACTERISTICS

Major (Must Be Present)

Expressed distress at potential loss

Minor (May Be Present)

Denial

Guilt

Anger

Sorrow

Change in eating habits

Change in sleep patterns

Change in social patterns

Change in communication patterns

Decreased libido

RELATED FACTORS

See *Grieving*.

OUTCOME CRITERIA

The person will:

1. Express grief
2. Participate in decision making for the future
3. Share concerns with significant others

⊕ GENERIC INTERVENTIONS

1. Encourage the person to share concerns, fears, effects on lifestyle.
2. Promote the integrity of person and family by acknowledging strengths and normalcy of reactions.
3. Prepare person and family for grief reactions.
4. Promote family cohesiveness.
5. Provide for the concept of hope by:
    a. Supplying accurate information
    b. Resisting the temptation to give false hope
    c. Discussing concerns willingly
6. Promote grief work with each response.
    a. Denial
        • Initially support and then strive to increase the development of awareness (when individual indicates readiness for awareness).
    b. Isolation
        • Listen and spend designated time consistently with person and family.
        • Offer person and family opportunity to explore their emotions.

    c. Depression
- Begin with simple problem solving, and move toward acceptance.
- Enhance self-worth through positive reinforcement.

    d. Anger
- Allow for crying to release this energy.
- Encourage concerned support from significant others and professional support.

    e. Guilt
- Allow for crying.
- Promote more direct expression of feelings.
- Explore methods to resolve guilt.

    f. Fear
- Help person and family recognize the feeling.
- Explore person's and family's attitudes about loss, death, etc.
- Explore person's and family's methods of coping.

    g. Rejection
- Allow for verbal expression of this feeling state to diminish the emotional strain.
- Recognize that expression of anger may create a rejection of self to significant others.

7. Caution against the use of sedatives and tranquilizers, which may prevent or delay emotional expressions of loss.
8. Teach signs of pathological responses and referrals needed.
9. Encourage person and family to engage in life review.
   a. Focus on and support the social network relationships.
   b. Reevaluate life experiences, and integrate them into a new meaning.
10. Encourage to continue usual schedule or activities (work and play).

Grieving, Dysfunctional

DEFINITION

Dysfunctional Grieving: The state in which an individual or group experiences prolonged unresolved grief and engages in detrimental activities.

Author's Note:
How one responds to loss is highly individual. Responses to acute loss should not be labeled Dysfunctional regardless of the severity. Dysfunctional Grieving is characterized by its sustained or prolonged detrimental response. The validation of Dysfunctional Grieving cannot occur until several months to 1 year after the loss. In many clinical settings, the diagnosis of Risk for Dysfunctional Grieving for individuals at risk for unsuccessful reintegration after a loss may be more useful.

DEFINING CHARACTERISTICS

Major (Must Be Present, One or More)

Unsuccessful adaptation to loss
Prolonged denial, depression
Delayed emotional reaction
Inability to assume normal patterns of living

Minor (May Be Present)

Social isolation or withdrawal
Failure to develop new relationships/interests
Failure to restructure life after loss

RELATED FACTORS

Situational (Personal, Environmental)

Related to:
  Unavailable (or lack of) support system
  Negation of the loss by others
  History of a difficult relationship with the lost person or
    object
  Multiple past or present losses
  History of ineffective coping strategies
  Unexpected death
  Expectations to "be strong"
  History of unresolved losses
  Thwarted grieving response secondary to:
    Role, work responsibilities

OUTCOME CRITERIA

The person will:

1. Acknowledge the loss
2. Demonstrate a lessening response of the pain of grief
3. Identify treatments available

GENERIC INTERVENTIONS

1. Teach the normal tasks of mourning (Worden, 1982), and help person recognize at which task he or she is:
   a. Acknowledging the loss
   b. Experiencing the pain
   c. Adjusting to the loss
   d. Reinvesting and goal setting
2. Encourage person to share perceptions of the situation.
   a. Review relationship with lost concept, person.
   b. Empathetically point out misrepresentations.
   c. Discuss the appropriateness of guilt, anger, or sorrow.
   d. Encourage expressions of anger or rage.
3. If denial persists, see *Ineffective Denial*.
4. Help identify activities that have been ignored or abandoned since loss. Encourage the selection of one to resume.
5. Encourage participation in large motor activities (*e.g.*, brisk walks, exercise bicycle).
6. Emphasize past successful coping.
7. Share community resources available for sharing experiences with others.
8. Refer for counseling if indicated.

✿ Growth and Development, Altered

Development, Risk for Altered
Growth, Risk for Altered
Adult Failure to Thrive

Growth and Development, Altered

DEFINITION

Altered Growth and Development: The state in which an individual has or is at risk for an impaired ability to perform tasks of his or her age group or impaired growth.

Author's Note:

The focus of this diagnosis will be children and adolescents. When an adult has not accomplished a developmental task, the nurse should assess for the altered functioning that has resulted from the failure to meet a developmental task, for example, Impaired Social Interactions or Ineffective Individual Coping.

DEFINING CHARACTERISTICS

Major (Must Be Present, One or More)

Inability to perform or difficulty performing skills or behaviors typical of age group, for example, motor, personal/social, language/cognition *and/or*

Altered physical growth: Weight lagging behind height by 2 standard deviations; pattern of height and weight percentiles indicating a drop in pattern

Minor (May Be Present)

Inability to perform self-care or self-control activities appropriate for age

Flat affect, listlessness, decreased responses, slow social responses, limited signs of satisfaction to caregiver, limited eye contact, difficulty feeding, decreased appetite, lethargic, irritable, negative mood, regression in self-toileting, regression in self-feeding

Infants: watchfulness, interrupted sleep pattern

RELATED FACTORS

Pathophysiological

Related to compromised physical ability and dependence secondary to:

(Circulatory impairment)

    Congenital heart defects   Congestive heart failure

(Neurological impairment)

    Cerebral damage   Cerebral palsy

    Congenital defects   Microcephaly

(Gastrointestinal impairment)

    Malabsorption syndrome   Cystic fibrosis

    Gastroesophageal reflux

(Endocrine or renal impairment)

    Hormonal disturbance

(Musculoskeletal impairments)

    Congenital anomalies of extremities

    Muscular dystrophy

    Acute illness

    Prolonged pain

    Repeated acute illness, chronic illness

    Inadequate caloric or nutritional intake

Treatment-Related

Related to separation from significant others, school, or inadequate sensory stimulation secondary to:

Prolonged, painful treatments

Repeated or prolonged hospitalization

Traction or casts

Prolonged bed rest

Isolation due to disease processes

Confinement for ongoing treatment

Situational (Personal, Environmental)

Related to:

Parental lack of knowledge

Stress (acute, transient, or chronic)
Change in usual environment
Separation from significant others (parents, primary care-
 giver)
Inadequate, inappropriate parental support (neglect, abuse)
Inadequate sensory stimulation (neglect, isolation)
Parent–child conflict
School-related stressors
Maternal or parental anxiety
Loss of significant other
Loss of control over environment (established rituals,
 activities, established hours of contact with family)

Maturational

(Infant–toddler; birth to 3 years)
 Related to limited opportunities to meet social, play, or
  educational needs secondary to:
   Separation from parents/significant others
   Restriction of activity secondary to (specify)
   Inadequate parental support
   Inability to trust significant other
   Inability to communicate (deafness)
   Multiple caregivers
(Preschool age; 4–6 years)
 Related to limited opportunities to meet social, play, or
  educational needs secondary to:
   Loss of ability to communicate
   Lack of stimulation
   Lack of significant other
 Related to loss of significant other (death, divorce)
 Related to loss of peer group
 Related to removal from home environment
(School age; 6–11 years)
 Related to loss of significant other
 Related to loss of peer group
 Related to strange environment
(Adolescent; 12–18 years)
 Related to loss of independence and autonomy secondary to
  (specify)
 Related to disruption of peer relationships
 Related to disruption in body image
 Related to loss of significant other

OUTCOME CRITERIA

The child will:

1. Demonstrate an increase in behaviors in personal, social, language, cognition, or motor activities appropriate to age group (specify the behaviors)

INTERVENTIONS

1. Teach parents the age-related developmental tasks (Table I-1).
2. Carefully assess child's level of development in all areas of functioning by using specific assessment tools (*e.g.*, Brazelton Assessment Table, Denver Developmental Screening Tool).
3. Provide opportunities for an ill child to meet age-related developmental tasks.
   a. Birth to 1 year
      • Provide increased stimulation using variety of colored toys in crib (*i.e.*, mobiles, musical toys, stuffed toys of varied textures, frequent periods of holding and speaking to infant).
      • Hold while feeding; feed slowly and in relaxed environment.
      • Provide periods of rest prior to feeding.
      • Observe mother and child during interaction, especially during feeding.
      • Investigate crying promptly and consistently.
      • Assign consistent caregiver.
      • Encourage parental visits/calls and involvement in care if possible.
      • Provide buccal experience if infant desires (*i.e.*, thumb, pacifier).
      • Allow hands and feet to be free if possible.
   b. 1 to 3½ years
      • Assign consistent caregiver.
      • Encourage self-care activities (*i.e.*, self-feeding, self-dressing, bathing).
      • Reinforce word development by repeating words child uses, naming objects by saying words, and speaking to child often.
      • Provide frequent periods of play with peers present and with a variety of toys (puzzles, books with pictures, manipulative toys, trucks, cars, blocks, bright colors).

- Explain all procedures as you do them.
- Provide safe area where the child can loco-mote; use walker, provide creeping area, and hold hand while taking steps.
- Encourage parental visits/calls and involve-ment in care if possible.
- Provide comfort measures after painful proce-dures.

c. 3½ to 5 years

- Encourage self-care: self-grooming, self-dressing, mouth care, hair care.
- Provide frequent play time with others and with variety of toys (*e.g.*, models, musical toys, dolls, puppets, books, mini-slide, wagon, tricycle).
- Read stories aloud.
- Ask for verbal responses and requests.
- Say words for equipment, objects, and people, and ask the child to repeat.
- Allow time for individual play and explo-ration of play environment.
- Encourage parental visits/calls and involve-ment in care if possible.
- Monitor television, and use television as means to help child understand time ("After Sesame Street, your mother will come.").

d. 5 to 11 years

- Talk with child about care provided.
- Request input from child (*e.g.*, diet, clothes, routine).
- Allow child to dress in clothes instead of pajamas.
- Provide periods of interaction with other chil-dren on unit.
- Provide craft project that can be completed each day or week.
- Continue school work at intervals each day.
- Praise positive behaviors.
- Read stories, and provide variety of indepen-dent games, puzzles, books, video games, painting, or other activity.
- Introduce child by name to persons on unit.

(Text continues on p. 170)

TABLE I-1.
Age-Related Developmental Needs

Developmental Tasks/Needs

BIRTH TO 1 YEAR

PERSONAL/SOCIAL

Learns to trust and anticipate satisfaction

Sends cues to mother/caretaker

Begins understanding self as separate from others (body image)

MOTOR

Responds to sound

Social smile

Reaches for objects

Begins to sit, creep, pull up, and stand with support

Attempts to walk

1–3½ YEARS

PERSONAL/SOCIAL

Establishes self-control, decision-making, self-independence (autonomy)

Extremely curious, prefers to do things independently

Demonstrates independence through negativism

Very egocentric: believes he or she controls the world

Learns about words through senses

MOTOR

Begins to walk and run well

Drinks from cup, feeds self

3½–5 YEARS

PERSONAL/SOCIAL

Attempts to establish self as like parents but independent

Explores environment on own initiative

Boasts, brags, has feelings of indestructibility

Family is primary group

Peers increasingly important

Assumes sex roles

Aggressive

LANGUAGE/COGNITION
Learns to signal wants/needs with sounds, crying
Begins to vocalize with meaning (two syllable words: dada, mama)
Comprehends some verbal/nonverbal messages (no, yes, bye-bye)
Learns about words through senses

FEARS
Loud noises
Falling

Develops fine-motor control
Climbs
Begins self-toileting

LANGUAGE/COGNITION
Has poor time sense
Increasingly verbal (4–5 word sentences by age 3½)
Talks to self/others
Misconceptions about cause/effect

FEARS
Loss/separation from parents
Darkness
Machines/equipment
Intrusive procedures
Unknown
Inanimate, unfamiliar objects

MOTOR
Locomotion skills increase, and coordinates easier
Rides tricycle/bicycle
Throws ball, but has difficulty catching

LANGUAGE/COGNITION
Egocentric
Language skills flourish
Generates many questions: how, why, what?
Simple problem-solving; uses fantasy to understand, problem-solve

FEARS
Mutilation
Castration

(Continued)

TABLE I-1. *(Continued)*

Developmental Tasks/Needs

5–11 YEARS

PERSONAL/SOCIAL

Learns to include values and skills of school, neighborhood, peers

Peer relationships important

Focuses more on reality, less on fantasy

Family is main base of security and identity

Sensitive to reactions of others

Seeks approval, recognition

Enthusiastic, noisy, imaginative, desires to explore

Likes to complete a task

Enjoys helping

11–15 YEARS

PERSONAL/SOCIAL

Family values continue to be significant influence

Peer group values have increasing significance

Early adolescence: outgoing and enthusiastic

Emotions are extreme, mood swings, introspection

Sexual identity fully mature

Wants privacy/independence

Develops interests not shared with family

Concern with physical self

Explores adult roles

MOTOR
Moves constantly
Physical play prevalent (sports, swimming, skating, etc.)

LANGUAGE/COGNITION
Organized, stable thought
Concepts more complicated
Focuses on concrete understanding

FEARS
Rejections, failure
Immobility
Mutilation
Death

MOTOR
Well developed
Rapid physical growth
Secondary sex characteristics

LANGUAGE/COGNITION
Plans for future career
Able to abstract solutions and problem-solve in future tense

FEARS
Mutilation
Disruption in body image
Rejection from peers

- Encourage visits and telephone calls from parents, siblings, and peers.
  e. 11 to 15 years
    - Speak frequently with child about feelings, ideas, concerns about condition or care.
    - Provide opportunity for interaction with others of the same age on unit.
    - Identify interest or hobby that can be supported on unit in some manner, and support it daily.
    - Allow hospital routine to be altered to suit child's schedule.
    - Allow child to dress in own clothes if possible.
    - Involve in decisions about care.
    - Provide opportunity for involvement in variety of activities (*i.e.*, reading, video games, movies, board games, art, trips outside or to other areas).
    - Encourage visits and telephone calls from parents, siblings, and peers.
4. Refer to community programs specific to contributing factors (*e.g.*, social services; family services, counseling).

Development, Risk for Altered

DEFINITION

Risk for Altered Development: The state in which an individual is at risk for an impaired ability to perform tasks of his or her age group.

RISK FACTORS

Refer to *Altered Growth and Development*

OUTCOME CRITERIA

1. Continue to demonstrate appropriate behavior in personal, social, language, cognition, or motor activities

INTERVENTIONS

Refer to *Altered Growth and Development.*

Growth, Risk for Altered

DEFINITION

Risk for Altered Growth: The state in which an individual is at risk for an impaired growth.

RISK FACTORS

Refer to *Altered Growth and Development*

OUTCOME CRITERIA

The child/adolescent will:

1. Continue to demonstrate appropriate growth for his or her age.

INTERVENTIONS

Refer to *Altered Growth and Development.*

Adult Failure to Thrive

DEFINITION

Adult Failure to Thrive: The state in which an individual experiences insidious and progressive deterioration with loss of appetite, weight loss, diminishing social competence, concentration, initiative, and drive (Hodkinson, 1973; Newbern, 1994).

DEFINING CHARACTERISTICS

Major

Declining physical functioning
Declining cognitive functioning
Depression
Weight loss
Anorexia

RELATED FACTORS

The cause of failure to thrive in adults, usually the elderly, is unknown. Researchers have identified some factors that may contribute to this condition.

Situational (Personal, Environmental)

Related to diminished coping abilities
Related to limited ability to adapt to effects of aging
Related to loss of social skills and the resulant social isolation
Related to loss of social relatedness
Related to increasing dependency and feelings of helplessness

OUTCOME CRITERIA

The person will:

1. Maintain present level of functioning
2. Maintain or increase present weight
3. Increase social relatedness

INTERVENTIONS

1. Consult with therapist to evaluate for depression and medication therapy as indicated.
2. Evaluate pattern of socialization (refer to *Risk for Loneliness*).
3. Provide opportunities to increase social relatedness:
   a. Music therapy
   b. Recreation therapy
   c. Reminiscence therapy
4. Maintain standards of empathic, respectful care.
5. Attempt to obtain information that will provide useful and meaningful topics for conversations (likes, dislikes; interests, hobbies; work history). Interview early in day.
6. Encourage significant others and caregivers to speak slowly with a low voice pitch and at an average volume (unless hearing deficits are present), as one adult to another, with eye contact, and as if expecting person to understand.
7. Provide respect and promote sharing.
   a. Pay attention to what person is saying.
   b. Pick out meaningful comments and continue talking.
   c. Call person by name and introduce yourself each time contact is made; use touch if welcomed.

Health Maintenance, Altered

DEFINITION

Altered Health Maintenance: The state in which an individual or group experiences or is at risk of experiencing a disruption in health because of an unhealthy lifestyle or lack of knowledge to manage a condition.

Author's Note:

Altered Health Maintenance can describe a person or persons who desire to change an unhealthy lifestyle (obesity, tobacco use). Ineffective Management of Therapeutic Regimen can be used for those who need teaching for self-management of a disease or condition.

DEFINING CHARACTERISTICS
(In The Absence of Disease)

Major (Must Be Present, One or More)

Reports or demonstrates an unhealthy practice or lifestyle, *e.g:*
Reckless driving of vehicle	Overeating
Substance abuse	High-fat diet

Minor (May Be Present)

Reports or demonstrates:
Skin and nails
Malodorous	Sunburn
Skin lesions (pustules,	Unusual color, pallor
rashes, dry or scaly skin)	Unexplained scars

Respiratory system
Frequent infections	Dyspnea with exertion
Chronic cough	

Oral cavity
Frequent sores (on tongue, buccal mucosa)
Loss of teeth at early age
Lesions associated with lack of oral care or substance abuse (leukoplakia, fistulas)

Gastrointestinal system and nutrition

Obesity	Chronic anemia
Anorexia	Chronic bowel irregularity
Cachexia	Chronic dyspepsia

Musculoskeletal system
    Frequent muscle strain, backaches, neck pain
Diminished flexibility and muscle strength
Genitourinary system
    Frequent venereal lesions and infections
    Frequent use of potentially unhealthful over-the-counter
      products (*e.g.*, chemical douches, perfumed vaginal
      products, nasal sprays)
Constitutional
    Chronic fatigue, malaise, apathy
Neurosensory
    Presence of facial tics (nonconvulsant)
    Headaches
Psychoemotional
    Emotional fragility
    Behavior disorders (compulsiveness, belligerence)
    Frequent feelings of being overwhelmed

RELATED FACTORS

A variety of factors can produce altered health maintenance. Some common causes are listed below.

Situational (Personal, Environmental)

Related to:
    Lack of motivation
    Lack of education or readiness
    Lack of access to adequate health care services
    Inadequate health teaching
    Impaired ability to understand secondary to (specify)

Maturational

Related to lack of education of age-related factors. Examples
    include:
Child

Sexuality and sexual development	Substance abuse
Safety hazards	Nutrition

Adolescent
    Same as children
    Cycle, automobile safety practices
    Substance abuse (alcohol, other drugs, tobacco)
Adult
    Parenthood   Safety practices
    Sexual function
Older adult
    Effects of aging
    Sensory deficits
See Table I-2 for age-related conditions.

OUTCOME CRITERIA

The person will:

1. Describe lifestyles that promote health
2. Describe/demonstrate health behaviors needed to manage condition
3. Describe signs and symptoms that need reporting

⊕ GENERIC INTERVENTIONS

1. Assess knowledge of primary prevention.
   a. Safety—accident prevention (*e.g.*, car, machinery, outdoor safety, occupational)
   b. Healthful diet (*e.g.*, "basic four," low fat and salt, high complex carbohydrate, sufficient intake of vitamins, minerals, 2–3 quarts of water daily)
   c. Weight control
   d. Avoidance of substance abuse (*e.g.*, alcohol, drugs, tobacco)
   e. Avoidance of sexually transmitted diseases
   f. Dental/oral hygiene (*e.g.*, daily, dentist)
   g. Immunizations
   h. Regular exercise pattern
   i. Stress management
   j. Lifestyle counseling (*e.g.*, safe sex, family planning, parenting skills, financial planning)
2. Teach importance of secondary prevention (Refer to Table I-2.)

(Text continues on p. 184)

TABLE I-2.
Primary and Secondary Prevention for Age-Related Conditions

Developmental Level	Primary Prevention	Secondary Prevention

Infancy (0–1 y)	Parent education
	Infant safety
	Nutrition
	Breastfeeding
	Sensory stimulation
	Infant massage and touch
	Visual stimulation
	  Activity
	  Colors
	Auditory stimulation
	  Verbal
	  Music
	Immunizations
	  DPT, hepatitis B ⎫ at 2, 4, and 6
	  TOPV ⎭ mo
	  Influenza (for high-risk >6 months)
	Oral hygiene
	Teething biscuits
		Complete physical examination every 2–3 mo
		Screening at birth
		  Congenital hip
		  Phenylketonuria (PKU)
		  Sickle cell disease
		  Cystic fibrosis
		  Vision (startle reflex)
		  Hearing (response to and localization of sounds)
		Tuberculin test at 12 mo
		Developmental assessments
		Screen and intervene for high risk
		  Low birth weight
		  Maternal substance abuse during pregnancy
		  Alcohol: fetal alcohol syndrome
		  Cigarettes: sudden infant death syndrome (SIDS)
		  Drugs: addicted neonate
		  Maternal infections during pregnancy

| Preschool (1–5 y) | Fluoride
Avoid sugared food and drink
Parent education
  Teething
  Discipline
  Nutrition
  Accident prevention
  Normal growth and development
Child education
  Dental self-care
  Dressing
  Bathing with assistance
  Feeding self-care
Immunizations
  DTap } at 18 mo
  TOPV }
  MMR at 12–15 mo
  HIB at 24 mo
  Influenza (for high risk)
Dental/oral hygiene
  Fluoride treatments
  Fluoridated water
  Dietary counsel | Complete physical examination between 2 and 3 y and preschool (urinalysis, CBC)
Tuberculin test at 3 y
Developmental assessments (annual)
  Speech development
  Hearing
  Vision
Screen and intervene
  Lead poisoning
  Developmental lag
  Neglect or abuse
  Strabismus
  Hemoglobin or hematocrit
  Vision, hearing deficit
Strong family history of arteriosclerotic disease (*e.g.,* MI, CVA, peripheral vascular disease), diabetes, hypertension, gout, or hyperlipidemia—fasting serum cholesterol at age 2 years, then every 3–5 years if normal. |

(Continued)

TABLE I-2. *(Continued)*

Developmental Level	Primary Prevention	Secondary Prevention
School age (6–11 y)	Health education of child Food pyramid Accident prevention Outdoor safety (*e.g.*, helmets) Substance abuse counsel Anticipatory guidance for physical changes at puberty Immunizations Tetanus at 10 y DTap⎫ Boosters between TOPV⎭ 4 and 6 y MMR Professional dental hygiene every 6–12 mo Continue fluoridation Complete physical examination (yearly)	Complete physical examination Tuberculin test every 3 y (at ages 6 and 9) Developmental measurements Language Vision: Snellen charts at school 6–8 y, use "E" chart Over 8 y, use alphabet chart Hearing: audiogram
Adolescence (12–19 y)	Health education Proper nutrition and healthful diets	Complete physical examination (prepuberty or age 13) Blood pressure

	Sex education (abstinence, family planning, sexually transmitted diseases)	Cholesterol profile
	Safe driving skills	Tuberculin test at 12, 15, 18 y
	Adult challenges	RPR, CBC, urinalysis
	Seeking employment and career choices	Female: breast self-examination, monthly
	Dating and marriage	Male: testicular self-examination, weekly
	Confrontation with substance abuse	Female, if sexually active: Papanicolaou test and pelvic examination, yearly (*Chlamydia* and cervical gonorrhea cultures with pelvic examination)
	Safety in athletics, water	Screening and interventions if high risk
	Skin care, sunscreens	Depression
	Professional dental hygiene every 6–12 mo	Suicide
	Immunization	Substance abuse
	Hepatitis B series (if needed)	Pregnancy
	TOPV booster at 12–14 y	Family history of alcoholism or domestic violence
Young Adult (20–39 y)	Health education	HIV infection
	Weight management with good nutrition as basal metabolic rate changes	Complete physical examination at about 20 y, then every 5–6 y
	Lifestyle counseling	Cancer checkup every 3 y
	Stress management skills	Female: breast self-examination monthly
		Gynecologic exam—same as adolescent 12–19 if high risk
		Male: testicular self-examination weekly

(Continued)

179

TABLE I-2. *(Continued)*

Developmental Level	Primary Prevention	Secondary Prevention
	Injury prevention "Safe sex" Parenting skills Substance abuse Environmental health choices Professional dental hygiene every 6–12 mo Immunization Tetanus at 20 y and every 10 y Female: rubella, if zero negative for antibodies Hepatitis B series if needed	All females: baseline mammography at age 40 then every 1–2 y Parents-to-be: high-risk screening for Down syndrome, Tay-Sachs disease Pregnant female: screen for sexually transmitted diseases, rubella titer, Rh factor Annual screening and interventions if high risk Female with previous breast cancer: annual mammography at 35 y and after Female with mother or sister who has had breast cancer, same as above Family history of colorectal cancer or high risk: annual stool guaiac, digital rectal examination, and sigmoidoscopy PPD if exposed to tuberculosis Glaucoma screening at 35 years along with routine physical exams Cholesterol profile every 5 years if normal Cholesterol profile every 1–2 years if borderline

Middle-aged adult (40–59 y)	Health education: continue with young adult, perimenopausal	Complete physical examination every 5–6 y with complete laboratory evaluation (serum/urine tests, x-ray, ECG)
	Midlife changes, male and female counseling	Cancer checkup every year
	"Empty-nest syndrome"	Female: breast self-examination monthly
	Anticipatory guidance for retirement	Male: testicular self-examination monthly
	Grandparenting	All females: mammography every 1–2 y 50 years and over
	Professional dental hygiene every 6–12 mo	Eye examination every 1–2 y
	Immunizations	Pregnant female: perinatal screening by amniocentesis if desired
	Tetanus every 10 years	Sigmoidoscopy at 50 and 51, then every 4 y if negative
	Influenza—annual if high risk (*i.e.,* major chronic disease [COPD, CAD])	Stool guaiac annually at 50 and thereafter
	Pneumococcal—single dose	Screening and intervention if high risk
		Endometrial cancer: have endometrial sampling at menopause
		Oral cancer: screen more often if substance abuser
		Skin cancer
Older adult (60–74 y)	Health education: continue with previous counseling	Complete physical examination every 2 y with laboratory assessments

(Continued)

181

TABLE I-2. *(Continued)*

Developmental Level	Primary Prevention	Secondary Prevention
	Home safety	Annual cancer checkup
	Retirement	Blood pressure annually
	Loss of spouse	Female: breast self-examination monthly
	Special health needs	Male: testicular self-examination monthly
	Nutritional changes	Female: annual mammogram
	Changes in hearing or vision	Annual stool guaiac
	Professional dental/oral hygiene every 6–12 mo	Sigmoidoscopy every 4 y
	Immunizations	Complete eye examination yearly
	Tetanus every 10 y	Podiatric evaluation with foot care PRN

Influenza—annual if high risk
Pneumococcal (one time only)

Old-age adult
(75 y and over)

Health education: continue counsel
Anticipatory guidance
  Dying and death
  Loss of spouse
  Increasing dependency on others
Professional dental/oral hygiene every
  6–12 mo
Immunizations
  Tetanus every 10 y
  Influenza—annual
  Pneumococcal—if not already
    received

Screen for high risk
  Depression
  Suicide
Complete physical examination annually
  Laboratory assessments
  Cancer checkup
  Blood pressure
  Stool guaiac
  Alcohol/drug abuse
  Elder abuse
Female: mammogram every 1–2 y sigmoidoscopy
  every 5 y
Complete eye examination yearly
Podiatrist PRN

(Source: U.S. Department of Health and Human Services [1994]. *Clinician's handbook of preventive services: Putting preven-tion into practice.* Washington, DC: U.S. Government Printing Office.)

3. Determine knowledge needed to manage condition.
   a. Causes
   b. Treatments
   c. Medications
   d. Diet
   e. Activity
   f. Risk factors
   g. Signs/symptoms of complications
   h. Restrictions
   i. Follow-up care
4. Assess if needed at-home resources are available.
   a. Caregiver
   b. Finances
   c. Equipment
5. Determine if referrals are indicated (*e.g.*, social services, housekeeping, home health).

Health Seeking Behaviors (Specify)

DEFINITION

Health Seeking Behaviors: The state in which an individual in stable health actively seeks ways to alter personal health habits and/ or the environment to move toward a higher level of wellness.*

Author's Note:

This diagnosis can be used to describe the individual/family that desires health teaching related to the promotion and maintenance of health (*e.g.*, preventive behavior, age-related screening, optimal nutrition). This diagnosis should be used to describe an asymptomatic person. However, it can be used for a person with a chronic

(Continued)

*Stable health is defined as a condition in which the client's well-being is maximized; signs and symptoms of disease, if present, are controlled; and disabilities are following a predictable, nonacute course.

Author's Note (Continued):
disease to help that person attain a higher level of wellness. For example, a woman with lupus erythematosus can have the diagnosis Health Seeking Behaviors: related to initiation of a regular exercise program.

DEFINING CHARACTERISTICS

Major (Must Be Present)

Expressed or observed desire to seek information for health promotion

Minor (May Be Present)

Expressed or observed desire for increased control of health
Expression of concern about current environmental conditions on health status
Stated or observed unfamiliarity with community wellness resources
Demonstrated or observed lack of knowledge in health-promotion behaviors

RELATED FACTORS

Situational (Personal, Environmental)

Related to anticipated role changes, for example, marriage, parenthood, "empty nest syndrome," retirement
Related to lack of knowledge of:
    Preventive behavior (disease)
    Screening practices for age and risk
    Optimal nutrition and weight control
    Regular exercise program
    Constructive stress management
    Supportive social networks

Maturational

See Table I-2.

OUTCOME CRITERIA

The person will:

1. Describe health promotion that is appropriate for age and risk factors
2. Plan for life cycle events and challenges
3. Participate in a regular physical exercise program
4. State an intent to use positive coping mechanisms and constructive stress management
5. Agree with self-responsibility for wellness and health promotion

⬇ GENERIC INTERVENTIONS

1. Determine the person's or family's knowledge or perception of:
   a. Life cycle challenges (*e.g.,* marriage, parenting, aging, finances)
   b. Need to maintain responsible relationships with health care providers
   c. Ability to attain a higher level of health through anticipatory planning for life cycle events (*e.g.,* financial planning)
   d. Need to provide and nurture reciprocity in social support
2. Determine the person's or family's past patterns of health care.
   a. Expectations
   b. Interactions with health care system or providers
   c. Influences of family, cultural group, peer group, mass media
3. Provide specific information concerning age-related health promotion (refer to Table I-2).
4. Discuss client's food choices, and assist as he or she identifies new goals for health promotion.
   a. Assist in the selection of foods to sustain life and facilitate body functioning.
   b. Provide information, when needed, about developmental considerations for dependents.
5. Discuss the benefits of a regular exercise program.
6. Discuss the elements of constructive stress management.
   a. Assertiveness training

b. Problem solving
c. Relaxation techniques
7. Discuss strategies for developing positive social networks.
8. Promote self-actualization in the client who is seeking to promote health.
   a. Demonstrate an interested but nonjudgmental attitude.
   b. View the client–nurse relationship as collaborative; the client remains in control of choices, actions, and evaluations.
   c. Facilitate adoption of new behaviors rather than defining them.
   d. Listen, reflect, and converse to clarify the client's current behavior patterns and desired goals.
   e. Enhance the client's strengths, empower with choices and self-control, and always demonstrate respect for those choices.

Home Maintenance Management, Impaired

DEFINITION

Impaired Home Maintenance Management: The state in which an individual or family experiences or is at risk to experience difficulty in maintaining a safe, hygienic, growth-producing home environment.

Author's Note:

This diagnosis can describe situations in which the individual or family needs specific support or instruction to manage home care of a family member or activities of daily living.

DEFINING CHARACTERISTICS

Major (Must Be Present, One or More)

Expressions or observations of:
  Difficulty in maintaining home hygiene
  Difficulty in maintaining a safe home
  Inability to keep home up
  Lack of sufficient finances

Minor (May Be Present)

Repeated infections
Accumulated wastes
Overcrowding
Infestations

Unwashed cooking and
  eating equipment
Offensive odors

RELATED FACTORS

Pathophysiological

Related to compromised functional ability secondary to
  chronic debilitating disease
    Diabetes mellitus
    Chronic obstructive
      pulmonary disease
    Congestive heart failure
    Cancer

Arthritis
Multiple sclerosis
Muscular dystrophy
Parkinson's disease
CVA

Situational (Personal, Environmental)

Related to change in functional ability of (specify family
  member) secondary to:
    Injury (fractured limb, spinal cord injury)
    Surgery (amputation, ostomy)
    Impaired mental status (memory lapses, depression, severe
      anxiety, panic)
    Substance abuse (alcohol, other drugs)
Related to unavailable support system
Related to loss of family member
Related to lack of knowledge
Related to insufficient finances

Maturational

Infant
  Related to multiple care requirements secondary to high-
    risk newborn

Older adult
Related to multiple care requirements secondary to family
member with deficits (cognitive, motor, sensory)

OUTCOME CRITERIA

The person or caretaker will:

1. Identify factors that restrict self-care and home management
2. Demonstrate the ability to perform skills necessary for the care of the individual or home
3. Express satisfaction with home situation

◆ GENERIC INTERVENTIONS

1. Determine with the person and family the information needed to be taught and learned.
2. Determine the type of equipment needed, considering availability, cost, and durability.
3. Determine the type of assistance needed (*e.g.*, meals, housework, transportation), and assist the individual to obtain them.
4. Discuss the implications of caring for a chronically ill family member (refer to Caregiver Role Strain).
   a. Amount of time
   b. Effects on other role responsibilities (spouse, children, job)
   c. Physical requirements (lifting)
5. Arrange for a home visit.
6. Allow the caretaker opportunities to share problems and feelings.
7. Refer to community agencies as indicated (*e.g.*, nursing, social service, meals).

Hopelessness

DEFINITION

Hopelessness: A sustained subjective emotional state in which an individual sees no alternatives or personal choices available to

solve problems or to achieve what is desired and cannot mobilize
energy on own behalf to establish goals.

Author's Note:

Hopelessness differs from Powerlessness in that a hopeless person
sees no solution to the problem or way to achieve what is desired,
even if he or she has control of his or her life. A powerless person
may see an alternative or answer to the problem yet be unable to
do anything about it because of perceived lack of control and resources.

DEFINING CHARACTERISTICS

Major (Must Be Present, One or More)

Expresses profound, overwhelming, sustained apathy in
response to situations perceived as impossible verbal cues of
dependency
Examples of expressions are:
"I might as well give up because I can't make things
better."
"My future seems awful to me."
"I can't imagine what my life will be like in 10 years."
"I've never been given a break, so why should I in the
future?"
"Life looks unpleasant when I think ahead."
"I know I'll never get what I really want."
"Things never work out how I want them to."
"It's foolish to want to get anything because I never do."
"It's unlikely that I'll get satisfaction in the future."
"The future seems vague and uncertain."
Physiological
Slowed responses to stimuli
Lack of energy
Increased sleep
Emotional
The hopeless person often has difficulty experiencing feel-
ings but may feel:
Unable to seek good fortune, luck, or God's favor
Lack of meaning or purpose in life
"Empty" or "drained"
A sense of loss and deprivation

    Helpless
    Incompetent
    Entrapped
Person exhibits:
  Passiveness, lack of involvement in care
  Decreased verbalization
  Decreased affect
  Lack of ambition, initiative, and interest
  "Giving up–given up complex"
  Inability to accomplish anything
  Impaired interpersonal relationship
  Slowed thought processes
  Does not take responsibility for own decisions and life
Cognitive
  Decreased problem-solving and decision-making capabilities
  Deals with past and future, not here and now
  Decreased flexibility in thought processes
  Rigidity (*e.g.*, "all or none" thinking)
  Lacks imagination and wishing capabilities
  Unable to identify and/or accomplish desired objectives
    and goals
  Unable to plan, organize, or make decisions
  Unable to recognize sources of hope
  Suicidal thoughts

Minor (May Be Present)

Physiological
  Anorexia
  Weight loss
Emotional
  Person feels:
    "A lump in the throat"
    Discouraged with self and others
    "At the end of his or her rope"
    Tense
    Overwhelmed (feels he just "can't . . ")
    Loss of gratification from roles and relationships
    Vulnerable
Person exhibits:
  Poor eye contact; turns away from speaker; shrugs in re-
  sponse to speaker
  Decreased motivation
  Sighing

    Regression
    Resignation
    Depression
  Cognitive
    Decreased ability to integrate information received
    Loss of time perception for past, present, and future
    Decreased ability to recall the past
    Confusion
    Inability to communicate effectively
    Distorted thought perceptions and associations
    Unreasonable judgment

RELATED FACTORS

Pathophysiological

Any chronic and/or terminal illness can cause or contribute to hopelessness (*e.g.*, heart disease, kidney disease, cancer, AIDS).

Related to:
  Failing or deteriorating physiological condition
  New and unexpected signs or symptoms of previous disease process
  Prolonged pain, discomfort, weakness
  Impaired functional abilities (walking, elimination, eating)

Treatment-Related

Related to:
  Prolonged treatments (*e.g.,* chemotherapy, radiation) that cause discomfort (pain, nausea, vomiting)
  Prolonged treatments with no positive results
  Treatments that alter body image (*e.g.*, surgery, chemotherapy)
  Prolonged diagnostic studies with no significant results
  Prolonged dependence on equipment for life support (*e.g.*, dialysis, ventilator)
  Prolonged dependence on equipment for monitoring bodily functions (telemetry)

Situational (Personal, Environmental)

Related to:
  Prolonged activity restriction (*e.g.*, fractures, spinal cord injury)

Prolonged isolation due to disease processes (*e.g.*, infectious diseases, reverse isolation for suppressed immune system)

Abandonment of or separation from significant others (parents, spouse, children, others)

Inability to achieve goals that one values in life (marriage, education, children)

Inability to participate in activities one desires (walking, sports)

Loss of something or someone valued (spouse, children, friend, financial resources)

Prolonged caretaking responsibilities (spouse, child, parent)

Exposure to long-term physiological or psychological stress

Loss of belief in transcendent values/God

Stressful stimuli or major decisions

History of physical or sexual abuse

Maturational

Related to:

(Child)

Loss of caregivers

Loss of trust in significant other (parents, sibling)

Rejection or abandonment by caregivers

Loss of autonomy related to illness (*e.g.*, fracture)

Loss of bodily functions

Inability to achieve developmental tasks (trust, autonomy, initiative, industry)

Rejection by family

(Adolescent)

Loss of significant other (peer, family)

Loss of bodily functions

Change in body image

Inability to achieve developmental task (role identity)

(Adult)

Impaired bodily functions, loss of body part

Impaired relationships (separation, divorce)

Loss of job, career

Loss of significant others (death of children, spouse)

Inability to achieve developmental tasks (intimacy, commitment, productivity)

Older adult

Sensory deficits

Motor deficits
Cognitive deficits
Loss of independence
Loss of significant others, things
Inability to achieve developmental tasks (integrity)

OUTCOME CRITERIA

Short-Term

The person will:

1. Share suffering openly and constructively with others
2. Reminisce and review life positively
3. Consider values and the meaning of life
4. Express feelings of optimism about the present
5. Express feelings of positive relationships with significant others
6. Express confidence in a desired outcome
7. Express confidence in self and others
8. Verbalize realistic goals

Long-Term

The person will:

1. Demonstrate an increase in energy level as evidenced by activities (*e.g.*, self-care, exercise, hobbies)
2. Express positive expectations about the future
3. Demonstrate initiative, self-direction, and autonomy in decision making and activities

GENERIC INTERVENTIONS

1. Convey empathy to promote verbalization of doubts, fears, and concerns.
2. Encourage verbalization of why and how hope is significant in client's life.
3. Encourage expressions of how hope is uncertain and areas in which hope has failed.
4. Teach how to deal with the hopeless aspects by separating them from the hopeful aspects.
5. Assess and mobilize the person's internal resources (autonomy, independence, rationale, cognitive thinking, flexibility, spirituality).

6. Assist with identification of sources of hope (*e.g.*, relationships, faith, things to accomplish).
7. Create an environment in which spiritual expression is encouraged.
8. Assist with development of realistic short- and long-term goals (progress from simple to more complex; may use a "goals poster" to indicate type and time for achieving specific goals).
9. Teach how to anticipate pleasurable experiences (*e.g.*, walking, reading favorite book, writing letter).
10. Assess and mobilize person's external resources (significant others, health care team, support groups, God or higher powers).
11. Help person to recognize that he or she is loved, cared about, and important in the lives of others regardless of failing health.
12. Encourage sharing of concerns with others who have had a similar problem or disease and have had positive experiences from coping effectively with it.
13. Assess belief support system (value, experiences with, religious activities, relationship with God, meaning and purpose of prayer; refer to *Spiritual Distress*).
14. Allow time and opportunities to reflect on the meaning of suffering, death, and dying.
15. Initiate referrals as indicated (*e.g.*, counseling, spiritual leader).

CHILD FOCUS INTERVENTIONS
(Adolescent) (Hinds, 1988)

1. Provide truthful explanations.
2. Engage in activities.
3. If appropriate, discuss knowledge of survivors.
4. Focus on future.
5. Discuss topics interesting to the child.
6. Use humor if appropriate.

♋ Infant Behavior, Disorganized

DEFINITION

Disorganized Infant Behavior: The state in which the neonate has an alteration in integration and modulation of the physiological and behavioral systems of adaptation (autonomic, motor, state, organizational, self-regulatory, and attention–interactional).

> **Author's Note:**
> This diagnosis describes an infant who has difficulty regulating and adapting to external stimuli. This difficulty is due to immature neurobehavioral development and increased environmental stimuli associated with neonatal units. When an infant is overstimulated or stressed, she or he uses energy to adapt, which depletes the supply of energy needed for physiological growth. The goal of nursing care is to assist the infant with energy conservation by reducing environmental stimuli, allowing the infant sufficient time to adapt to handling, and providing sensory input when appropriate to the infant's physiological and neurobehavioral status.

DEFINING CHARACTERISTICS
(Vandenberg, 1990)

Autonomic system
Cardiac
Increased rate
Respiration
Pauses, tachypnea, gasping
Color changes
Paling around nostrils, perioral duskiness, mottled, cyanotic, gray, flushed, ruddy
Visceral
Hiccups, gagging, grunting, spitting up
Straining as if actually producing a bowel movement
Motor
Seizures   Sneezing
Tremoring/startling   Yawning

Twitching   Sighing
Coughing
Motor system
  Fluctuating tone
    Flaccidity of:
      Trunk   Face
      Extremities
    Hypertonicity
      Leg extensions   Arching
      Salutes   Finger splays
      Airplaning   Tongue extensions
      Sitting on air   Fisting
    Hyperflexions
      Trunk   Fetal tuck
      Extremities
  Frantic diffuse activity
State system (range)
  Diffuse states
    Sleeping
      Twitches   Whimpers
      Sound   Grimacing
      Jerky moves   Fussy in sleep
      Irregular respirations
    Awake
      Eye floating   Panicked, worried,
      Glassy eyed   or dull look
      Strained fussy   Weak cry
      Staring   Irritability
      Gaze aversion   Abrupt state changes
Attention–interaction system
  Imbalance of withdrawal versus engaging behaviors
  Impaired ability to orient, attend, engage in reciprocal
    social interactions
  Difficult to console
Self-regulatory system
  Limited or absent use of self-regulatory behaviors to main-
    tain or regain control
    Postural changes
    Foot, leg bracing
    Sucking fists
    Finger folding
    Hand to mouth
  Stressed with more than one mode of stimuli

RELATED FACTORS

Pathophysiological

Related to immature or impaired CNS secondary to:
  Prematurity
  Prenatal exposure to drugs
  Congenital anomalies
  Hypoglycemia
  Infection
  Hyperbilirubinemia
  Decreased oxygen saturation
Related to nutritional deficits secondary to: reflux emesis,
  colic, swallowing problems, or feeding intolerances
Related to excess stimulation secondary to: pain, hunger, oral
  hypersensitivity, or temperature variation

Treatment-Related

Related to excess stimulation secondary to, for example,
  invasive procedures, chest physical therapy, restraints, lights
  (*e.g.*, bililights), tubes, tape, medication administration,
  movement, feeding, noise (*e.g.*, prolonged, alarms)
Related to inability to see caregivers secondary to eye patches

Situational (Personal, Environmental)

Related to multiple caregivers
Related to imbalance of task touch and consoling touch
Related to decreased ability to self-regulate secondary to
  sudden movement, noise, fatigue, or insufficient sleep

OUTCOME CRITERIA (Blackburn, 1993)

The infant will:

1. Experience minimal fluctuation of tone and muscle extensions
2. Demonstrate organized sleep states and calm quiet alerting
3. Demonstrate improvement of respiratory regularity and color during handling

The parent(s)/caregiver(s) will:

1. Describe techniques to reduce environmental stress in agency or at home

INTERVENTIONS

1. Assess for causative/contributing factors
   a. Pain
   b. Fatigue
   c. Disorganized sleep–wake pattern
   d. Feeding problems
2. Reduce or eliminate contributing factors if possible.
   a. Pain:
   - Determine the baseline behavioral manifestations of the infant and document.
   - Observe for responses different from baseline that have been associated with neonatal pain responses (Grunau & Craig, 1987; Bozzette, 1993).
     ○ Facial responses (open mouth, brow bulge, grimace, chin quiver, nasolabial furrow, taut tongue)
     ○ Motor responses (flinch, muscle rigidity, clenched hands, withdrawal)
   - If unsure whether behavior indicates pain but pain is suspected, consult with physician for an analgesic trial. Evaluate the infant's response.
   - Aggressively manage obvious pain stimuli (*e.g.*, postsurgical, lack of feeding, painful procedures, hyperglycemia; Acute Pain Management Guideline Panel, 1992).
     ○ Consult with physician for an analgesic.
     ○ Provide analgesic before painful procedures.
     ○ Consider topical analgesia for frequent painful procedures (*e.g.*, heelstick, venipuncture).
   - When administering analgesics (Acute Pain Management Guideline Panel, 1992):
     ○ Reduce initial dose and monitor respiratory response cautiously.
     ○ Determine optimal dose and interval.
     ○ Monitor when pain breaks through.
     ○ Determine if infant appears comfortable after the dose.

- When indicated, wean infant slowly over a period of days from the drug. Assess response to withdrawal. Consult with physician to manage withdrawal symptoms if indicated.
  b. Fatigue/disorganized sleep–wake patterns:
    - Evaluate the need and if needed, the frequency of each intervention.
    - Organize care plan for every-4-hour interventions.
  c. Feeding problems (Flandermeyer, 1993):
    - Reduce the stress of feeding.
      ○ Initiate contact slowly.
      ○ Touch the infant's back lightly.
      ○ Swaddle infant with hands crossing midline.
      ○ When this is tolerated, pick infant up facing out toward room to eliminate visual stimulation.
      ○ Prevent auditory stimulation (*e.g.*, do not talk).
      ○ Give bottle; provide jaw support if needed.
      ○ After infant is settled, use soothing techniques, hand holding, vertical rocking.
    - Allow infant's behavioral cues to set the pace and tone of the interaction.
    - Position to facilitate feeding.
3. Provide comfort measures when infant is in a nonarousal state (Blackburn, 1993).
   a. Tactile stimulation (*e.g.*, kangaroo care, massage)
   b. Music, intrauterine sounds (Callins, 1991)
      - Play music, and evaluate response.
   c. Swaddling, rocking
4. Reduce environmental stimuli.
   a. Noise (Thomas, 1989)
      - Do not tap on incubator.
      - Place a folded blanket on top of incubator if it is the only work surface available.
      - Slowly open and close portholes.
      - Pad incubator doors to reduce banging.
      - Remove water from ventilator tubing.
      - Speak softly at the bedside and only when necessary.
      - Slowly drop the head of the mattress.

- Position the infant's bed away from sources of noise (*e.g.*, telephone, intercom, unit equipment).
- Evaluate the effectiveness of a quiet hour each shift. Collect data before and after to evaluate effects on staff, infants, and parents (Blackburn, 1993).

b. Lights
- Use full-spectrum light instead of white light at bedside.
- Cover cribs, incubators, and radiant warmers completely during sleep periods, partially during awake times.
- Shade infant's eyes with a blanket tent or cutout box.

5. Position in postures that permit flexion and minimize flailing, arching, and squirming.

6. Reduce the stress associated with handling.
   a. When moving or lifting the infant, contain the infant with your hands by wrapping or placing rolled blankets around his or her body.
   b. Maintain containment during procedures and caregiving activities.
   c. Handle slowly and gently.
   d. Initiate all interactions and treatments with one sense stimulus at a time (*e.g.*, touch), then slowly progress to visual, auditory, movement.
   e. Assess for cues for readiness, impending disorganization, or stability; respond to cues.
   f. Allow to be protected and undisturbed for 2- to 3-hour intervals.
   g. Use suctioning or postural drainage as needed instead of routinely.

7. Reduce disorganized neurobehavior during transport (transfer) (Little et al., 1994).
   a. Have a plan for transport with assigned roles for each team member.
   b. Establish behavior cues of stress for this infant with primary nurse before transport.
   c. Swaddle infant or place in a nest made of blankets.
   d. Ensure the transport equipment is ready (*e.g.*, ventilator). Warm mattress or use sheepskin.
   e. Carefully and smoothly move infant. Avoid talking if possible.

201

       f. If stress behaviors manifest, stop and allow infant to return to a stable state.

8. Enhance parent participation.

    a. Encourage parents to share their feelings, fears, and expectations. Gently correct misconceptions.

    b. Teach the behavioral cues and signs of stress in their infant.

    c. Assist the parent(s) to interact with their infant as appropriate to status and maturity.

9. Initiate health teaching and referrals as indicated.

    a. Prepare for discharge. Provide parent(s) with teaching related to (Johnson-Crowley, 1993):

- Health concerns:
  - Feeding, hygiene
  - Safety, temperature
  - Illness, infection
  - Growth and development
- State modulation
  - Appropriate stimulation
  - Sleep–wake patterns
- Parent–infant interaction
  - Behavior cues
  - Signs of stress
- Infant's environment
  - Animate, inanimate stimulation
  - Role of father and siblings
  - Playing with infant
- Parental coping and support

    b. Refer for follow-up home visits.

♋ Infant Behavior, Risk for Disorganized

DEFINITION

Risk for Disorganized Infant Behavior: The state in which the neonate is at risk for an alteration in integration and modulation of the physiological and behavioral systems of adaption (autonomic, motor, state, organizational, self-regulatory, and attentional–interactional).

RISK FACTORS

Refer to Related Factors.

RELATED FACTORS

Refer to *Disorganized Infant Behavior.*

INTERVENTIONS

Refer to *Disorganized Infant Behavior.*

✿ Infant Behavior, Potential for Enhanced Organized

DEFINITION

Potential for Enhanced Organized Infant Behavior: A pattern of modulation of the physiological and behavioral systems of functioning of an infant (*i.e.*, autonomic, motor, state, organizational, self-regulatory, and attentional–interactional) that is satisfactory but can be improved, resulting in higher levels of integration in response to environmental stimuli.

Author's Note:

This diagnosis describes an infant who is responding to the environment with stable and predictable autonomic, motoric, and state cues. The focus of interventions is to promote continued stable development and to reduce excess environmental stimuli that may stress the infant.

(Continued)

> **Author's Note (Continued):**
>   Because this is a wellness diagnosis, the use of related factors is not needed. The diagnostic statement can be written as Potential for Enhanced Organized Infant Behavior as evidenced by ability to regulate autonomic, motor, and state systems to environmental stimuli.

DEFINING CHARACTERISTICS
(Blackburn & Vandenberg, 1993)

Autonomic system
  Able to regulate color and respiration
  Reduction of tremors, twitches
  Reduction of visceral signals (*e.g.*, smooth)
  Digestive functioning, feeding tolerance
Motor system
  Smooth, well-modulated posture and tone
  Synchronous smooth movements with:
    Hand/foot clasping
    Grasping
    Hand-to-mouth activity
    Suck/suck searching
    Hand holding
    Tucking
State system
  Well-differentiated range of states
  Clear, robust sleep states
  Active self-quieting/consoling
  Focused, shiny eyed alertness with intent or animated facial expressions
  "Ooh" face
  Cooing
  Attentional smiling

RELATED FACTORS

Because this is a diagnosis of effective functioning, the use of related factors is not warranted.

OUTCOME CRITERIA

The infant will:

1.   Continue age-appropriate growth and development
2.   Not experience excessive environmental stimuli

The parent(s) will:

1. Demonstrate handling that promotes stability
2. Describe developmental needs of infant
3. Describe signs of stress or exhaustion
4. Demonstrate (Reeder et al., 1992):
   a. Gentle, soothing touch
   b. Melodic tone of voice, coos
   c. Mutual gazing
   d. Rhythmic movements
   e. Acknowledgment of all baby's vocalizations
   f. Recognition of soothing qualities of actions

✎ CHILD FOCUS INTERVENTIONS

1. Explain developmental needs of infants.
   a. Stimulation (visual, auditory, vestibular, tactile, olfactory, gustatory)
   b. Periods of alertness
   c. Sleep requirements
2. Explain the effects of excess environmental stress on the infant.
   a. Provide a list of signs of stress for their infant.
   b. Teach to terminate stimulation if infant shows signs.
   c. When providing developmental intervention(s):
      • Offer only when infant is alert.
      • If possible, show parents examples of their infant when alert and not alert.
      • Begin with one stimulus at a time (touch, voice).
      • Provide intervention for a short time.
      • Increase interventions according to infant's cues.
      • Provide frequent, short-duration interventions instead of infrequent, long-term ones.
3. Explain role model, and observe parent engaging in developmental interventions.
   a. Visual (Reeder et al., 1992):
      • Eye-to-eye contact
      • Face-to-face experiences
      • Provide with high-contrast colors, geometric shapes (*e.g.*, black-and-white shapes on paper mobile)

      b. Auditory:
- Use high-pitched vocalization.
- Play classical music softly.
- Avoid loud talking.
- Call infant by name.
- Avoid monotone speech patterns.

      c. Tactile:
- Use firm, gentle touch as initial approach.
- Use skin-to-skin contact in a warm room.
- For a massage, stroke skin very slowly and gently in head-to-toe direction. Begin at trunk.
- Provide alternative textures (*e.g.*, sheep-skin, velvet, satin).

      d. Vestibular (movement):
- Rock in chair; provide head support.
- Place in sling and rock.
- Slowly change position during handling.

      e. Olfactory:
- Wear a light perfume.

      f. Gustatory:
- Allow non-nutritive sucking (*e.g.*, pacifier, hand in mouth).

4. Promote adjustment and stability to caregiving activities (Blackburn & Vandenberg, 1993).

      a. Waking
- Enter room slowly.
- Turn on light; open curtains slowly.
- Avoid waking if asleep.

      b. Changing
- Keep room warm.
- Gently change position; contain limbs during movement.
- Stop changing if infant is irritable.

      c. Feeding
- Time feedings with alert states.
- Hold infant close, and if needed, swaddle in blanket.

      d. Bathing
- Ventral openness may be stressful.
- Cover body parts not being bathed.
- Proceed slowly; allow for rest.
- Offer a pacifier or hand to suck.
- Eliminate unnecessary noise.
- Use soft, soothing voice.

5. Explain the need to reduce environmental stimuli when taking infant outside home.
   a. Shelter eyes from light.
   b. Swaddle infant so hands can reach mouth.
   c. Protect from loud noises.
6. Praise parent(s) on their interaction patterns. Point out infant's engaging responses.
7. Initiate health teaching and referrals if needed.
   a. Explain that developmental interventions will change as child develops. Refer to *Altered Growth and Development* for specific age-related developmental needs.
   b. Provide parent(s) with resources for assistance at home (*e.g.*, community resources).

Infection, Risk for

Infection Transmission, Risk for

Infection, Risk for

DEFINITION

Risk for Infection: The state in which an individual is at risk to be invaded by an opportunistic or pathogenic agent (virus, fungus, bacterium, protozoan, or other parasite) from endogenous or exogenous sources.

Author's Note:
Risk for Infection describes a situation when host defenses are compromised, making the host more susceptible to environmental pathogens. Nursing interventions focus on minimizing introduction of organisms or increasing resistance to infection (*e.g.*, improving nutritional status).

RISK FACTORS

Presence of risk factors (see Related Factors)

RELATED FACTORS

A variety of health problems and situations can create favorable conditions that would encourage the development of infections. Some common factors are listed below.

Pathophysiological

Related to compromised host defenses secondary to:
Chronic diseases

Cancer	Arthritis
Renal failure	AIDS
Hematological disorders	Hepatic disorders
Diabetes mellitus	Respiratory disorders
Collagen diseases	
Heritable disorders	
Alcoholism	
Immunosuppression	
Immunodeficiency	
Altered or insufficient leukocytes	
Blood dyscrasias	
Altered integumentary system	
Periodontal disease	

Related to compromised circulation secondary to:
Lymphedema
Obesity
Peripheral vascular disease

Treatment-Related

Related to a site for organism invasion secondary to:

Surgery	Presence of invasive lines
Dialysis	Intubation
Total parenteral nutrition	Enteral feedings

Related to compromised host defenses secondary to:
Radiation therapy
Organ transplant
Medication therapy (specify, *e.g.*, chemotherapy, immunosuppressants)

Situational (Personal, Environmental)

Related to compromised host defenses secondary to:

Prolonged immobility	Stress
Increased length of	Smoking
hospital stay	History of infections
Malnutrition	

Related to a site for organism invasion secondary to:

Trauma (accidental, intentional)

Postpartum period

Bites (animal, insect, human)

Thermal injuries

Warm, moist, dark environment (skin folds, casts)

Related to contact with contagious agents (nosocomial or community acquired)

Maturational

(Newborn)

Related to increased vulnerability of infant secondary to:

Lack of maternal antibodies (dependent on maternal exposure)

Lack of normal flora

Open wounds (umbilical, circumcision)

Immature immune system

(Infant/child)

Related to increased vulnerability secondary to lack of immunization

(Older adults)

Related to increased vulnerability of elder secondary to: debilitated condition, decreased immune response, or multiple chronic diseases

OUTCOME CRITERIA

The person will:

1. Demonstrate meticulous handwashing technique by the time of discharge
2. Be free from nosocomial infectious processes during hospitalization
3. Demonstrate knowledge of risk factors associated with infection and practice appropriate precautions to prevent infection

🔋 GENERIC INTERVENTIONS

1. Identify individuals at risk for nosocomial infections.
   a. Assess for predictors.
      - Infection (preoperatively)
      - Abdominal or thoracic surgery
      - Surgery longer than 2 hours
      - Genitourinary procedure
      - Instrumentation (ventilator, suction, catheters, nebulizers, tracheostomy, invasive monitoring)
      - Anesthesia
   b. Assess for confounding factors.
      - Age younger than 1 year or older than 65 years
      - Obesity
      - Underlying disease conditions (chronic obstructive pulmonary disease, diabetes, cardiovascular blood dyscrasias)
      - Substance abuse
      - Medications (steroids, chemotherapy, antibiotic therapy)
      - Nutritional status (intake less than minimum daily requirements)
      - Smoker
2. Reduce the entry of organisms into individuals.
   a. Meticulous handwashing
   b. Aseptic technique
   c. Isolation measures
   d. No unnecessary diagnostic or therapeutic procedures
   e. Reduction of airborne microorganisms
3. Protect the immune-deficient individual from infection.
   a. Instruct individual to ask all visitors and personnel to wash their hands before approaching individual.
   b. Limit visitors when appropriate.
   c. Restrict invasive devices (intravenous line, laboratory specimens) to those that are absolutely necessary.
   d. Teach individual and family members signs and symptoms of infection.
4. Reduce individual's susceptibility to infection.
   a. Encourage and maintain caloric and protein intake in diet (see *Altered Nutrition*).

    b. Monitor use or overuse of antimicrobial therapy.
    c. Administer prescribed antimicrobial therapy within 15 minutes of scheduled time.
    d. Minimize length of stay in hospital.
5. Observe for clinical manifestations of infection (*e.g.*, fever, cloudy urine, purulent drainage).
6. Instruct individual and family regarding the causes, risks, and communicability of the infection.
7. Report communicable diseases as appropriate to public health department.

🏵 CHILD FOCUS INTERVENTIONS

1. Monitor for signs of infection (*e.g.*, lethargy, feeding difficulties, vomiting, temperature instability, and subtle color changes).
2. Provide umbilical cord care. Teach cord care and signs of infection (*e.g.*, increased redness, purulent drainage).
3. Teach the signs of infection of circumcised area (*e.g.*, bleeding, increased redness, or unusual swelling).

🈯 MATERNAL FOCUS INTERVENTIONS

1. Explain the increased vulnerability to infection during pregnancy.
2. Teach how to prevent urinary tract infections during pregnancy.
    a. Drink at least eight 8-oz glasses of water.
    b. Void frequently.
    c. Void before and after intercourse (Reeder et al, 1997).
3. Teach how to prevent infection postpartum:
    a. Wipe from front to back.
    b. Clean perineal area after voiding or defecating (*e.g.*, sitz bath, squirt bottle).
    c. Change perineal pads after each voiding.
    d. Teach proper breast care.
4. Identify risk factors for postpartum infections:
    a. Anemia
    b. Poor nutrition
    c. Lack of prenatal care
    d. Obesity
    e. Intercourse after membrane rupture
    f. Immunosuppression
    g. Prolonged labor

    h. Prolonged membrane rupture
    i. Intrauterine fetal monitoring (in high-risk mothers)
    j. Hemorrhage
5. Instruct on signs and symptoms of infection (*e.g.*, fever, purulent drainage), and report promptly.

OLDER ADULT FOCUS INTERVENTIONS

1. Explain that the usual signs of infection may not be present (*e.g.*, fever, chills).
2. Assess for anorexia, weakness, change in mental status, or hypothermia.
3. Monitor skin and urinary system for signs of fungal, viral, or mycobacterial pathogens.

Infection Transmission,*
Risk for

DEFINITION

Risk for Infection Transmission: The state in which an individual is at risk for transferring an opportunistic or pathogenic agent to others.

RISK FACTORS

Presence of risk factors (see Related Factors)

RELATED FACTORS

Pathophysiological

Related to:
    Colonization with highly antibiotic-resistant organism
    Airborne transmission exposure
    Contact transmission exposure (direct, indirect, contact droplet)

*This diagnosis is not currently on the NANDA list but has been included for clarity or usefulness.

Treatment-Related

Related to contaminated wound
Related to devices with contaminated drainage (urinary and
chest tubes, suction equipment, endotracheal tubes)

Situational (Personal, Environmental)

Related to:
Disaster with hazardous infectious material
Unsanitary living conditions (sewage, personal hygiene)
Areas considered high risk for vector-borne diseases
(malaria, rabies, bubonic plague, natural disasters)
Areas considered high risk for vehicle-borne diseases
(hepatitis A, shigella, *Salmonella*)
Lack of knowledge of sources or prevention of infection
Intravenous drug use
Multiple sexual partners
Unprotected sexual intercourse
Natural disaster (*e.g.*, flood, hurricane)

Maturational

Newborn
Related to birth outside a hospital setting in an uncontrolled
environment
Related to exposure during prenatal or perinatal period to
communicable disease via mother

OUTCOME CRITERIA

The person will:

1. Relate the need to be isolated until noninfectious
2. Describe the mode of transmission of disease
3. Demonstrate meticulous handwashing during hospitalization

GENERIC INTERVENTIONS

1. Identify susceptible host individuals based on focus assessment for risk factors and history of exposure.
2. Identify the mode of transmission based on infecting agent.
   a. Airborne

      b. Contact
- Direct
- Indirect
- Contact droplet

      c. Vehicle-borne (*e.g.*, food, water, blood, body fluids)

      d. Vector-borne (insects, animals)

3. Initiate appropriate isolation precautions. Consult with infection control practitioner.
4. Secure appropriate room assignment, depending on the type of infection and hygienic practices of the infected person.
5. Adhere to the Universal Infection Precautions.
6. Refer to infection control practitioner for follow-up with the health department concerning family exposure and cause of exposure and assist in appropriate isolation of the client.
7. Teach client regarding the chain of infection and patient responsibility in the hospital and at home.

Injury, Risk for

Aspiration, Risk for

Poisoning, Risk for

Suffocation, Risk for

Trauma, Risk for

Injury, Risk for

DEFINITION

Risk for Injury: The state in which an individual is at risk for harm because of a perceptual or physiological deficit, a lack of awareness of hazards, or maturational age.

Author's Note:
This diagnosis has four subcategories: Risk for Aspiration, Poisoning, Suffocation, and Trauma. Should the nurse choose to isolate interventions only for prevention of poisoning, then the diagnosis Risk for Poisoning would be useful.

RISK FACTORS

Presence of risk factors (see Related Factors for specific factors)

RELATED FACTORS

Pathophysiological

Related to altered cerebral function secondary to, for example, tissue hypoxia, vertigo, syncope
Related to altered mobility secondary to:

Unsteady gait	Cerebrovascular accident
Amputation	Parkinsonism
Arthritis	Loss of limb

Related to impaired sensory function (*e.g.*, vision, hearing, thermal/touch, smell)
Related to fatigue
Related to orthostatic hypotension
Related to vertebrobasilar insufficiency
Related to vestibular disorders
Related to carotid sinus syncope
Related to lack of awareness of environmental hazards secondary to, for example, confusion, hypoglycemia, depression, electrolyte imbalance
Related to tonic-clonic movements secondary to seizures
Related to carotid sinus syncope

Treatment-Related

Related to effects of (specify) on mobility or sensorium:

Medications

Sedatives	Diuretics
Vasodilators	Phenothiazines

Antihypertensives   Psychotropics
Hypoglycemics
Related to casts/crutches, canes, walkers

Situational (Personal, Environmental)

Related to decrease in or loss of short-term memory
Related to faulty judgment secondary to, for example, dehydration (*e.g.,* summer), stress, alcohol
Related to prolonged bed rest
Related to vasovagal reflex
Related to household hazards (specify)

Unsafe walkways   Stairs
Unsafe toys   Slippery floors
Inadequate lighting   Faulty electric wires
Bathrooms (tubs, low   Improperly stored poisons
toilets)

Related to automotive hazards
Related to fire hazards
Related to unfamiliar setting (hospital, nursing home)
Related to improper footwear
Related to inattentive caretaker
Related to improper use of aids (crutches, canes, walkers, wheelchairs)
Related to history of accidents

Maturational

Infant/child
Related to lack of awareness of hazards
Older adult
Related to faulty judgment secondary to:
Sensory deficits
Medication (accidental overdose)
Cognitive deficits

OUTCOME CRITERIA

The person will:

1. Identify factors that increase the risk for injury
2. Relate an intent to use safety measures to prevent injury (*e.g.,* remove throw rugs or anchor them)
3. Relate an intent to practice selected prevention measures (*e.g.,* wear sunglasses to reduce glare)

⊞ GENERIC INTERVENTIONS

1. Orient each new admission to surroundings, explain the call system, and assess the person's ability to use it.
2. Closely supervise the person during the first few nights to assess safety.
3. Use night light.
4. Encourage the person to request assistance during the night.
5. Keep bed at lowest level during the night.
6. Teach proper use of crutches, canes, walkers, prosthesis.
7. Instruct person to wear shoes that fit properly and have nonskid soles.
8. Assess for the presence of side effects of drugs that may cause vertigo.
9. Teach person to:
   a. Eliminate throw rugs, litter, and highly polished floors
   b. Provide nonslip surfaces in bathtub or shower by applying commercially available traction tapes
   c. Provide hand grips in bathroom
   d. Provide railings in hallways and on stairs
   e. Remove protruding objects (*e.g.*, coat hooks, shelves, light fixtures) from stairway walls
10. Institute safety precautions for confused persons (Evans, 1992).
    a. Observe frequently.
    b. Ask roommate, if capable, to alert nurses of a problem.
    c. Use low bed, with side rails up.
    d. Use mattress on floor.
    e. Place bedside table or commode chair in front of patient when sitting in a chair.
    f. Consider an alarm system.
    g. Place person in room near traffic (*e.g.*, nurses' station).
    h. Provide a distraction: music, companion, simple craft, pet therapy.

⊛ CHILD FOCUS INTERVENTIONS

1. Teach parents to expect frequent changes in infants' and children's ability and to take precautions (*e.g.*, infant who

suddenly rolls over for the first time might be on a changing table unattended).

2. Discuss with parents the necessity of constant monitoring of small children.

3. Provide parents with information to assist them in selecting a babysitter.
   a. Determine previous experiences and knowledge of emergency measures.
   b. Observe the interaction of the sitter with the child.

4. Teach parents to expect children to mimic them and to teach children what they can do with or without supervision (seat belts, helmets, safe driving).

5. Explain and expect compliance with certain rules (depending on age) concerning
   a. Streets
   b. Playground equipment
   c. Water (pools, bathtubs)
   d. Bicycles
   e. Fire
   f. Animals
   g. Strangers

6. Instruct how to "child-proof" the home.

7. Explain why children should not ride in front (air bags).

8. Refer to local fire department for assistance in staging home fire drills.

9. Encourage parents to learn basic life-saving skills (CPR, Heimlich maneuver).

10. Teach children how to dial 911.

11. Teach parents to assist their children in handling peer pressure that involves risk-taking behavior.

OLDER ADULT FOCUS INTERVENTIONS

1. Assess for orthostatic hypotension. Compare brachial blood pressure (supine, standing).

2. Discuss physiology of orthostatic hypotension with client.

3. Teach techniques to reduce orthostatic hypotension.
   a. Change positions slowly.
   b. Move from lying to an upright position in stages.
   c. During day, rest in a recliner rather than in bed.
   d. Avoid prolonged standing.

4. Teach to avoid dehydration and vasodilation (*e.g.*, hot tubs)

Aspiration, Risk for

DEFINITION

Risk for Aspiration: The state in which a person is at risk for entry of secretions, solids, or fluids into the tracheobronchial passages.

RISK FACTORS

Presence of favorable conditions for aspiration (see Related Factors)

RELATED FACTORS

Pathophysiological

Related to reduced level of consciousness secondary to:

Anesthesia	Coma
Head injury	Presenile dementia
Cerebrovascular accident (CVA)	Seizures

Related to depressed cough and gag reflexes
Related to increased intragastric pressure secondary to:

Lithotomy position	Obesity
Enlarged uterus	Ascites

Related to delayed gastric emptying secondary to:

Intestinal obstruction	Gastric outlet syndrome
Ileus	

Related to impaired swallowing or decreased laryngeal and glottic reflexes secondary to:

Achalasia	Catatonia
Scleroderma	Myasthenia gravis
Esophageal strictures	Guillain-Barré syndrome
CVA	Multiple sclerosis
Parkinson's disease	Muscular dystrophy
Debilitating conditions	

Related to tracheoesophageal fistula
Related to impaired protective reflexes secondary to:
facial/oral/neck surgery or trauma
Paraplegia or hemiplegia

Treatment-Related

Related to depressed laryngeal and glottic reflexes secondary to:

Presence of tracheostomy/endotracheal tube
Sedation
Tube feedings

Related to impaired ability to cough secondary to:

Wired jaw
Imposed prone position

Situational (Personal, Environmental)

Related to inability/impaired ability to elevate upper body
Related to eating when intoxicated

Maturational

Premature
Related to impaired sucking/swallowing reflexes
Neonate
Related to decreased muscle tone of inferior esophageal sphincter
Older adult
Related to poor dentition

OUTCOME CRITERIA

The person will:

1. Not experience aspiration
2. Relate measures to prevent aspiration

⊞ GENERIC INTERVENTIONS

1. Reduce the risk of aspiration in:
   a. Individuals with decreased strength, decreased sensorium, or autonomic disorders
      • Maintain a side-lying position if not contraindicated by injury.
      • Assess for position of the tongue, ensuring that it has not dropped backward, occluding the airway.
      • Keep the head of the bed elevated if not contraindicated.

- Clear secretions from mouth and throat with a tissue or gentle suction.
- Reassess frequently for presence of obstructive material in mouth and throat.

b. For persons with tracheostomies or endotracheal tubes
- Inflate cuff (during continuous mechanical ventilation, during and after eating, during and 1 hour after tube feeding, during intermittent positive-pressure breathing treatments).
- Suction every 1 to 2 hours and as needed.

c. For persons with gastrointestinal tubes and feedings
- Verify that feeding tube has not moved upward since insertion.
- Aspirate for residual contents before each feeding for tubes positioned gastrically.
- Elevate head of bed for 30 to 45 minutes during feeding period and 1 hour after to prevent reflux by use of reverse gravity.
- Administer feeding if residual contents are less than 150 mL (intermittent), or
- Administer feeding if residual is not greater than 150 mL at 10% to 20% of hourly rate (continuous).
- Regulate gastric feedings using an intermittent schedule, allowing periods of stomach emptying between feeding intervals.

d. Assure emergency management of obstructions is known.

🌀 CHILD FOCUS INTERVENTIONS

1. Position infant in side-lying position or supine, not prone.
2. Teach parents:
   a. Not to prop bottle
   b. To keep small objects out of reach (*e.g.*, coins)
   c. To remove all plastic bags
   d. To inspect toys for removable parts or long strings
3. Teach what foods to avoid for young children (*e.g.*, fruits with pits, nuts, gum, whole grapes, hot dogs, popcorn kernels).

4. Teach emergency management of airway obstruction.
   a. Back blows and chest thrusts (infants)
   b. Heimlich maneuver (children)

Poisoning, Risk for

DEFINITION

Risk for Poisoning: The state in which an individual is at risk of accidental exposure to or ingestion of drugs or dangerous substances.

RISK FACTORS

Presence of risk factors (see Related Factors under Risk for Injury)

Suffocation, Risk for

DEFINITION

Risk for Suffocation: The state in which an individual is at risk for smothering and asphyxiation.

RISK FACTORS

Presence of risk factors (see Related Factors under Risk for Injury)

Trauma, Risk for

DEFINITION

Risk for Trauma: The state in which an individual is at risk of accidental tissue injury (*e.g.*, wound, burns, fracture).

RISK FACTORS

Presence of risk factors (see Related Factors under Risk for Injury)

Injury, Risk for Perioperative Positioning

DEFINITION

Risk for Perioperative Positioning Injury: The state in which an individual is at risk for harm as a result of positioning requirements for surgery and loss of usual protective responses secondary to anesthesia.

Author's Note:

This diagnosis focuses on identifying the vulnerability for tissue, nerve, and joint injury resulting from required positions for surgery. The addition of the term "perioperative positioning" to the Risk for Injury diagnosis adds etiology to the label.

If a client has no preexisting risk factors that make him or her more vulnerable to injury, this diagnosis could be used with no related factors because they are evident. If related factors are desired, the statement could read, for example, Risk for Perioperative Positioning Injury related to position requirements for surgery and loss of usual sensory protective measures secondary to anesthesia. When a client has preexisting risk factors, the statement should include them, for example, Risk for Perioperative Positioning Injuries related to compromised tissue perfusion secondary to peripheral arterial disease.

RISK FACTORS

Presence of risk factors (see Related Factors)

RELATED FACTORS

Pathophysiological

Related to increased vulnerability secondary to:

Chronic disease	Radiation therapy
Renal, hepatic dysfunction	Cancer
Osteoporosis	Infection
Compromised immune system	Thin body frame

Related to compromised tissue perfusion secondary to:

Diabetes mellitus	Cardiovascular disease

Peripheral vascular disease	Anemia
Hypothermia	History of thrombosis
Ascites	Dehydration
Edema	

Related to vulnerability of stoma during positioning
Related to preexisting contractures or physical impairments
  secondary to: for example, rheumatoid arthritis, polio

Treatment-Related

*Related to position requirements and loss of usual sensory
  protective responses secondary to anesthesia
Related to surgical procedures of 2 hours or longer
Related to vulnerability of implants or prostheses (*e.g.*, pace-
  makers) during positioning

Situational (Personal, Environmental)

Related to compromised circulation secondary to:

Obesity	Pregnancy
Tobacco use	

Maturational

Related to increased vulnerability to tissue injury secondary to
decreased circulatory volume (infant, elder).

OUTCOME CRITERIA

The person will:

1. Have no evidence of neuromuscular damage or injury re-
    lated to the surgical position

🔁 GENERIC INTERVENTIONS

1. Determine if client has preexisting risk factors (refer to
    Risk Factors). Communicate findings to the surgical
    team.
2. Prior to positioning, assess and document the following:
    a. Range-of-motion ability

---

*This risk factor is always present and may be deleted from the diag-
nostic statement.

     b. Physical abnormalities
     c. External/internal prostheses or implants
     d. Neurovascular status
     e. Circulatory status

3. Move the person from the stretcher to the operating room bed according to protocol. Lift; do not pull or drag. Do not leave unattended.

4. Discuss the surgical position desired with the surgeon. Advise if any preexisting factors exist. Determine if the position will be arranged before or after anesthesia.

5. Always ask the anesthesiologist's or nurse anesthetist's permission before moving or repositioning an anesthetized person.

6. Reduce vulnerability to tissue injury.
     a. Align neck and spine at all times.
     b. Gently manipulate joints. Do not abduct more than 90 degrees.
     c. Do not let limbs extend off the operating room bed. Reposition slowly and gently.
     d. Use a draw sheet above the elbows to tuck in arms at side or abduct arm on an arm board with padding.

7. Protect eyes and ears from pressure. Ensure that ears are not bent. Use eye shields if needed.

8. Depending on the surgical position, pad areas vulnerable to injury. Refer to unit protocols.

9. If feasible, ask client if he or she feels pain, burning, pressure, or any discomforts after positioning.

10. Continually assess that team members are not leaning on the client, especially on the limbs.

11. Ensure that the head is lifted slightly every 30 minutes.

12. When repositioning or returning the person to a supine position after certain surgical positions (*e.g.*, Trendelenburg, lithotomy, reverse Trendelenburg, jack-knife, lateral), slowly change position to prevent severe hypotension.

13. Assess client's skin condition when surgery is completed, and document findings. Inform postanesthesia nurses whether preexisting risk factors are present that increase vulnerability postoperatively.

Knowledge Deficit

DEFINITION

Knowledge Deficit: The state in which an individual or group experiences a deficiency in cognitive knowledge or psychomotor skills concerning the condition or treatment plan.

Author's Note:

Knowledge Deficit does not represent a human response, alteration, or pattern of dysfunction; rather, it is an etiological or contributing factor (Jenny, 1987). Lack of knowledge can contribute to a variety of responses (*e.g.*, anxiety, self-care deficits). All nursing diagnoses have related client/family teaching as a part of nursing interventions (*e.g.*, Altered Bowel Elimination, Impaired Verbal Communication). When the teaching directly relates to a specific nursing diagnosis, incorporate the teaching into the plan. When specific teaching is indicated prior to a procedure, the diagnosis Anxiety related to unfamiliar environment or procedure can be used. When information is given to assist a person or family with self-care at home, the diagnosis Ineffective Management of Therapeutic Regimen may be indicated.

DEFINING CHARACTERISTICS

Major (Must Be Present, One or More)

Verbalizes a deficiency in knowledge or skill or requests information
Expresses an inaccurate perception of health status
Does not correctly perform a desired or prescribed health behavior

Minor (May Be Present)

Lack of integration of treatment plan into daily activities
Exhibits or expresses psychological alteration (*e.g.*, anxiety, depression) resulting from misinformation or lack of information

Latex Allergy

Latex Allergy, Risk for

Latex Allergy

DEFINITION

Latex Allergy: The state in which an individual experiences an immunoglobin E (lgE)–mediated allergic response to latex.

DEFINING CHARACTERISTICS

Major

Positive skin test to NRL extract

Minor

Allergic conjunctivitis	Rhinitis
Urticaria	Asthma

RELATED FACTORS
Biopathophysiological

Related to hypersensitivity
Response to the protein component of natural rubber latex

OUTCOME CRITERIA

The person will:

1. Describe products of natural rubber latex
2. Describe strategies to avoid exposure

◆ GENERIC INTERVENTIONS

1. Explain the importance of completely avoiding direct contact with all NRL products.
2. Advise that a person with a history of a mild skin reaction to latex is at risk for anaphylaxis.

3. Instruct patient to wear a medical alert bracelet stating "Latex Allergy" and to carry auto-injectable epinephrine.
4. Instruct to warn all health care providers (*e.g.*, dental, medical, surgical) of the allergy.
5. Use non-latex alternative supplies:
   a. Clear disposable amber bags
   b. Silicone baby nipples
   c. 2 × 2 gauze pads with silk tape in place of adhesive bandages
   d. Clear plastic or Silastic catheters
   e. Vinyl or neoprene gloves
   f. Use silk or plastic tape, not plastic or adhesive
6. Protect from exposure to latex:
   a. Cover skin with cloth before applying BP cuff.
   b. Do not allow rubber stethoscope tubing to touch person.
   c. Do not inject through rubber parts (*e.g.*, heparin locks); use syringe and stopcock.
   d. Change needles after each puncture of rubber stopper.
   e. Cover rubber parts with tape.
7. Teach what products are commonly made of latex:
   a. Healthcare equipment:
      - Natural latex rubber gloves, powdered or unpowdered, including those labeled "hypoallergenic"
      - Blood pressure cuffs
      - Stethoscopes
      - Tourniquets
      - Electrode pads
      - Airways, endotracheal tubes
      - Syringe plunges, bulb syringes
      - Masks for anesthesia
      - Rubber aprons
      - Catheters, wound drains
      - Injection ports
      - Tops of multidose vials
      - Adhesive tape
      - Ostomy pouches
      - Wheelchair cushions
      - Briefs with elastic
      - Pads for crutches
   b. Office/household products:
      - Erasers
      - Rubber bands

- Dishwashing gloves
- Balloons
- Condoms, diaphragms
- Baby bottle nipples, pacifiers
- Rubber balls and toys
- Racquet handles and cycle grips
- Tires
- Hot water bottles
- Carpeting
- Shoe soles
- Elastic in underwear
- Rubber cement

Latex Allergy, Risk for

DEFINITION

Risk for Latex Allergy: The state in which an individual is at risk for experiencing an immunoglobin E (lgE)–mediated allergic response to latex.

RISK FACTORS
Biopathophysiological

Related to history of atopic eczema
Related to history of allergic rhinitis
Related to history of asthma

Treatment-Related

Related to frequent urinary catheterizations
Related to frequent rectal disimpaction removal
Related to frequent surgical procedures

Situational (Personal, Environmental)

Related to history of food allergy to banana, kiwi, avocado, tomato, raw potato, peach, chestnuts, mango, papaya, passion fruit
Food handler
History of allergy to gloves, condoms, etc.
Frequent occupational exposure to natural rubber latex, such as:
    Health care workers
    Housekeepers

Food handlers
Greenhouse workers
Workers making NRL products

Loneliness, Risk for

DEFINITION

Risk for Loneliness: The state in which an individual is at risk for experiencing discomfort associated with a desire or need for contact with others.

Author's Note:

Risk for Loneliness was added to the NANDA list in 1994. Presently Social Isolation is also on the NANDA list. Social Isolation is a conceptually incorrect diagnosis because it does not represent a response but instead is the cause. Loneliness and Risk for Loneliness better describe the negative state of aloneness.

Loneliness is a subjective state that exists whenever a person says it does and is perceived as imposed by others. Loneliness is *not* the result of voluntary solitude that is necessary for personal renewal, nor is it the creative aloneness of the artist or the initial aloneness one may experience as a result of seeking individualism and independence (*e.g.*, moving to a new city, going away to college).

RISK FACTORS

See Related Factors.

RELATED FACTORS

Pathophysiological
    Related to fear of rejection secondary to:
        Obesity
        Cancer (disfiguring surgery of head or neck, superstitions of others)
        Physical handicaps (paraplegia, amputation, arthritis, hemiplegia)
        Emotional handicaps (extreme anxiety, depression, paranoia, phobias)

Incontinence (embarrassment, odor)
Communicable diseases (AIDS, hepatitis)
Psychiatric illness (schizophrenia, bipolar affective disor-
der, personality disorders)
Related to difficulty accessing social events secondary to:
Debilitating diseases
Physical disabilities

Treatment-Related

Related to therapeutic isolation

Situational (Personal, Environmental)

Related to insufficient planning for retirement
Related to death of a significant other
Related to divorce
Related to disfiguring appearance
Related to fear of rejection secondary to: for example,
obesity, extreme poverty, hospitalization or terminal illness
(dying process), or unemployment
Related to moving to another culture (*e.g.*, unfamiliar lan-
guage)
Related to history of unsatisfying social experiences sec-
ondary to: drug abuse, alcohol abuse, immature behavior,
unacceptable social behavior or delusional thinking
Related to loss of usual means of transportation
Related to change in usual residence secondary to long-term
care or relocation

Maturational

Child
Related to protective isolation or a communicable disease
Older adult
Related to loss of usual social contacts secondary to retire-
ment, relocation, death of (specify), or loss of driving
ability

OUTCOME CRITERIA

The person will:

1. Identify the reasons for feelings of isolation
2. Discuss ways of increasing meaningful relationships
3. Identify appropriate diversional activities

⚡ GENERIC INTERVENTIONS

The nursing interventions for a variety of contributing factors that might be associated with a diagnosis of *Risk for Loneliness* are very similar.

1. Identify causative and contributing factors.
2. Reduce or eliminate causative and contributing factors.
   a. Promote social interaction.
      - Support the individual who has experienced a loss as he or she works through grief (see *Grieving*).
      - Validate the normalcy of grieving.
      - Encourage person to talk about feelings of loneliness and the reasons they exist.
      - Mobilize person's support system of neighbors and friends.
      - Discuss the importance of quality socialization rather than a great number of interactions.
      - Refer to social skills teaching (see *Social Interaction, Impaired*).
      - Offer feedback on how the person presents himself or herself to others (see *Social Interactions, Impaired*).
   b. Decrease barriers to social contact.
      - Determine available transportation in the community (public, church-related, volunteer).
      - Determine if person must be taught how to use alternate transportation (*e.g.*, drive a car).
      - Identify activities that help keep people busy, especially during times of high risk of loneliness (see *Diversional Activity Deficit*).
      - Assist with the development of alternate means of communication for persons with compromised sensory ability (*e.g.*, amplifier on phone; see *Impaired Communication*).
      - Assist with the management of esthetic problems (*e.g.*, consult enterostomal therapist if odor is a problem).
      - Assist person in locating stores that sell clothing especially made for those who have had disfiguring surgery (*e.g.*, mastectomy).
      - Refer to *Altered Patterns of Urinary Elimination* for specific interventions to control incontinence.

c. For individuals with poor or offensive social skills:
- Engage in one-to-one social dialogue. Explain the difference between casual and meaningful conversation.
- Discuss the characteristics of meaningful conversation (Durham, 1983):
  - Initiating interactions
  - Being spontaneous
  - Being alert
  - Showing interest
  - Giving and receiving compliments
  - Showing interest in others, in activities
  - Requesting help when needed
  - Using increased eye contact
  - Using appropriate speech tone and nonverbal behavior
- Allow person opportunities to observe others engaged in meaningful conversation.
- Observe the person socializing, and discuss the interactions after. Offer praise. Gently discuss alternative approaches. Role play skills.

3. Initiate referrals as indicated.
   a. Community-based groups that contact the socially isolated
   b. Self-help groups for clients isolated due to specific medical problems (Reach to Recovery, United Ostomy Association)
   c. Wheelchair groups
   d. Psychiatric consumer rights associations

🏛 OLDER ADULT FOCUS INTERVENTIONS

1. Discuss the anticipatory effects of retirement on person's life. Assist with preplanning (Stanley & Beare, 1994).
   a. Plan to ensure adequate income.
   b. Decrease time at work the last 2 to 3 years (*e.g.*, shorter days, longer vacations).
   c. Cultivate friends outside of work.
   d. Develop routines at home to replace work structure.
   e. Rely on others rather than spouse for leisure activities.
   f. Cultivate leisure activities that are realistic (energy, cost).
   g. Prepare self for ambivalent feelings and short-term negative impact on self-esteem.

2. Identify strategies to expand the world of the isolated.
   a. Senior centers and church groups
   b. Foster grandparent program
   c. Day care centers for the elderly
   d. Retirement communities
   e. House sharing, group homes
   f. College classes opened to older persons
   g. Pets
   h. Telephone contact
   i. Psychiatric day hospital or activity program
3. Identify community sources for socialization.
4. Refer to transportation services if needed.

Management of Therapeutic Regimen, Effective: Individual

DEFINITION

Effective Management of Therapeutic Regimen: Individual: A pattern in which the individual integrates into daily living a program for treatment of illness and its sequelae that is satisfactory for meeting health goals.

Author's Note:

Effective Management of Therapeutic Regimen describes an individual who is successfully managing an illness or condition. The concept of enhanced is appropriate. The nurse can assist the person to enhance his or her management. The focus would be one of anticipatory guidance (*e.g.*, teaching the person what events could negatively impact his or her management and how to reduce the negative impact).

This diagnosis does not need related factors. Writing related factors would only repeat the characteristics of persons who manage their conditions well (*e.g.*, motivated, knowledgeable).

234

DEFINING CHARACTERISTICS

Appropriate choices of daily activities for meeting the goals of a treatment or prevention program

Illness symptoms within a normal range of expectation

Verbalization of desire to manage the treatment of illness and prevention of sequelae

Verbalization of intent to reduce risk factors for progression or illness and sequelae

RELATED FACTORS

Refer to Author's Note for an explanation.

OUTCOME CRITERIA

The person will:

1. Describe strategies to address progression or complications of his or her condition if they arise
2. Discuss situations that can challenge his or her continued successful management

◆ GENERIC INTERVENTIONS

1. Discuss possible changes in person's condition that may impact the usual management:
   a. Exacerbation
   b. Complications
   c. Side effects of medication
2. Advise early contact with care provider to discuss possible changes in management regimen.
3. Discuss how increased levels of stress can negatively impact previous successful management and possibly decrease resistance to colds or influenza.
4. Explore with the person his or her evaluation of the level of stress with which he or she usually lives:
   a. Usual level of stress
   b. Signs of overload
5. Discuss that stress comes with favorable and unfavorable life events (*e.g.*, marriage, divorce, birth, death, vacations, work).
6. When faced with upcoming additional stresses, plan to:
   a. Reduce stress in other aspects of one's life, if possible

    b. Increase adherence to healthy habits
- Sleep 7 to 8 hours.
- Eat breakfast.
- Exercise daily (at least a 30-minute brisk walk).
- Eliminate or minimize alcohol intake.
- Increase intake of complex carbohydrates/fiber.
- Decrease intake of fat.
- Decrease caffeine intake.

    c. Increase spiritually related activities.
- Meditation
- Listening to relaxing music
- Nature walking (*e.g.*, woods, near water, mountains)
- Reading poetry

7.   Initiate health teaching and referrals regarding stress-reduction techniques.

Management of Therapeutic Regimen, Ineffective

Management of Therapeutic Regimen, Ineffective: Families

Management of Therapeutic Regimen, Ineffective: Community

Management of Therapeutic Regimen, Ineffective

DEFINITION

Ineffective Management of Therapeutic Regimen: A pattern in which the individual experiences or is at risk to experience difficulty integrating into daily living a program for treatment of illness and the sequelae of illness and reduction of risk situations (*e.g.*, unsafe, pollution).

Author's Note:

Ineffective Management of Therapeutic Regimen is a useful diagnosis for nurses in most settings. Individuals and families experiencing a variety of health problems, acute or chronic, are usually faced with treatment programs that require changes in previous functioning or lifestyle. These regimens are activities or habits of medication therapy, treatments, diet, exercise, stress management, problem solving, symptom management, and other strategies that improve health and well-being.

This diagnosis describes individuals or families who are experiencing difficulty in achieving positive outcomes. The nurse is the primary professional who, with the client, determines what choices are available and how success can be achieved. The primary nursing interventions are exploring available options with the client and family and teaching the client how to implement the selected option.

When an individual is faced with a complex regimen to follow or has compromised functioning that impedes successful management, the diagnosis Risk for Ineffective Management of Therapeutic Regimen is appropriate. In addition to teaching the client how to manage the regimen, the nurse must also assist him or her to identify the adjustments needed because of a functional deficit. Risk for Ineffective Management of Therapeutic Regimen is a useful diagnosis for discharge teaching.

DEFINING CHARACTERISTICS

Major (Must Be Present, One or More)

Verbalized desire to manage the treatment of illness and prevention of sequelae
Verbalized difficulty with regulation/integration of one or more prescribed regimens for treatment of illness and its effects or for prevention of complications

Minor (May Be Present)

Acceleration (expected or unexpected) of illness symptoms
Verbalization that client did not take action to include treatment regimens in daily routines
Verbalization that client did not take action to reduce risk factors for progression of illness and sequelae

RELATED FACTORS

Treatment-Related

Related to:
Complexity of therapeutic regimen
Financial cost of regimen
Complexity of health care system
Side effects of therapy
Unfamiliar treatments or techniques

Situational (Personal, Environmental)

Related to:
Decisional conflicts
Insufficient knowledge
Family conflicts
Mistrust of regimen
Mistrust of health care personnel
Health belief conflicts
Questions about seriousness of problem
Questions about susceptibility
Questions about benefits of regimen
Insufficient social support
Insufficient confidence
Previous unsuccessful experiences
Related to barriers to comprehension secondary to:

Cognitive deficits	Fatigue
Hearing impairments	Motivation
Anxiety	Memory problems

Maturational

Child, adolescent
Related to fear of being different

OUTCOME CRITERIA

The person will:

1. Relate less anxiety about fear of the unknown, fear of loss of control, or misconceptions
2. Describe disease process, causes and factors contributing to symptoms, and the regimen for disease or symptom control
3. Relate an intent to practice health behaviors needed or desired for recovery from illness and prevention of recurrence or complications

⬇ GENERIC INTERVENTIONS

1. Identify causative or contributing factors that impede effective management.
   a. Lack of trust
   b. Insufficient confidence (self-efficacy)
   c. Insufficient knowledge
   d. Insufficient resources
2. Build trust and strength (Zerwich, 1992).
   a. Gain entrance to family system. Do not take over.
   b. Avoid impression of pressuring.
   c. Listen to discover concerns, not to impose expectations.
   d. Attempt to discover a match between expressed needs and services the nurse can provide.
   e. Discover and affirm strengths.
   f. Accept persons where they are.
   g. Demonstrate persistence, but proceed slowly.
   h. Demonstrate honesty, consistency, stability.
   i. Maintain preestablished contacts in person or by phone.
3. Promote confidence and positive self-efficacy (Bandura, 1982).
   a. Explore with person(s) past successful management of problems.
   b. Tell stories of other "successes."
   c. If appropriate, encourage opportunities to witness others successfully coping in a similar situation.
   d. Encourage participation in self-help groups.
   e. If high autonomic response (*e.g.*, rapid pulse, diaphoresis) is reducing feeling of confidence, teach short-term anxiety interrupters (Grainger, 1990).
      - Look up
      - Control breathing
      - Lower shoulders
      - Slow thoughts
      - Alter voice
      - Give self-directions (out loud, if possible)
      - Exercise
      - "Scruff your face"—change facial expression
      - Change perspective (imagine watching the situation from a distance)

4. Identify factors that influence learning.
   a. Perception of seriousness
   b. Susceptibility to complications
   c. Prognosis
   d. Perception of control of progression
   e. Level of anxiety
   f. Financial status
   g. Support system
   h. Past experiences
   i. Physical status
   j. Emotional status
   k. Cognitive ability
5. Promote a positive attitude and active participation of the person and family.
   a. Solicit expressions of feelings, concerns, and questions from person and family.
   b. Encourage person/family to seek information and make informed decisions.
   c. Explain responsibilities of person/family and how these can be assumed.
6. Explain and discuss (Rakel, 1992):
   a. Disease process
   b. Treatment regimen (medications, diet, procedures, exercises, equipment use)
   c. Rationale of regimen
   d. Expectations (client, family) of regimen
   e. Side effects of regimen
   f. Lifestyle changes needed
   g. Methods to monitor condition
   h. Follow-up care needed
   i. Signs or symptoms of complications
   j. Resources, support available
   k. Home environment alterations needed
7. Explain that changes in lifestyle and needed learning will take time to integrate.
   a. Provide printed material.
   b. Explain whom to contact with questions.
8. Identify referrals or community services needed for follow-up.

🏛 OLDER ADULT FOCUS INTERVENTIONS

1. To promote learning:
   a. Avoid times of day when fatigued.
   b. Reduce distractions.

      c. Relate information to prior experiences.

      d. Use visual cues.

      e. Provide outlines prior to class.

2. Allow person to self-pace the learning.
3. Create a list of cues to organize activities.

Management of Therapeutic Regimen, Ineffective: Families

DEFINITION

Ineffective Management of Therapeutic Regimen, Families: A pattern in which the family experiences or is at risk to experience difficulty integrating into daily living a program for treatment of illness and the sequelae of illness and reduction of risk situations (*e.g.*, unsafe, pollution).

Author's Note:
Refer to Ineffective Management of Therapeutic Regimen.

DEFINING CHARACTERISTICS

Major

Inappropriate family activities for meeting the goals of a treatment or prevention program

Minor

Acceleration (expected or unexpected) of illness symptoms of a family member

Lack of attention to illness and its sequelae

Verbalization of desire to manage the treatment of illness and prevention of sequelae

Verbalization of difficulty with regulation/integration of one or more prescribed regimens for treatment of illness and its effects or prevention of complications

Verbalization that family did not take action to reduce risk factors for progression of illness and sequelae

RELATED FACTORS

Refer to *Ineffective Management of Therapeutic Regimen.*

GENERIC INTERVENTIONS

Refer to *Ineffective Management of Therapeutic Regimen.*

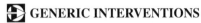 Management of Therapeutic Regimen, Ineffective: Community

DEFINITION

Ineffective Management of Therapeutic Regimen: Community: A pattern in which the community experiences or is at high risk to experience difficulty integrating a program for prevention/treatment of illness and the sequelae of illness and reduction of risk situations (*e.g.*, safety, pollution).

> **Author's Note:**
> This diagnosis describes a community that has evidence that a population is underserved because of insufficient availability of, access to, or knowledge of health care resources. The community nurse using the results of a community assessment can identify at-risk groups and overall community needs. In addition, the nurse will assess health systems, transportation, social services, and access.

DEFINING CHARACTERISTICS

Major

Verbalized difficulty in meeting health needs in communities
Acceleration (expected or unexpected) of illness(es)
Morbidity, mortality rates above the norm

RELATED FACTORS

Situational (Environmental)

Related to availability of community programs for (specify):
  Prevention of diseases   Screening for diseases

Immunizations	Dental care
Accident prevention	Fire safety
Smoking cessation	Substance abuse
Alcohol abuse	Child abuse

Related to problem accessing program secondary to, for example, inadequate communication, limited hours, no transportation, insufficient funds

Related to complexity of population's needs

Related to lack of awareness of availability

Related to presence of environmental or occupational health hazards

Related to multiple needs of vulnerable groups (specify):
　　Homeless
　　Pregnant teenagers
　　Persons living below poverty level
　　Home-bound individuals

Related to unavailable or insufficient health care agencies

OUTCOME CRITERIA

The community will:

1. Identify community resources that are needed
2. Promote the use of community resources for health problems

INTERVENTIONS

1. Create a survey to determine:
   a. Health problem identification
   b. Awareness of health services
   c. Use of health services
   d. Interest in health-promotion programs
   e. Recommendation for funding sources
2. Survey samples of the target population
   a. Mail survey
   b. One-to-one survey at community center, sports field, supermarket
   c. Group survey (*e.g.*, church groups, clubs)
   d. Survey of key community leaders
3. Design the survey for easy reading and answering (*e.g.*, circle the number that best describes your answer: 1—no concern; 2—medium; 3—high).
   a. How concerned are you about, *e.g.*:
      • Hypertension
      • Stress

- Alcohol misuse
- Violence
- Nutrition
- HIV

4. Organize the response data.
5. Analyze the findings.
   a. What are the overall health problems reported?
   b. What are the health concerns of:
      - Elderly population
      - Households with children up to age 20
      - Single-parent households
      - Respondents younger than 45 years
      - Individuals below the poverty level
6. Evaluate community resources.
   a. What resources are available for the health problems identified?
   b. Are there use or access problems with the services?
   c. How does the population know of services?
   d. Identify problems that do not have community services available.
7. If services are available but are underused, evaluate:
   a. Hours of operation (convenient?)
   b. Location of services (access, esthetics)
   c. Efficiency and atmosphere
   d. Advertising strategies
8. If services are unavailable, pursue program development.
   a. Examine and evaluate similar programs in other communities.
      - Basic information
      - Purpose, goals
      - Services available
      - Funding
      - Cost to participants
      - Availability of services
      - Accessibility of services
      - Satisfaction (citizen, employees)
   b. Meet with appropriate persons to discuss findings (survey, on-site visits).
   c. Address the following:
      - Presence of community support
      - Available expertise and technology in community
      - Financial support

    d. Identify appropriate community sources of assistance (*e.g.*, hospital departments, schools of nursing, private foundations).

    e. Plan the program (refer to *Effective Community Coping* for interventions for community planning).

9. Evaluate vulnerable population's access to health care and knowledge of risk factors:
   a. Rural families, elderly
   b. Migrant workers
   c. New immigrants
   d. Homeless
   e. Individuals and groups below the poverty level

10. Make a priority of ensuring that basic needs for food, shelter, clothing, and safety are met before attempting to address higher health needs.

11. Provide information regarding illness prevention, health promotion, and health services to vulnerable populations.

Mobility, Impaired Physical

Bed Mobility, Impaired
Walking, Impaired
Wheelchair Mobility, Impaired
Wheelchair Transfer Ability, Impaired

Mobility, Impaired Physical

DEFINITION

Impaired Physical Mobility: The state in which an individual experiences or is at risk of experiencing limitation of physical movement but is not immobile.

Author's Note:
Impaired Physical Mobility describes an individual with limited use of arm(s) or leg(s) or limited muscle strength. Impaired Physical Mobility should not be used to describe complete immobility; instead, Disuse Syndrome is more applicable. Limitation of physical movement can also be the etiology of other nursing diagnoses, such as Self-Care Deficit or Risk for Injury.

Nursing Interventions for Impaired Physical Mobility focus on strengthening and restoring function and preventing deterioration.

DEFINING CHARACTERISTICS
(Levin et al., 1989)

Major (80%–100%)

Compromised ability to move purposefully within the environment (*e.g.*, bed mobility, transfers, ambulation)
ROM limitations

Minor (50%–80%)

Imposed restriction of movement
Reluctance to move

RELATED FACTORS

Pathophysiological

Related to decreased strength and endurance secondary to:
  (Neuromuscular impairment)
    Autoimmune alterations (*e.g.*, multiple sclerosis, arthritis)
    Nervous system diseases (*e.g.*, parkinsonism, myasthenia gravis)
    Muscular dystrophy
    Partial or total paralysis (*e.g.*, spinal cord injury, stroke)
    CNS tumor
    Increased ICP
    Sensory deficits
  (Musculoskeletal impairment)
    Fractures
    Connective tissue disease (systemic lupus erythematosus)
Related to edema (increased synovial fluid)

Treatment-Related

Related to external devices (casts or splints, braces,
  intravenous tubing)
Related to insufficient strength and endurance for ambulation
  with (specify; *e.g.,* prosthesis, crutches, walker)

Situational (Personal, Environmental)

Related to fatigue, decreased motivation, or pain

Maturational

Children
  Related to abnormal gait secondary to:
    Congenital skeletal deficiencies
    Osteomyelitis
    Congenital hip dysplasia
    Legg-Calvé-Perthes disease
Older Adults
  Related to decreased motor agility or muscle weakness

OUTCOME CRITERIA

The person will:

1. Demonstrate the use of adaptive devices to increase
   mobility
2. Use safety measures to minimize potential for injury
3. Demonstrate measures to increase mobility
4. Report an increase in mobility

⊠ GENERIC INTERVENTIONS

1. Refer to *Disuse Syndrome* for interventions to prevent the
   complications of immobility.
2. Teach to perform active ROM exercises on unaffected
   limbs at least four times a day.
   a. Perform passive ROM exercises on affected limbs.
      • Perform slowly.
      • Support the extremity above and below the
        joint.
   b. Gradually progress from active ROM to functional
      activities.

3. Position in alignment to prevent complications.
   a. Use a foot board.
   b. Avoid prolonged periods of sitting or lying in the same position.
   c. Change position of the shoulder joints every 2 to 4 hours.
   d. Use a small pillow or no pillow when in Fowler's position.
   e. Support the hand and wrist in natural alignment.
   f. If the client is supine or prone, place a rolled towel or small pillow under the lumbar curvature or under the end of the rib cage.
   g. Place a trochanter roll or sandbags alongside the hips and upper thighs.
   h. If the client is in the lateral position, place pillow(s) to support the leg from groin to foot and a pillow to flex the shoulder and elbow slightly; if needed, support the lower foot in dorsal flexion with a sandbag.
   i. Use hand and wrist splints.
4. Provide progressive mobilization.*
   a. Assist the person slowly to sitting position.
   b. Allow the person to dangle legs over the side of the bed for a few minutes before standing.
   c. Limit the time to 15 minutes, three times a day, the first few times out of bed.
   d. Increase the person's time out of bed, as tolerated, by 15-minute increments.
   e. Progress to ambulation, with or without assistive devices.
   f. If unable to walk, assist the person out of bed to a wheelchair or chair.
   g. Encourage ambulation for short frequent walks (at least three times daily), with assistance if unsteady.
   h. Increase lengths of walks progressively each day.
5. Observe and teach the use of:
   a. Crutches
      • No pressure should be exerted on axilla; hand strength should be used.
      • Type of gait varies with individual's diagnosis.
      • Measure crutches 2 to 3 in below axilla and tips 6 in away from feet.

*This may require a primary care professional's order.

b. Walkers
- Use arm strength to support weakness in lower limbs.
- Gait varies with individual's problems.

c. Wheelchairs
- Practice transfers.
- Practice maneuvering around barriers.

d. Prostheses
- Stump wrapping before application of the prosthesis
- Application of the prosthesis
- Principles of stump care
- Importance of cleaning the stump, keeping it dry, and applying the prosthesis only when the stump is dry

e. Slings
- Assess for correct application; sling should be loose around neck and should support elbow and wrist above level of the heart.
- Remove slings for ROM.*

f. Ace bandages
- Observe for correct position.
- Apply with even pressure, wrapping distally to proximally.
- Observe for "bunching."
- Observe for signs of skin irritation (redness, ulceration) or tightness (compression).
- Rewrap Ace bandages b.i.d. or as needed unless contraindicated (*e.g.*, if bandage is postoperative compression dressing, check physician's orders).

6. Teach the individual safety precautions.
   a. Protect areas of decreased sensation from extremes of heat and cold.
   b. Practice falling and how to recover from falls while transferring or ambulating.
   c. For decreased perception of lower extremity (post-CVA "neglect"), instruct the individual to check where limb is placed when changing positions or going through doorways; check to make sure both shoes are tied, that affected leg is dressed with trousers, and that pants are not dragging.
   d. Instruct individuals who are confined to wheelchair to shift position and lift up buttocks every 15 minutes to relieve pressure; maneuver curbs, ramps,

inclines, and around obstacles; and lock wheel-chairs before transferring.

7. Encourage use of affected arm when possible.
    a. Encourage the person to use affected arm for self-care activities (*e.g.*, feeding, dressing, brushing hair).
    b. For post-CVA neglect of upper limb, see also *Unilateral Neglect*.
    c. Instruct the person to use unaffected arm to exercise the affected arm.
    d. Use appropriate adaptive equipment to enhance the use of arms.
        • Universal cuff for feeding in individuals who have poor control in both arms, hands
        • Large-handled or padded silverware to assist individuals with poor fine-motor skills
        • Dishware with high edges to prevent food from slipping
        • Suction-cup aids to hold dishes in place and prevent sliding of plate
    e. Use a warm bath to alleviate early morning stiffness and improve mobility.
8. Have person demonstrate:
    a. Strengthening exercises
    b. ROM exercises
    c. Care of adaptive devices
    d. Safety precautions

Impaired Bed Mobility

DEFINITION

Impaired Bed Mobility: The state in which an individual experiences, or is at risk of experiencing, limitation of movement in bed.

Author's Note:

Impaired Bed Mobility would be a clinically useful diagnosis when an individual is a candidate for rehabilitation to improve strength, range of motion, and movement. The nurse could consult with a physical therapist for a specific plan for the individual. This diagnosis would be inappropriate for an unconscious or terminally ill person.

DEFINING CHARACTERISTICS

Impaired ability to turn from side to side
Impaired ability to move from supine to sitting or sitting to supine
Impaired ability to "scoot" or reposition self in bed
Impaired ability to move from supine to prone or prone to supine
Impaired ability to move from supine to long sitting or long
  sitting to supine

RELATED FACTORS

Refer to *Impaired Physical Mobility*.

OUTCOME CRITERIA

Refer to *Impaired Physical Mobility*.

INTERVENTIONS

Refer to *Impaired Physical Mobility*.

Impaired Walking

DEFINITION

Impaired Walking: The state in which an individual experiences, or is at risk of experiencing, limitation in walking.

DEFINING CHARACTERISTICS

Impaired ability to climb stairs
Impaired ability to walk required distances
Impaired ability to walk on an incline
Impaired ability to walk on uneven surfaces
Impaired ability to navigate curbs

RELATED FACTORS

Refer to *Impaired Physical Mobility*.

OUTCOME CRITERIA

The person will:

1. Demonstrate safe mobility
2. Increase walking distance to (specify) by (specify)

🔁 GENERIC INTERVENTIONS

1. Explain that safe ambulation is a complete movement involving the muscoskeletal, neurological, and cardiovascular systems and cognitive factors such as mentation and orientation.

2. If the person is deconditioned, a progressive program of exercise is needed; consult with physical therapist for an evaluation and plan.

3. Ascertain that ambulatory aids are being used correctly and safely (*e.g.*, cane, walker, crutches):
   a. Wears well-fitting, firm shoes
   b. Can ambulate on inclines, uneven surfaces, and up and down stairs
   c. Is aware of hazards (*e.g.*, wet floors, throw rugs)

4. Provide progressive mobilization if indicated.
   a. Assist the person slowly to a sitting position.
   b. Allow the person to dangle legs over the side of the bed for a few minutes before standing.
   c. Limit the time to 15 minutes, three times a day, the first few times out of bed.
   d. Increase the person's time out of bed, as tolerated, by 15-minute increments.
   e. Progress to ambulation, with or without assistive devices.
   f. If unable to walk, assist the person out of bed to a wheelchair or chair.
   g. Encourage ambulation for short frequent walks (at least three times daily), with assistance if unsteady.
   h. Increase lengths of walks progressively each day.

5. Evaluate response to ambulation.
   a. Refer to *Activity Intolerance*.

Impaired Wheelchair Mobility

DEFINITION

Impaired Wheelchair Mobility: The state in which an individual experiences, or is at risk of experiencing, difficulty with wheelchair mobility and safety.

DEFINING CHARACTERISTICS

Impaired ability to operate manual or power wheelchair on even or uneven surface

Impaired ability to operate manual or power wheelchair on an incline

Impaired ability to operate wheelchair on curbs

RELATED FACTORS

Refer to *Impaired Physical Mobility*.

OUTCOME CRITERIA

The person will:

1. Demonstrate safe use of wheelchair
2. Demonstrate safe transfer to wheelchair

⊕ GENERIC INTERVENTIONS

1. Determine factors that are interfering with proper wheelchair use:
   a. Knowledge
   b. Strength
   c. Mentation
2. Consult with physical therapist if strengthening exercises are indicated.
3. Teach transfer techniques:
   a. Weight-bearing
   b. Non–weight-bearing
4. Have person demonstrate technique and evaluate effectiveness and safety.

Impaired Wheelchair Transfer Ability

DEFINITION

Impaired Wheelchair Transfer Ability: The state in which an individual experiences, or is at risk of experiencing, difficulty with transfer to and from the wheelchair.

253

DEFINING CHARACTERISTICS

Impaired ability to transfer from bed to chair and chair to bed
Impaired ability to transfer on or off a toilet or commode
Impaired ability to transfer in and out of tub or shower
Impaired ability to transfer between uneven levels
Impaired ability to transfer from chair to car or car to chair
Impaired ability to transfer from chair to floor or floor to chair
Impaired ability to transfer from standing to floor or floor to
    standing

RELATED FACTORS

Refer to *Impaired Physical Mobility.*

OUTCOME CRITERIA

The person will:

1. Demonstrate safe transfer to and from the wheelchair
2. Identify when assistance is needed

⊞ GENERIC INTERVENTIONS

1. Explain that safe ambulation is a complete movement involving the muscoskeletal, neurological, and cardiovascular systems and cognitive factors such as mentation and orientation.
2. If the person is deconditioned, a progressive program of exercise is needed; consult with physical therapist for an evaluation and plan.
3. Explain that one should always transfer toward the unaffected side.
4. Determine whether an assisted device is needed (*e.g.*, walking belt with handles, mechanical lift, transfer sheets).
5. Consult with physical therapist to determine how much assistance is needed:
    a. Requires no assistance
    b. Requires only verbal cuing
    c. Support by clinician's hand if additional help is needed
    d. Requires physical assistance
    e. Needs mechanical device to execute transfer (*e.g.*, lifts)
6. Advise that ability may fluctuate and to request assistance in order to prevent injury.

Neurovascular Dysfunction, Risk for Peripheral

DEFINITION

Risk for Peripheral Neurovascular Dysfunction: A state in which an individual is at risk of experiencing a disruption in circulation, sensation, or motion of an extremity.

> **Author's Note:**
> This diagnosis represents a situation that nurses can prevent by identifying who is at risk and implementing measures to reduce or eliminate the causative or contributing factors. If undetected, compromised neurovascular function can lead to compartmental syndrome. Compartmental syndrome requires medical intervention (*e.g.*, fasciotomy and nursing care before and after surgery).

RISK FACTORS

Presence of risk factors (see Related Factors)

RELATED FACTORS

Pathophysiological

Related to increased volume of (specify extremity) secondary to:
  Bleeding (*e.g.*, trauma, fractures)
  Coagulation disorder
  Venous obstruction/pooling
  Arterial obstruction
Related to increased capillary filtration secondary to:
  Trauma
  Severe burns (thermal, electrical)
  Hypothermia
  Frostbite
  Allergic response (*e.g.*, insect bites)
  Venomous bites (*e.g.*, snake)
  Nephrotic syndrome

Related to restrictive envelope secondary to:
    Circumferential burns of extremities
    Excessive pressure

Treatment-Related

Related to increased volume secondary to:
    Infiltration of intravenous infusion
    Excessive movement
    Dislocated prosthesis (knee, hip)
    Nonpatent wound drainage system
Related to increased capillary filtration secondary to:
    Total knee replacement
    Total hip replacement
Related to restrictive envelope secondary to:
    Tourniquet
    Blood pressure cuff
    Cast
    Brace
    Restraints
    Antishock trousers
    Excessive traction
    Circumferential dressings, Ace wraps
    Air splints
    Premature or tight closure of fascial defects

OUTCOME CRITERIA

The individual will continue to demonstrate:

1. Palpable peripheral pulses
2. Warm extremities
3. Capillary refill <3 seconds

GENERIC INTERVENTIONS

1. Assess and evaluate neurovascular status at least every hour for first 24 hours. Compare with unaffected limb if possible.
   a. Peripheral pulses
   b. Skin color, temperature
   c. Capillary refill time
2. For injured arms (Ross, 1991):
   a. Assess for ability:
      - To hyperextend thumbs, wrist, and four fingers

- To abduct (fanning out) all fingers
- To touch thumb to small finger

    b. Assess sensation with pressure from a sharp point:
- Web space between thumb and index finger
- Distal fat pad of small finger
- Distal surface of the index finger

3. For injured legs (Ross, 1991):

    a. Assess for ability to:
- Dorsiflex (upward movement) ankle and extend toes at metatarsal phalangeal joints
- Plantarflex (downward movement) ankle and toes

    b. Assess sensation with pressure from a sharp point:
- Web space between great toe and second toe
- Medial and lateral surfaces of the sole (upper third)

4. Instruct to report unusual, new, or different sensations (*e.g.*, tingling, numbness, or decreased ability to move toes or fingers; pain with passive stretch; unrelieved pain).

5. Reduce edema or its effects on function.

    a. Remove jewelry from affected limb.

    b. Elevate limbs unless contraindicated.

    c. Advise to move fingers or toes of affected limb two to four times per hour.

    d. Apply ice bags around injured site. Place a cloth between ice bag and skin.

    e. Monitor drainage (characteristics, amount) from wounds or incisional site.

    f. Maintain patency of the wound drainage system.

6. Notify the physician if the following occur:

    a. Change in sensation

    b. Movement ability

    c. Pale, mottled, or cyanotic skin

    d. Slowed capillary refill >3 seconds

    e. Diminished or absent pulse

    f. Increasing pain or pain not controlled by medication

    g. Pain with passive stretching of muscle

    h. Pain increased with elevation

7. If previous signs or symptoms occur, discontinue elevation and ice application.

8. Promote circulation in affected limb.

    a. Ensure hydration is optimal to maximize circulation.

      b. Monitor traction apparatus and splints for pressure on vessels or nerves.

      c. If wrist or ankle restraints are used, monitor for pressure on vessels or nerves. Remove at least every hour, and perform ROM exercises.

      d. Encourage active ROM exercises of unaffected body parts and ambulation if permissible.

9. After hip or knee joint replacement, maintain correct positioning to prevent prosthetic dislocation.

10. Initiate health teaching as indicated.

      a. Teach the client and family to watch for and report the following symptoms:
- Severe pain
- Numbness or tingling
- Swelling
- Skin discoloration
- Paralysis or reduced movement
- Cool, white toes or fingertips
- Foul odor, warm spots, soft areas, or cracks in the cast

      b. Emphasize the importance of follow-up evaluations.

Noncompliance

DEFINITION

Noncompliance: The state in which an individual or group desires to comply, but factors are present that deter adherence to agreed upon health-related advice given by health professionals.

Author's Note:

Noncompliance describes the individual who desires to comply, but the presence of certain factors prevents him or her from doing so. The nurse must attempt to reduce or eliminate these factors for the interventions to be successful. However, the nurse is cautioned

(Continued)

DEFINING CHARACTERISTICS

Major (Must Be Present)

Verbalization of difficulty with compliance or confusion about therapy *or*

Minor (May Be Present)

Missed appointments
Partially used or unused medications
Persistence of symptoms
Progression of disease process
Occurrence of undesired outcomes (postoperative morbidity, pregnancy, obesity, addiction, regression during rehabilitation)

RELATED FACTORS

Pathophysiological

Related to impaired ability to perform tasks because of disability secondary to: (*e.g.*, poor memory, motor and sensory deficits)
Related to increasing amount of disease-related symptoms despite adherence to advised regimen

Treatment-Related

Related to:
  Side effects of therapy
  Previous unsuccessful experiences with advised regimen
  Impersonal aspects of referral process
  Nontherapeutic environment
  Duration of therapy
  Cost of therapy
  Complexity of plan

Situational (Personal, Environmental)

Related to barriers to access secondary to:
  Mobility problems
  Financial issues
  Lack of child care
  Transportation problems
  Inclement weather
Related to concurrent illness of family member
Related to nonsupportive family, peers, community
Related to hopelessness
Related to barriers to comprehension secondary to:
  Cognitive deficits
  Visual deficits
  Hearing deficits
  Poor memory
  Anxiety
  Fatigue
  Decreased attention span
  Motivation
Related to perception of seriousness and susceptibility

OUTCOME CRITERIA

The person will:

1. Verbalize fears related to health needs
2. Identify factors that are contributing to anxiety
3. Identify alternatives to present coping patterns

⬕ GENERIC INTERVENTIONS

1. Using open-ended questions, encourage person to talk about experiences with health care (*e.g.*, hospitalizations, family deaths, diagnostic tests, blood tests, x-rays).
2. Ask client directly, "What are your concerns about:
   a. taking this drug?"
   b. following this diet?"
   c. having a blood test?"
   d. going through the cystoscopy?"
   e. having your gallbladder removed?"
   f. using a diaphragm?"
   g. paying for the operation?"
3. Explore the person's understanding of the problem and his or her expectations of treatment and of outcomes. Determine if beliefs are realistic and correct.

4. Assess problematic factors of prescribed therapy (*e.g.*, time, cost, complexity, convenience, adverse effects).
5. Assess person for recent changes in lifestyle (personal, work, family, health, financial).
6. Assist to reduce side effects, if possible.
   a. For gastric irritation, suggest that drug be taken with milk or food; it may be advisable to eat yogurt (unless contraindicated).
   b. For drowsiness, take medication at bedtime or late in afternoon; consult physician for dose reduction.
7. Discuss the risks and benefits of adhering to the prescribed regimen.
8. Affirm client's right to refuse all or part of the prescribed regimen.

Nutrition, Altered: Less Than Body Requirements

Altered Dentition

Impaired Swallowing

Ineffective Infant Feeding Pattern

Nutrition, Altered: Less Than Body Requirements

DEFINITION

Altered Nutrition: Less than body requirements: The state in which an individual, who is not NPO, experiences or is at risk for inadequate intake or metabolism of nutrients for metabolic needs with or without weight loss.

261

Author's Note:

This diagnosis describes individuals who can ingest food but have an intake of less-than-adequate amounts. This diagnosis should not be used to describe individuals who are NPO or cannot ingest food. These situations should be described by the collaborative problems of

Potential Complication:
Electrolyte imbalances
Negative nitrogen balance

Nurses monitor to detect complications of an NPO state and confer with physicians for parenteral therapy. Some nursing diagnoses that may relate to an individual who is NPO are Risk for Altered Oral Mucous Membrane and Altered Comfort.

DEFINING CHARACTERISTICS

Major (Must Be Present)

One who is not NPO reports or has: inadequate food intake less than recommended daily allowance with or without weight loss *or*
Actual or potential metabolic needs in excess of intake

Minor (May Be Present)

Weight 10% to 20% or more below ideal for height and frame
Triceps skin fold, midarm circumference, and midarm muscle circumference less than 60% standard measurement
Muscle weakness and tenderness
Mental irritability or confusion
Decreased serum prealbumin
Decreased serum transferrin or iron-binding capacity

RELATED FACTORS

Pathophysiological

Related to increased caloric requirements and difficulty in ingesting sufficient calories secondary to burns (postacute phase), infection, chemical dependence, cancer, or trauma
Related to dysphagia secondary to:
Cerebrovascular accident   Parkinson's disease

Amyotrophic lateral	Neuromuscular disorders
sclerosis	Muscular dystrophy
Cerebral palsy	

Related to decreased absorption of nutrients secondary to Crohn's disease, cystic fibrosis, or lactose intolerance

Related to decreased desire to eat secondary to altered level of consciousness

Related to self-induced vomiting, physical exercise in excess of caloric intake, or refusal to eat secondary to anorexia nervosa

Related to reluctance to eat for fear of poisoning secondary to paranoid behavior

Related to anorexia, excessive physical agitation secondary to bipolar disorder

Related to anorexia and diarrhea secondary to protozoal infection

Related to vomiting, anorexia, and impaired digestion secondary to pancreatitis

Related to anorexia, impaired protein and fat metabolism, and impaired storage of vitamins secondary to cirrhosis

Treatment-Related

Related to increased protein and vitamin requirements for wound healing and decreased intake secondary to: surgery, medications (cancer chemotherapy), surgical reconstruction of the mouth, wired jaw, or radiation therapy

Related to inadequate absorption as a side effect of (specify)

Colchicine	Neomycin
Pyrimethamine	*para*-Aminosalicylic acid
Antacid	

Related to decreased oral intake, mouth discomfort, nausea, vomiting secondary to: radiation therapy, chemotherapy, or tonsillectomy

Situational (Personal, Environmental)

Related to decreased desire to eat secondary to: anorexia, depression, stress, social isolation, nausea and vomiting, or allergies

Related to inability to procure food (physical limitations, financial or transportation problems)

Related to inability to chew (damaged or missing teeth, ill-fitting dentures)

Related to diarrhea secondary to (specify)

Maturational

Infant/child

Related to inadequate intake secondary to: lack of emotional/sensory stimulation or lack of knowledge of caregiver

Related to malabsorption, dietary restrictions and anorexia secondary to celiac disease, lactose intolerance, or cystic fibrosis

Related to sucking difficulties (infant) and dysphagia secondary to: cerebral palsy or cleft lip and palate

Related to inadequate sucking, fatigue, and dyspnea secondary to: congenital heart disease or prematurity

Older adult

Related to effects of declining metabolic rate, estrogen levels, and bone mineral density (women)

Related to degeneration of periodontal membrane with loose teeth

OUTCOME CRITERIA

The person will:

1. Increase oral intake as evidenced by (specify)
2. Describe causative factors when known
3. Describe rationale and procedure for treatments

➡ GENERIC INTERVENTIONS

1. Determine the daily caloric requirements that are realistic and adequate. Consult with dietitian.
2. Weigh daily; monitor laboratory results.
3. Explain the importance of adequate nutrition. Negotiate with client intake goals for each meal and snacks.
4. Teach person to use spices to help improve the taste and aroma of food (lemon juice, mint, cloves, basil, thyme, cinnamon, rosemary, bacon bits).
5. Encourage individual to eat with others (meals served in dining room or group area or at local meeting place, such as community center, by church groups).
6. Plan care so that unpleasant or painful procedures do not take place before meals.
7. Provide pleasant, relaxed atmosphere for eating (no bedpans in sight; do not rush); try a "surprise" (*e.g.*, flowers with meal).

8. Arrange plan of care to decrease or eliminate nauseating odors or procedures near mealtimes.

9. Teach or assist individual to rest before meals.

10. Teach person to avoid cooking odors—frying foods, brewing coffee—if possible (take a walk; select foods that can be eaten cold).

11. Maintain good oral hygiene (brush teeth, rinse mouth) before and after ingestion of food.

12. Offer frequent small feedings (six per day plus snacks) to reduce the feeling of a distended stomach.

13. Arrange to have highest protein/calorie nutrients served at the time individual feels most like eating (*e.g.,* if chemotherapy is in early morning, serve in late afternoon).

14. Instruct person with decreased appetite to:
    a. Eat dry foods (toast, crackers) on arising.
    b. Eat salty foods if permissible.
    c. Avoid overly sweet, rich, greasy, or fried foods.
    d. Try clear, cool beverages.
    e. Sip slowly through straw.
    f. Take whatever can be tolerated.
    g. Eat small portions low in fat, and eat more frequently.

15. Try commercial supplements available in many forms (liquids, powder, pudding).

16. If person has an eating disorder (Townsend, 1994):
    a. Establish intake goals with client, physician, and nutritionist.
    b. Discuss the benefits of compliance and the consequences of nonadherence.
    c. If intake is refused, notify physician.
    d. Sit with person during meals. Limit meal times to 30 minutes.
    e. Observe person for at least 1 hour after meals. Accompany to bathroom.
    f. Weigh on arising and after first voiding.
    g. Provide reinforcement for improvement, but do not focus discussions on food or eating.
    h. As person improves, explore issues of body image, weight gain, and control.

17. For a hyperactive person (Townsend, 1994):
    a. Provide high-protein, high-calorie finger foods and drinks.

b. Offer frequent snacks. Avoid empty calories (*e.g.*, soda).
c. Walk or pace with person as finger foods are eaten.

⛪ OLDER ADULT FOCUS INTERVENTIONS

1. Evaluate ability to process and prepare food.
   a. Finances
   b. Transportation
   c. Mobility
   d. Manual dexterity
2. Explain community resources available.
   a. Meals on Wheels
   b. Senior centers
   c. Supermarkets that deliver
3. For women over age 50, advise to:
   a. Increase calcium intake to 1200 mg/d (1500 mg/d if not in hormone replacement therapy).
   b. Reduce calorie intake to 1700–1800.
   c. Balance intake and exercise.
   d. Include beta-carotene and vitamin C and E supplements daily.

Altered Dentition

DEFINITION

Altered Dentition: The state in which an individual experiences a disruption in tooth development/eruption patterns or structural integrity of individual teeth.

Author's Note:

Altered Dentition describes a multitude of problems with teeth. It is unclear how this diagnosis would be used by nurses or any health care professional. If the client has caries, abscesses, or misaligned or malformed teeth, the nurse would refer him or her to a dental professional. If the tooth problem is affecting comfort or nutrition, Altered Comfort or Altered Nutrition would be the appropriate nursing diagnosis.

DEFINING CHARACTERISTICS

Excessive plaque
Crown or root caries
Halitosis
Tooth enamel discoloration
Toothache
Loose teeth
Excessive calculus
Incomplete eruption for age (may be primary or permanent
 teeth)
Malocclusion or tooth misalignment
Premature loss of primary teeth
Worn down or abraded teeth
Tooth fracture(s)
Missing teeth or complete absence
Erosion of enamel
Asymmetrical facial expression

Impaired Swallowing

DEFINITION

Impaired Swallowing: The state in which an individual has decreased ability to voluntarily pass fluids or solid foods from the mouth to the stomach.

DEFINING CHARACTERISTICS

Major (Must Be Present)

Observed evidence of difficulty swallowing *or*
Stasis of food in oral cavity

Minor (May Be Present)

Coughing
Choking
Apraxia (ideational, constructional, or visual)

RELATED FACTORS

Pathophysiological

Related to decreased/absent gag reflex, mastication difficulties, or decreased sensations secondary to:
  Neurological/neuromuscular disorders
  Cerebrovascular accident
  Right or left hemispheric damage to the brain
  Damage to the 5th, 7th, 9th, 10th, or 11th cranial nerves
    Cerebral palsy   Myasthenia gravis
    Muscular dystrophy   Guillain-Barré syndrome
    Amyotrophic lateral   Poliomyelitis
      sclerosis   Parkinsonism
Related to tracheoesophageal tumors, edema

Treatment-Related

Related to surgical reconstruction of the mouth, throat, jaw and/or nose
Related to mechanical obstruction secondary to tracheostomy tube
Related to esophagitis secondary to radiotherapy
Related to decreased consciousness secondary to anesthesia
Related to increased viscosity and diminished quantity of saliva (*e.g.*, secondary to medications, radiation)

Situational (Personal, Environmental)

Related to altered level of consciousness
Related to fatigue
Related to limited awareness, distractibility
Related to irritated oropharyngeal cavity
Related to decreased saliva

Maturational

Infant/children
  Related to decreased sensations or difficulty with mastication
  Refer to Ineffective Infant Feeding Pattern

OUTCOME CRITERIA

The person will:

1. Report improved ability to swallow

The person or family will:

1. Describe causative factors when known
2. Describe rationale and procedures for treatment

⏩ GENERIC INTERVENTIONS

1. Reduce the possibility of aspiration.
   a. Before beginning feeding, assess that person is adequately alert and responsive, is able to control mouth, has cough/gag reflex, and can swallow own saliva.
   b. Have suction equipment available and functioning properly.
   c. Position correctly.
      • Sit upright (60–90 degrees) in chair or dangle feet at side of bed if possible (prop pillows if necessary).
      • Assume position 10 to 15 minutes before eating, and maintain position for 10 to 15 minutes after finishing eating.
      • Flex head forward on the midline about 45 degrees to keep esophagus patent.
   d. Keep individual focused on task by giving directions until he or she has finished swallowing each mouthful.
   e. Start with small amounts, and progress slowly as person learns to handle each step.
      • Ice chips
      • Part of eyedropper filled with water
      • Use juice in place of water
      • $1/4$, $1/2$, 1 teaspoon semisolid
      • Pureed food or commercial baby foods
      • One-half cracker
      • Soft diet–regular diet
2. Assist the individual with moving the bolus of food from the anterior to the posterior of mouth.
   a. Place food in the posterior mouth where swallowing can be assured.
3. Prevent/decrease thick secretions.
4. Progress to ice chips, water, and then food when danger of aspiration is decreased.
5. For individuals with impaired cognition or awareness:
   a. Concentrate on solids rather than liquids, because liquids are generally less well tolerated.

 b. Keep extraneous stimuli at minimum while eating (e.g., no television or radio, no verbal stimuli unless directed at task).
 c. Have person concentrate on task of swallowing.
 d. Have person sit up in chair with neck slightly flexed.
 e. Instruct person to hold breath while swallowing.
 f. Observe for swallowing and check mouth for emptying.
 g. Avoid overloading mouth, because this decreases swallowing effectiveness.
 h. Give solids and liquids separately.
 i. Reinforce behaviors with simple one-word commands.

6. Feed slowly, making certain previous bite has been swallowed.
7. Consult with speech pathologist.
8. Teach family emergency interventions for obstruction (*e.g.*, Heimlich maneuver).

♥ Ineffective Infant Feeding Pattern

DEFINITION

Ineffective Infant Feeding Pattern: A state in which an infant (birth to 9 months) demonstrates an impaired ability to suck or coordinate the suck–swallow response, resulting in inadequate oral nutrition for metabolic needs.

Author's Note:

This diagnosis represents a specific type of nutritional problem of infants grouped under the more general diagnosis Altered Nutrition: Less than body requirements. The nursing role is to provide or assist caregivers to provide appropriate calories to gain weight. Specific feeding techniques and energy expenditure reduction are used to achieve oral feedings for all nutrition. Some infants with sucking or such swallow-response difficulties can meet nutritional needs unless additional factors that increase caloric needs are present (*e.g.*, infection).

DEFINING CHARACTERISTICS

Major (Must Be Present, One or More)

Inability to initiate or sustain an effective suck; inability to
coordinate sucking, swallowing, and breathing

Actual metabolic needs in excess of oral intake with weight
loss or need for enteral feeding supplement

Minor (May Be Present)

Inconsistent oral intake (volume, time interval, duration)
Oral motor developmental delay
Tachypnea with increased respiratory effort
Regurgitation or vomiting after feeding

RELATED FACTORS

Pathophysiological

Related to increased caloric need secondary to:

Body temperature
instability

Growth needs

Tachypnea with increased
respiratory effort

Wound healing

Infection

Major organ system disease
or failure

Related to muscle weakness/hypotonia secondary to:

Malnutrition

Prematurity

Acute/chronic illness

Lethargy

Congenital defects

Major organ system disease
or failure

Neurological impairment/
delay

Treatment-Related

Related to hypermetabolic state and increase caloric needs
secondary to: surgery or painful procedures

Related to muscle weakness and lethargy secondary to sleep
deprivation or medications (muscle relaxants, *e.g.*, anti-
seizure medications, paralyzing agents in past, sedatives,
narcotics)

Related to oral hypersensitivity

Related to previous prolonged NPO state

Situational (Personal, Environmental)

Related to inconsistent caretakers (feeders)

Related to lack of knowledge of or commitment of caretaker
(feeder) to special feeding needs or regimen

Related to presence of noxious facial or absence of oral stimuli

OUTCOME CRITERIA

The infant will:

1. Receive adequate nutrition for growth appropriate to age
   and need
2. Demonstrate increasing skill in oral feedings appropriate
   for developmental ability

🔊 CHILD FOCUS INTERVENTIONS

1. Assess the infant's feeding pattern and nutritional needs.
   a. Assess volume, duration, and effort during feed-
      ing; respiratory rate and effort; signs of fatigue.
   b. Assess past caloric intake, weight gain, trends in
      intake and output, renal function, fluid retention.
2. Collaborate with clinical dietitian to set calorie, volume,
   and weight gain goals.
3. Collaborate with parent(s) about effective techniques
   used with this infant.
4. Provide specific interventions to promote effective oral
   feeding:
   a. Non-nutritive sucking
   b. Nutritive sucking for identified amount of time
   c. Consistency in approach to feeding
   d. Specific interventions for oral motor delays (posi-
      tion, equipment, jaw/mouth manipulation)
   e. Control of adverse environmental stimuli and
      noxious stimuli to face and mouth
5. Promote sleep and reduce unnecessary energy expenditure.
6. If needed, plan for enteral feeding includes guidelines for
   increasing oral feeding and decreasing enteral feeding as
   the infant eats more effectively by mouth.
7. Establish partnership with parent(s) in all stages of plan.
8. Provide ongoing information to parent(s) about special
   needs, and assist them in establishing needed resources
   (equipment, nursing care, other caretakers).

Nutrition, Altered: More Than Body Requirements

DEFINITION

Altered Nutrition: More than body requirements: The state in which an individual experiences or is at risk of experiencing weight gain related to an intake in excess of metabolic requirements.

Author's Note:

Obesity is a complex condition with sociocultural, psychological, and metabolic implications. This diagnosis, when used to describe obesity or overweight conditions, focuses on them as nutritional problems. The focus of treatment is behavioral modification and lifestyle changes. It is recommended that Altered Health Maintenance related to intake in excess of metabolic requirements be used in place of this diagnosis. In addition, *Ineffective Individual Coping* related to increased food consumption secondary to response to external stressors may be used. When weight gain is the result of physiological conditions (*e.g.*, altered taste); pharmacological interventions, such as corticosteroid therapy; or history of excessive weight gain during pregnancy, this diagnosis can be clinically useful.

DEFINING CHARACTERISTICS

Major (Must Be Present, One or More)

Overweight (weight 10% over ideal for height and frame)
or
Obese (weight 20% or more over ideal for height and frame)
Triceps skin fold greater than 15 mm in men and 25 mm in women

Minor (May Be Present)

Reported undesirable eating patterns
Intake in excess of metabolic requirements
Sedentary activity patterns

RELATED FACTORS

Pathophysiological

Related to altered satiety patterns secondary to (specify)
Related to decreased sense of taste and smell

Treatment-Related

Related to altered satiety secondary to:
   Medications (corticosteroids, antihistamines)
   Radiation (decreased sense of taste and smell)

Situational (Personal, Environmental)

Related to risk of gaining more than 25 to 30 lb when
   pregnant
Related to lack of basic nutritional knowledge
Related to sendentary activity patterns

Maturational

Adult/older adult
   Related to decreased activity patterns and decreased
      metabolic needs

OUTCOME CRITERIA

The person will:

1. Experience increased activity expenditure with weight
   loss
2. Describe relationship between activity level and weight
3. Identify eating patterns that contribute to weight gain
4. Lose weight

⬗ GENERIC INTERVENTIONS

1. Increase individual's awareness of amount/type of food
   consumed.
      a. Instruct person to keep a diet diary for 1 week.
         • What, when, where, and why eaten
         • Whether doing anything else (*e.g.*, watching
            television, preparing dinner)
         • Emotions just before eating
         • Others present (spouse, children)

    b. Review diet diary with individual to point out patterns (*i.e.*, time, place, people, emotions, foods) that affect intake.

    c. Review high- and low-calorie food items.

2. Assist person to set realistic goals (*i.e.*, decreasing oral intake by 500 calories will result in a 1- to 2-lb loss each week).

3. Teach behavior modification techniques.

    a. Eat only at a specific spot at home (*e.g.*, kitchen table).

    b. Do not eat while doing other activities, such as reading or watching television; eat only when sitting.

    c. Drink an 8-oz glass of water immediately before eating.

    d. Use small plates (portions look bigger).

    e. Prepare small portions, just enough for a meal, and discard leftovers.

    f. Never eat from another person's plate.

    g. Eat slowly, and chew thoroughly.

    h. Put down utensils and wait 15 seconds between bites.

    i. Eat low-calorie snacks that need to be chewed to satisfy oral need (carrots, celery, apples).

    j. Decrease liquid calories; drink diet sodas or water.

4. Plan a daily walking program, and gradually increase rate and length of walk.

    a. Start out at 5 to 10 blocks for 0.5 to 1 mile per day; increase 1 block or 0.1 mile per week.

    b. Progress slowly.

    c. Avoid straining or pushing too hard and becoming overly fatigued.

    d. Stop immediately if any of the following signs occur:
- Tightness or pain in chest
- Severe breathlessness
- Lightheadedness
- Dizziness
- Loss of muscle control
- Nausea

    e. Establish a regular time of day for physical activity; the goal is three to five times a week for a duration of 15 to 45 minutes and with a heart rate of 80% of

> stress test or gross calculation (170 beats/min for 20–29 age group; decrease 10 beats/min for each additional decade of life; *e.g.*, 160 beats/min for ages 30–39, 150 beats/min for ages 40–49).
>
> f. Advise that intermittent physical activity that accumulates to 30 or more minutes daily is beneficial.
>
> g. Suggest to take every opportunity to increase activity (*e.g.*, walk down stairs instead of using elevator, park car further from store).

5. Refer to support groups (*e.g.*, Weight Watchers, Overeaters Anonymous, TOPS, trim clubs, The Diet Workshop, Inc.).

Nutrition, Altered: Potential for More Than Body Requirements

DEFINITION

Altered Nutrition: Potential for more than body requirements: The state in which an individual is at risk of experiencing an intake of nutrients that exceeds metabolic needs.

Author's Note:

This diagnosis is similar to Risk for Altered Nutrition: More than body requirements. It describes an individual who has a family history of obesity, who is demonstrating a pattern of higher weight, or who has had a history of excessive weight gain (*e.g.*, previous pregnancy). Until clinical research differentiates this diagnosis from other presently accepted diagnoses, use Altered Health Maintenance (Actual or Risk) or Risk for Altered Nutrition: More than body requirements to direct teaching to assist families and individuals to identify unhealthy dietary patterns.

DEFINING CHARACTERISTICS

Reported or observed obesity in one or both parents

Rapid transition across growth percentiles in infants or
children

Reported use of solid food as major food source before
5 months of age

Observed use of food as a reward or comfort measure

Reported or observed higher baseline weight at beginning of
each pregnancy

Dysfunctional eating patterns

Parenting, Altered

Parent–Infant Attachment, Risk for Altered

Parental Role Conflict

Parenting, Altered

DEFINITION

Altered Parenting: The state in which one or more caregivers
demonstrate real or potential inability to provide a constructive
environment that nurtures the growth and development of his,
her, or their child (children).

Author's Note:

A family's ability to function is at a high risk of developing problems when the child or parent has a condition that increases the stress of the family unit. The term *parent* refers to any individual(s) defined as the primary caregiver(s) for a child.

DEFINING CHARACTERISTICS

Major (Must Be Present)

Inappropriate or non-nurturing parenting behaviors or lack of parental attachment behavior

Minor (May Be Present)

Frequent verbalization of dissatisfaction or disappointment with infant or child

Verbalization of frustration of role

Verbalization of perceived or actual inadequacy

Diminished or inappropriate visual, tactile, or auditory stimulation of infant

Evidence of abuse or neglect of child

Growth and developmental delays in infant or child

RELATED FACTORS

Individuals or families who may be at risk for developing or experiencing parenting difficulties

Parent(s)

Single   Addicted to drugs

Adolescent   Terminally ill

Abusive   Acutely disabled

Emotionally disturbed   Accident victim

Alcoholic

Child

Of unwanted pregnancy

Of undesired gender

With undesired characteristics

Physically handicapped

Mentally handicapped

Hyperactive characteristics

Terminally ill

Situational (Personal, Environmental)

Related to interruption of bonding process secondary to: illness (child, parent), incarceration, or relocation

Related to separation from nuclear family

Related to inconsistent caregivers or techniques

Related to lack of knowledge

Related to lack of available role model

Related to relationship problems (specify)
  Marital discord
  Divorce
  Separation
  Step-parents
  Live-in partner
  Relocation
Related to ineffective adaptation to stressors associated with illness, new baby, elder care, economic problems, or substance abuse

Maturational

Adolescent
  Related to the conflict of meeting own needs over child's
  Related to history of ineffective relationships with own parents
  Related to parental history of abusive relationship with parents
  Related to unrealistic expectations of child by parent
  Related to unrealistic expectations of self by parent
  Related to unrealistic expectations of parent by child
  Related to unmet psychosocial needs of child by parent

OUTCOME CRITERIA

The person will:

1. Share feelings regarding parenting
2. Identify factors that interfere with effective parenting
3. Describe appropriate disciplinary measures
4. Share feelings regarding parenting
5. Identify resources available for assistance with parenting

GENERIC INTERVENTIONS

1. Encourage to share parenting difficulties and usual or recent stressors.
2. If abuse is suspected, notify appropriate authorities (see *Ineffective Family Coping: Disabling*).
3. Provide with information about:
    a. Age-related development needs
    b. Age-related problematic behavior

4. Observe the parent interacting with child.
   a. Support strengths.
   b. Role model in areas that are uncomfortable or problematic.
   c. Emphasize the child's strengths or unique characteristics.
5. Allow parent(s) to watch nurse care for child. Role model comfort measures, sensory stimulation (verbal, toys, touch).
6. Encourage parent to participate in care.
7. Explain all procedures and the associated discomforts.
8. Encourage parents to be present for procedures when possible and to comfort the child.
9. Explore parents' expectations of child and differentiate realistic from unrealistic.
10. Assess usual discipline methods for appropriateness and follow-through.
11. Explore with parent(s) the child's problem behavior (Herman-Staab, 1994).
    a. Frequency, duration
    b. Situational context (when, where, triggers)
    c. Consequences of problem behavior (parental attention, discipline, inconsistencies in response)
    d. Behavior desired by parents
12. Discuss positive parenting techniques (Herman-Staab, 1994).
    a. Convey to child that he or she is loved.
    b. Catch child being good; use good eye contact.
    c. Set aside "special time" when the parent guarantees a time with child without interruptions.
    d. Ignore minor transgressions by having no physical contact or eye contact or discussion about the behavior.
    e. Practice active listening. Describe what child is saying, reflect back the child's feelings, and do not judge.
    f. Use "I" statements when disapproving of behavior. Focus on the act as undesirable, not the child.
13. Discuss discipline methods:
    a. For small child—sit in chair 1 minute for each year of age (if child gets up, put back in chair, and reset timer).

      b. For older child—deprive of favorite pastime (*e.g.*, bicycle, television show).

      c. Avoid hitting except for one hand slap for a small child for dangerous touching (*e.g.*, stove, electric plug).

      d. Do not threaten. Clarify punishment, and follow through with it.

      e. Expect child to obey.

      f. Parents should jointly agree and follow through with consistency.

14. Discuss resources available (*e.g.*, counseling, community, social service, parenting classes).

15. Initiate a referral to community nursing service if indicated.

Parent–Infant Attachment, Risk for Altered

DEFINITION

Risk for Altered Parent–Infant Attachment: The state in which there is a risk for a disruption of a nurturing, protective, interactive process between a parent/primary caregiver and infant.

Author's Note:

This new diagnosis describes a parent or caregiver who is at risk for attachment difficulties with his or her infant. Barriers to attachment can be the environment, knowledge, anxiety, and health of the parent or infant. This diagnosis is appropriate as a risk or high-risk diagnosis. If the nurse diagnoses a problem in infant–parent attachment, the diagnosis Risk for Altered Parenting related to inadequate parent attachment would be more useful so that the nurse could focus on improving attachment and preventing destructive parenting patterns.

RISK FACTORS

Refer to Related Factors.

RELATED FACTORS

Pathophysiological

Related to interruption of bonding process secondary to:
Parental illness
Infant illness

Treatment-Related

Related to barriers to holding secondary to: bililights or intensive care monitoring

Situational (Personal, Environmental)

Related to unrealistic expectations (*e.g.*, of child or self)
Related to unwanted pregnancy
Related to disappointment with infant (*e.g.*, gender, appearance)
Related to ineffective adaption to stressors associated with new baby and other responsibilities secondary to:

Health problems	Substance abuse
Mental illness	Relationship problems
Economic problems	

Related to history of ineffective relationship with own parents
Related to lack of knowledge or available role model for parental role
Related to physical disabilities of parent (*e.g.*, blindness, paralysis, deafness)

Maturational

Adolescent
Related to difficulty delaying her own gratification for the gratification of the infant

OUTCOME CRITERIA

The parent will:

1. Demonstrate increased attachment behaviors, such as holding infant close, smiling and talking to infant, and seeking eye contact with infant
2. Request to be involved in infant's care
3. Begin to verbalize positive feelings regarding the infant

⬛ GENERIC INTERVENTIONS

1. Assess causative or contributing factors.
   a. Maternal
      - Unwanted pregnancy
      - Prolonged or difficult labor and delivery
      - Postpartum pain or fatigue
      - Lack of positive support system (mother, spouse, friends)
      - Lack of positive role model (mother, relative, neighbor)
   b. Parental inadequate coping patterns (one or both parents)
      - Alcoholic
      - Drug addict
      - Marital difficulties (separation, divorce, violence)
      - Change in lifestyle related to new role
      - Adolescent parent
      - Career change (*e.g.*, working woman to mother)
      - Illness in family
   c. Infant
      - Premature, defective, ill
      - Multiple birth
2. Eliminate or reduce contributing factors if possible.
   a. Illness, pain, fatigue
      - Establish with mother what infant-care activities are feasible.
      - Provide mother with uninterrupted sleep periods of at least 2 hours during the day and 4 hours during the night.
      - Provide relief for discomforts.
   b. Lack of experience or lack of positive mothering role model
      - Explore with mother her feelings and attitudes concerning her own mother.
      - Assist her to identify someone who is a positive mother, and encourage her to seek that person's aid.
      - Outline the teaching program available to her during hospitalization.

- Determine who will assist her at home initially.
- Identify community programs and reference material that can increase her learning about child care after discharge.

c. Lack of positive support system
- Identify parent's support system, and assess its strengths and weaknesses.
- Assess the need for counseling.
  - Encourage the parent(s) to express feelings about the experience and about the future.
  - Be an active listener to the parent(s).
  - Observe the parent(s) interacting with the infant.

3. Provide opportunities for the attachment process.
  a. Promote attachment in the immediate postdelivery phase.
  - Encourage mother to hold infant following birth (may need a short recovery period).
  - Provide skin-to-skin contact if desired; keep room warm (72°–76°F), or use a heat panel over the infant.
  - Provide mother with an opportunity to breast-feed if desired.
  - Delay the administration of silver nitrate to allow for eye contact.
  - Give family as much time as they need together with minimum interruption from the staff (the "sensitive period" lasts from 30–90 minutes).
  - Encourage father to hold infant.
  b. Facilitate the attachment process during the postpartum phase.
  - Check mother regularly for signs of fatigue, especially if she had anesthesia.
  - Offer flexible rooming-in to the mother; establish with her the amount of care she will assume initially, and support her requests for assistance.
  - Discuss the future involvement of the father in the infant's care. (If desired, discuss opportunities for father to participate in his child's care at home.)

  c. Provide support to the parent(s).
- Listen to the mother's replay of her labor and delivery experience.
- Allow for verbalization of feelings.
- Indicate acceptance of feelings.
- Point out the infant's strengths and individual characteristics to the parent(s).
- Demonstrate the infant's responses to the parents.
- Have a system of follow-up following discharge, especially for families considered at risk (*e.g.*, phone call or a home visit by the community health nurse).

  d. Assess the need for teaching.
- Observe the parent(s) interacting with the infant.
- Support each parent's strengths.
- Assist each parent in areas in which they are uncomfortable (role modeling).
- Offer classes in infant care.
- Have handouts and audiovisual aids available for parent(s) to view at odd hours.
- Assess for level of knowledge in the area of growth and development, and provide information as needed.
- Help parents understand infant's cues and temperament.
- See References/Bibliography for recommended printed material on parenting and child care.

  e. When immediate separation of the child from the parents is necessary due to prematurity or illness, provide for bonding or attachment experiences, as possible.
- Allow parents to see and touch infant prior to transport.
- Encourage father to visit the neonatal intensive care unit and bring back verbal reports of infant and pictures if possible (Brazelton, 1981).
- Encourage earliest visiting for mother as feasible, with frequent phone contact with infant's caregivers if visiting is not possible.

4. Initiate referrals as needed.
   a. Consult with community agencies for follow-up visits if indicated.
   b. Refer parents to pertinent organizations.

Parental Role Conflict

DEFINITION

Parental Role Conflict: The state in which a parent or primary caregiver experiences or perceives a change in role in response to external factors (*e.g.*, illness, hospitalization, divorce, separation).

Author's Note:

This diagnosis describes a parent or parents whose previously effective functioning ability is challenged by external factors. In certain situations, such as illness, role confusion and conflict are expected. This diagnosis differs from Altered Parenting, which describes a parent (or parents) who demonstrates or is at high risk of demonstrating inappropriate parenting behaviors or lack of parental attachment. If parents are not assisted in adapting their role to external factors, Parental Role Conflict can lead to Altered Parenting. The term *parent* refers to any individual(s) defined as the primary caregiver(s) for a child.

This diagnosis was developed by the Nursing Diagnosis Discussion Group, Rainbow Babies' and Children's Hospital, University Hospitals of Cleveland.

DEFINING CHARACTERISTICS

Major (Must Be Present, One or More)

Parent(s) expresses concerns about changes in parental role
Parent(s) demonstrates disruption in care and/or caretaking routines.

Minor (May Be Present)

Parent(s) expresses concerns/feelings of inadequacy to provide for child's physical and emotional needs during hospitalization or in the home.

Parent(s) expresses concern about effect of child's illness on other children.

Parent(s) expresses concerns about care of siblings at home.

Parent(s) expresses guilt about contributing to the child's illness through lack of knowledge, judgment, and so forth.

Parent(s) expresses concern about perceived loss of control over decisions relating to the child.

Parent(s) is reluctant, unable, or unwilling to participate in normal caregiving activities, even with encouragement and support.

Parent(s) verbalizes/demonstrates feelings of guilt, anger, fear, anxiety, or frustration.

RELATED FACTORS

Situational (Personal, Environmental)

Related to separation from child secondary to:
  Birth of a child with a congenital defect or chronic illness
  Hospitalization of a child with an acute or chronic illness
  Change in acuity, prognosis, or environment of care (*e.g.*, transfer to or from an intensive care unit)
Related to fear of involvement secondary to invasive or restrictive treatment modalities (*e.g.*, isolation, intubation, etc.)
Related to interruption of family life secondary to:
  Home care of a child with special needs (*e.g.*, apnea monitoring, postural drainage, hyperalimentation)
  Frequent visits to hospital
  Addition of new family member (aging relative, newborn)
Related to change in ability to parent secondary to:
  Illness of parent
  Travel requirements
  Work responsibilities
  Divorce
  Remarriage
  Dating
  Death

OUTCOME CRITERIA

The person will:

1. Identify source of role conflict
2. Define the parental role desired

3. Participate in decision making regarding health/illness care of child
4. Participate in care of child at level desired

🔁 GENERIC INTERVENTIONS

1. Discuss what has influenced a change in role (*e.g.*, divorce, remarriage, illness [child, parent], boarding away, family additions [newborn, aging parent]).
2. Allow person to share frustrations.
3. Assist person to determine the type of role desired and if realistic.
4. If indicated, refer for counseling for management of stressors and role changes.
5. For ill or hospitalized child:
   a. Help parent(s) adapt parenting behaviors to allow for continuation of parenting role during hospitalization or illness.
   b. Provide information about hospital routines and policies, such as visiting hours, mealtimes, division routines, medical and nursing routines, rooming-in.
   c. Explain procedures and tests to parent(s); help them interpret these activities to the child; discuss child's age-appropriate range of responses.
   d. Instruct parents to continue limit-setting strategies and demonstrations of caring behaviors (*e.g.*, touching, hugging despite hospitalization and equipment).
   e. Provide information to empower parent(s) to adapt parenting role to the situation of hospitalization or the event of chronic illness of the child.
   f. Foster open communication between self and parent(s), allowing time for questions, frequent repetition of information; provide direct and honest answers.
   g. Approach parent(s) with new information; do not make them assume the responsibility for seeking out the information.
   h. When parent(s) cannot be with their child, facilitate information-sharing through telephone calls; allow parent(s) to call primary nurse or nurse caring for child.

i. Support continued decision making of parent(s) regarding the child's care.
- Provide parent(s) opportunity to help formulate plan of care for their child.
- Use parent(s) as source of information about the child, child's usual behaviors, reactions, and preferences.
- Recognize parent(s) as "expert(s)" about their child.
- Allow parent(s) the choice to be present during treatments and procedures.

j. Allow parents to participate in caring for their child to the degree they desire.
- Provide for 24-hour rooming-in for at least one parent and extended visiting for other family members.
- Collaborate and negotiate with parent(s) about parental tasks they want to continue to do, tasks they want others to assume, tasks they want to share, and tasks they want to learn to do; continually assess changes in their desired involvement in care.
- Allow parent(s) to have uninterrupted time with the child.

k. Explore with parent(s) their personal responsibilities (*e.g.*, work schedule, sibling care, household responsibilities, responsibilities to extended family); assist them in establishing a schedule that allows sufficient caretaking time for the child or visiting time with the hospitalized child, without frustration in meeting other role responsibilities (*e.g.*, if visiting is not possible until evening hours, delay child's bath time, and allow parent to bathe child then).

l. Support parental ability to normalize the hospital/home environment for themselves and the child.
- Encourage parent(s) to bring clothing and toys from home.
- Allow parent(s) to prepare home-cooked food or bring food from home if desired.
- Encourage opportunities for families to eat meals together.

- Encourage opportunities for parent(s) to take the child on leaves from the hospital, including visits home, as possible.

m. Help parent(s) verbalize feelings about the child's illness or hospitalization and adaptation of the parenting role to the situation.

n. Provide for physical and emotional needs of parent(s).

- Assess and facilitate parental ability to meet self-care needs (*e.g.*, rest, nutrition, activity, privacy).
- Allow parent(s) an opportunity to determine the caregiving schedule to correspond with a schedule to meet their own needs.
- Assess support systems: parent to parent, family, friends, minister, etc.

o. Initiate referrals if indicated: chaplain, social service, community agencies (respite care), parent self-help groups.

Post-Trauma Response

Post-Trauma Response, Risk for

Rape-Trauma Syndrome

Post-Trauma Response

DEFINITION

Post-Trauma Response: The state in which an individual experiences a sustained painful response for more than 1 month to one or more overwhelming traumatic events that have not been assimilated.

DEFINING CHARACTERISTICS

Major (Must Be Present, One or More)

Reexperiencing the traumatic event, which may be identified
in cognitive, affective, or sensory–motor activities, such as:
  Flashbacks, intrusive thoughts
  Repetitive dreams/nightmares
  Excessive verbalization of the traumatic events
  Survival guilt or guilt about behavior required for survival
  Painful emotion, self-blame, shame, or sadness
  Vulnerability or helplessness, anxiety, or panic
  Fear of repetition, death, loss of bodily control
  Anger outburst/rage, startle reaction
  Hyperalertness or hypervigilance

Minor (May Be Present)

Psychic/emotional numbness
  Impaired interpretation of reality, impaired memory
  Confusion, dissociation, or amnesia
  Vagueness about traumatic event
  Narrowed attention or inattention/daze
  Feeling of numbness, constricted affect
  Feeling detached/alienated
  Reduced interest in significant activities
  Rigid role adherence or stereotyped behavior
Altered lifestyle
  Submissiveness, passiveness, or dependency
  Self-destructiveness (*e.g.*, alcohol/drug abuse, suicide at-
    tempts, reckless driving, illegal activities)
  Thrill-seeking activities
  Difficulty with interpersonal relationships
  Development of phobia regarding trauma
  Avoidance of situations or activities that arouse recollec-
    tion of the trauma
  Social isolation/withdrawal, negative self-concept
  Sleep disturbances, emotional disturbances
  Irritability, poor impulse control, or explosiveness
  Loss of faith in people or the world/feeling of meaningless-
    ness in life
  Feeling of not achieving normally expected life goals

Sense of foreshortened future or disturbance in orientation
of the future
Chronic anxiety or chronic depression
Somatic preoccupation/multiple physiological symptoms

RELATED FACTORS

Situational (Personal, Environmental)

Related to traumatic events of natural origin, including:

Floods	Epidemics (may be of
Earthquakes	human origin)
Volcanic eruptions	Other natural disasters,
Storms	which are overwhelming
Avalanches	to most people

Related to traumatic events of human origin, such as:

Wars	Concentration camp
Airplane crashes	confinement
Serious car accidents	Torture
Large fires	Assault
Bombing	Rape

Related to industrial disasters (nuclear, chemical, or other life-threatening accidents)

OUTCOME CRITERIA

Short-Term

The person will:

1. Report a lessening of reexperiencing numbing symptoms
2. Acknowledge the traumatic event and begin to work with the trauma by talking about the experience and expressing feelings, such as fear, anger, and guilt
3. Identify and make connection with support persons/resources

Long-Term

The person will:

1. Assimilate the experience into a meaningful whole and go on to pursue his or her life as evidenced by goal setting

The child will:

1. Describe the event.
2. Share feelings concerning the event.

⬢ GENERIC INTERVENTIONS

1. In a quiet room, explore with person what happened. If person is too anxious, discontinue assessment.
2. Communicate to the person that you are sorry that this happened, they are not to blame, you are glad they are alive, and they are safe here (Smith, 1987).
3. Assist the person to decrease extremes of reexperiencing or numbing symptoms.
   a. Provide a safe, therapeutic environment where the person can regain control.
   b. Stay with the person, and offer support during an episode of high anxiety.
   c. Assist the person to control impulsive acting-out behavior by setting limits, promoting ventilation, and redirecting excess energy into physical exercise activity (*e.g.*, going to the gym, walking, jogging).
4. Reassure the person that these feelings/symptoms are often experienced by individuals who underwent such traumatic events.
5. Assist person to acknowledge the traumatic event and begin to work through the trauma by talking about the experience and expressing feelings, such as fear, anger, and guilt.
6. Assist individual to make connections with support and resources according to his or her needs.
7. Encourage person to resume old activities and begin some new ones.
8. Assist family/significant others to understand what is happening to the victim.
   a. Encourage ventilation of their feelings.
   b. Provide counseling sessions, or link person with appropriate community resources as necessary.
9. Explain to person and significant others:
   a. Flashbacks, nightmares
   b. Avoidance behavior
   c. Detached behavior
   d. Hypervigilance
   e. Exaggerated startle reflex
   f. Angry outbursts
10. Provide or arrange follow-up treatment where person/family can continue to work through the trauma and integrate the experience into new ego synthesis.

🎗 CHILD FOCUS INTERVENTIONS

1. Assist child to understand and integrate the experience in accordance with their developmental stage.
   a. Assist to describe the experience and to express feelings (*e.g.*, fear, guilt, rage) in safe, supportive places, such as play therapy sessions.
   b. Provide accurate information and explanations to the child in terms child can understand.
   c. Provide family counseling to promote family members' understanding of the child's needs.
2. Assist family/significant others:
   a. Assist them to understand what is happening to the child.
   b. Encourage ventilation of their feelings.
   c. Provide family counseling and/or link them with appropriate community resources, as necessary.

Post-Trauma Response, Risk for

DEFINITION

Risk for Post-Trauma Response: A state in which the individual is at risk to experience a sustained painful response to one or more overwhelming traumatic events that have not been assimilated.

RISK FACTORS

Refer to Related Factors in *Post-Trauma Response*.

OUTCOME CRITERIA

The person will:

1. Identify signs or symptoms that necessitate professional consultation.
2. Continue to function appropriately after the traumatic event.

INTERVENTIONS

Refer to *Post-Trauma Syndrome.*

Rape-Trauma Syndrome

DEFINITION

Rape-Trauma Syndrome: The state in which an individual experiences a forced, violent sexual assault (vaginal or anal penetration) against his or her will and without his or her consent. The trauma syndrome that develops from this attack or attempted attack includes an acute phase of disorganization of the victim and family's lifestyle and a long-term process of reorganization of lifestyle (Holmstrom & Burgess, 1975).

DEFINING CHARACTERISTICS

Major (Must Be Present)

Reports or evidence of sexual assault

Minor (May Be Present)

If the victim is a child, parent(s) may experience similar responses.

    Acute phase
        Somatic responses
        Gastrointestinal irritability (nausea, vomiting, anorexia)
        Genitourinary discomfort (pain, pruritus)
        Skeletal muscle tension (spasms, pain)
    Psychological responses
        Denial
        Emotional shock
        Anger
        Fear of being alone or that the rapist will return (a child
            victim will fear punishment, repercussions, abandonment,
            rejection)
        Guilt
        Panic on seeing assailant or scene of attack
    Sexual responses
        Mistrust of men (if victim is a woman)
        Change in sexual behavior

Long-term phase
Any response of the acute phase may continue if resolution does not occur.
Psychological responses
Phobias
Nightmares or sleep disturbances
Anxiety
Depression

OUTCOME CRITERIA

Short-Term

The person will:

1. Share feelings
2. Describe rationale and treatment procedures
3. Identify members of support system, and use them appropriately

Long-Term

The person will:

1. Return to precrisis level of functioning

The child will:

1. Discuss the assault
2. Express feelings concerning the assault and the treatment

The parent(s), spouse, or significant other will:

1. Discuss their response to the assault
2. Return to precrisis level of functioning

⬛ GENERIC INTERVENTIONS

1. Promote trusting relationship, and stay with person during acute stage or arrange for other support.
2. Communicate:
   a. They are safe here.
   b. It was not their fault.
   c. You are sorry this happened.
   d. You are glad they are alive.
3. Provide this analogy: "Every time you think you are responsible for this rape, think instead that you were hit

over the head with a shovel (*e.g.*, 'I would not have been hit over the head with a shovel if I didn't wear that dress, drink too much, kiss him, walk home . . .'). This may help effect the realization that this was a crime of violence and control, not sex."

4. Explain the care and examination she or he will experience.
   a. Conduct the examinations in an unhurried manner.
   b. Explain every detail before action.
   c. If this is the person's first pelvic examination, explain the position and the instruments.
   d. Discuss the possibility of pregnancy and a sexually transmitted disease and treatments available.

5. Explain the legal issues and police investigation (Heinrich, 1987).
   a. Explain the need to collect specimens for future possible court use.
   b. Explain that the choice to report the rape is the victim's.
   c. If the police interview is permitted:
      • Negotiate with victim and police for an advantageous time.
      • Explain to victim what kind of questions will be asked.
      • Remain with the victim during the interview; do not ask questions or offer answers.

6. Record presence and location of bruises, lacerations, edema, or abrasion.

7. Whenever possible, provide crisis counseling within 1 hour of rape-trauma event.

8. Before person leaves hospital, provide card with information about follow-up appointments and names and telephone numbers of local crisis and counseling centers.

9. Encourage person to recognize positive responses or support from sexual partner or members of opposite sex.

CHILD FOCUS INTERVENTIONS

1. Addressing the child's developmental level, elicit the child's reaction.

2. Explain what happened. Reinforce that the child did not deserve this.

3. Use play therapy with puppets or dolls with genitalia.

4. Evaluate the risk for suicide, especially in adolescent boys.
5. For adolescents:
    a. Educate the individual and family that rape is a violent crime.
    b. Discourage focusing on what if . . . I should have . . . .
    c. Discourage violent, destructive, or irrational retribution toward rapist.
    d. Help family to be supportive of individual.
6. Refer child and caregivers for counseling.

Powerlessness

DEFINITION

Powerlessness: The state in which an individual or group perceives a lack of personal control over certain events or situations, which impacts outlook, goals, and lifestyle.

Author's Note:
Most individuals are subject to feelings of powerlessness in varying degrees in various situations. This diagnosis can be used to describe individuals who respond to loss of control with apathy, anger, or depression. Prolonged states of powerlessness may lead to hopelessness.

DEFINING CHARACTERISTICS

Major (Must Be Present)

Overt or covert expressions of dissatisfaction about inability to control situation (*e.g.*, work, illness, prognosis, care, recovery rate) that is negatively impacting outlook, goals, and lifestyle

Minor (May Be Present)

Apathy	Uneasiness
Anger	Resignation
Violent behavior	Acting-out behavior
Anxiety	Depression
Unsatisfactory dependence on others	Passivity

RELATED FACTORS

Pathophysiological

Any disease process—acute or chronic—can contribute to powerlessness. Some common sources are the following:

Related to inability to communicate secondary to:
Cerebrovascular accident
Guillain-Barré syndrome
Intubation

Related to inability to perform activities of daily living secondary to: cerebrovascular accident, cervical trauma, myocardial infarction, or pain

Related to inability to perform role responsibilities secondary to: surgery, trauma, or arthritis

Related to progressive debilitating disease secondary to: for example, multiple sclerosis, terminal cancer, AIDS

Related to substance abuse

Situational (Personal, Environmental)

Related to feeling of loss of control and lifestyle restrictions secondary to (specify)

Related to change from curative status to palliative status

Related to overeating patterns

Related to personal characteristics that highly value control (*e.g.*, internal locus of control)

Related to effects of hospital or institutional limitations

Related to lifestyle of helplessness

Related to fear of disapproval

Related to unmet dependency needs

Related to consistent negative feedback

Related to long-term abusive relationship

Maturational

Parents of adolescent children
Related to child rearing problems

Older adult
  Related to multiple losses secondary to aging, *e.g.*, retirement, sensory deficits, motor deficits, financial status, or significant others

OUTCOME CRITERIA

The person will:

1. Identify factors that can be controlled by self
2. Make decisions regarding own care, treatment, and future when possible

◆ GENERIC INTERVENTIONS

1. Explore the effects of condition on
   a. Occupation
   b. Leisure activities
   c. Role responsibilities
   d. Relationships
2. Allow to share losses (*e.g.*, independence, roles, income).
3. Assist to not see self as helpless. Help person to identify personal strengths and assets.
4. Explain all procedures, rules, and options to person. Allow time to answer questions; ask person to write questions down so as not to forget them.
5. Keep person informed about condition, treatments, and results.
6. Anticipate questions/interest, and offer information.
7. While being realistic, point out positive changes in person's condition.
8. Provide opportunities for individual to control decisions.
9. Allow person to manipulate surroundings, such as deciding what is to be kept where (shoes under bed, picture on window).
10. Record person's specific choices on care plan to ensure that others on staff acknowledge preferences ("Dislikes orange juice." "Takes showers." "Plan dressing change at 7:30 prior to shower.").
11. Provide daily recognition of progress.
12. For the person with chronic helplessness:
    a. Encourage to take responsibility for self-care.
    b. Assist to set realistic goals.

   c. Help to differentiate areas of life that she or he can and cannot control.
   d. Provide opportunities for person to be successful.

🌀 CHILD FOCUS INTERVENTIONS

1. Explore with child perceptions of the situation.
2. Use play therapy to help gain mastery of stressful situations.
3. Encourage personal possessions.
4. Explain all procedures. Allow the child some aspect of control or choices.
5. Actively encourage child to ask questions.
6. If possible, elicit information from the child rather than parent or caregiver.

🏛 OLDER ADULT FOCUS INTERVENTIONS

1. Involve in discussing plans and options early.
2. Provide time to adjust to changes.
3. Listen carefully to person's perceptions of the situation.

Protection, Altered

DEFINITION

Altered Protection: The state in which an individual experiences a decrease in the ability to guard against internal or external threats, such as illness or injury.

Author's Note:
Altered Protection represents a broad diagnostic category under which several specific nursing diagnoses are clustered: Impaired Tissue Integrity, Altered Oral Mucous Membrane, and Impaired Skin Integrity. These diagnoses are more clinically useful than Altered Protection.

(Continued)

Author's Note (Continued):
   The nurse should be cautioned concerning the substitution of Altered Protection as a new name for compromised immune system, AIDS, disseminated intravascular coagulation, diabetes mellitus, etc. The nurse should focus on the functional abilities of the individual that are or may be compromised because of altered protection, such as Fatigue, Risk for Infection, Risk for Social Isolation. The nurse should also focus on the physiological complications of altered protection that require nursing and medical interventions for management (*i.e.*, collaborative problems, such as Potential Complication: Thrombocytopenia or Potential Complication: Sepsis).

DEFINING CHARACTERISTICS

Major

Deficient immunity
Impaired healing
Altered clotting
Maladaptive stress response
Neurosensory alterations

Minor

Chilling
Perspiring
Dyspnea
Insomnia
Fatigue
Anorexia
Weakness

Cough
Itching
Restlessness
Immobility
Disorientation
Pressure sores

Tissue Integrity, Impaired

Skin Integrity, Impaired

Skin Integrity, Impaired, Risk for

Oral Mucous Membrane, Altered

Tissue Integrity, Impaired

DEFINITION

Impaired Tissue Integrity: The state in which an individual experiences or is at risk for altered integumentary, corneal, or mucous membranous tissues of the body.

Author's Note:

Impaired Tissue Integrity is the broad category under which the more specific nursing diagnoses of Impaired Skin Integrity and Altered Oral Mucous Membranes fall. Because tissue is composed of epithelium and connective muscle and nervous tissue, Impaired Tissue Integrity correctly describes some pressure ulcers that are deeper than dermal. Impaired Skin Integrity should be used to describe potential or actual disruptions of epidermal and dermal tissue only.

When a pressure ulcer is stage IV, necrotic, or infected, it may be more appropriate to label the diagnosis a collaborative problem as Potential Complication: Stage IV pressure ulcer. This would represent a situation a nurse manages with physician- and nurse-prescribed interventions. When a stage II or III pressure ulcer needs a dressing that requires a physician's order in an acute care setting, the nurse should continue to label the situation a nursing diagnosis because other than hospital regulation, it would be appropriate and legal for a nurse to treat the ulcer independently (*e.g.*, in the community).

(Continued)

Author's Note (Continued):

   If an individual is at risk for damage to corneal tissue, the nurse can use the diagnosis Risk for Impaired Corneal Tissue Integrity related to, for example, corneal drying and reduced lacrimal production secondary to unconscious state. If an individual is immobile and multiple systems—respiratory, circulatory, musculoskeletal, and integumentary—are threatened, the nurse can use Disuse Syndrome to describe the entire situation.

DEFINING CHARACTERISTICS

Major (Must Be Present, One or More)

Disruptions of corneal, integumentary, or mucous membranous tissue or invasion of body structure (incision, dermal ulcer, corneal ulcer, oral lesion)

Minor (May Be Present)

Lesions (primary, secondary)   Dry mucous membrane
Edema   Leukoplakia
Erythema   Coated tongue

RELATED FACTORS

Pathophysiological

Related to inflammation of dermal–epidermal junctions secondary to:
   Autoimmune alterations
      Lupus erythematosus   Scleroderma
   Metabolic and endocrine alterations
      Diabetes mellitus   Jaundice
      Hepatitis   Cancer
      Cirrhosis   Thyroid dysfunction
      Renal failure
Bacterial (impetigo, folliculitis, cellulitis)
Viral (herpes zoster [shingles], herpes simplex, gingivitis, AIDS)
Fungal (ringworm [dermatophytosis], athlete's foot, vaginitis)

Related to decreased blood and nutrients to tissues secondary to:

Diabetes mellitus	
Peripheral vascular alterations	Anemia
Venous stasis	Cardiopulmonary disorders
Arteriosclerosis	
Hyperthermic	
Nutritional alterations	Edema
Obesity	Emaciation
Dehydration	Malnutrition

Treatment-Related

Related to decreased blood and nutrients to tissues secondary to: NPO status, therapeutic extremes in body temperature, or surgery

Related to imposed immobility related to sedation

Related to mechanical trauma (*e.g.*, therapeutic fixation devices, wired jaw, traction, casts, orthopedic devices/braces)

Related to effects of radiation on epithelial and basal cells

Related to effects of mechanical irritants or pressure secondary to:

Inflatable or foam "donuts"	External urinary catheters
Tourniquets	Nasogastric tubes
Foot boards	Endotracheal tubes
Restraints	Oral prostheses/braces
Dressings, tape, solutions	Contact lenses

Situational (Personal, Environmental)

Related to chemical trauma secondary to: excretions, secretions, or noxious agents/substances

Related to environmental irritants secondary to:

Radiation—sunburn	Bites (insect, animal)
Temperature	Inhalants
Humidity	Poisonous plants
Parasites	

Related to the effects of pressure or immobility secondary to pain, fatigue, motivation, cognitive, sensory, or motor deficits

Related to inadequate personal habits (hygiene, dental, dietary, sleep)

Related to impaired mobility secondary to (specify)

Related to thin body frame

Maturational

Older adult
Related to dry, thin skin and decreased dermal vascularity
secondary to aging

Skin Integrity, Impaired

DEFINITION

Impaired Skin Integrity: The state in which an individual experiences or is at risk for altered epidermis and/or dermis.

DEFINING CHARACTERISTICS

Major (Must Be Present)

Disruptions of epidermal and dermal tissue

Minor (May Be Present)

Denuded skin
Erythema
Lesions (primary, secondary)
Pruritus

RELATED FACTORS

See *Impaired Tissue Integrity*.

OUTCOME CRITERIA

The person will:

1. Identify causative factors for pressure ulcers
2. Identify rationale for prevention and treatment
3. Participate in the prescribed treatment plan to promote wound healing
4. Demonstrate progressive healing of dermal ulcer

⬖ GENERIC INTERVENTIONS

1. Identify the stage of pressure ulcer development.
   a. Stage I: Nonblanchable erythema of intact skin
   b. Stage II: Ulceration of epidermis or dermis
   c. Stage III: Ulceration involving subcutaneous fat

    d. Stage IV: Extensive ulceration penetrating muscle bone or supporting structure

2. Wash reddened area gently with a mild soap; rinse area thoroughly to remove soap, and pat dry.
3. Gently massage healthy skin around the affected area to stimulate circulation; do not massage if reddened.
4. Protect the healthy skin surface with one or a combination of the following:
   a. Apply a thin coat of liquid copolymer skin sealant.
   b. Cover area with moisture-permeable film dressing.
   c. Cover area with a hydrocolloid wafer barrier, and secure with strips of 1-in microscope tape; leave in place for 2 to 3 days.
5. Increase protein and carbohydrate intake to maintain a positive nitrogen balance; weigh the person daily, and determine serum albumin level weekly to monitor status.
6. Devise plan for pressure ulcer management using principles of moist wound healing.
   a. Assess status of pressure ulcer (color, odor, amount of drainage from wound and surrounding skin).
   b. Débride necrotic tissue (collaborate with physician).
   c. Flush ulcer base with sterile saline solution.
   d. Protect granulating wound bed from trauma.
   e. Cover pressure ulcer with a sterile dressing that maintains a moist environment over the ulcer base (*e.g.*, film dressing, hydrocolloid wafer dressing, moist gauze dressing).
   f. Avoid the use of drying agents (heat lamps, magnesium hydroxide [Maalox], Milk of Magnesia).
   g. Monitor for clinical signs of wound infection.
7. Consult with nurse specialist or physician for treatment of stage IV pressure ulcers.
8. Refer to community nursing agency if additional assistance at home is needed.

Risk for Impaired Skin Integrity

DEFINITION

Refer to *Impaired Skin Integrity.*

RISK FACTORS

Refer to Related Factors—*Impaired Skin Integrity.*

OUTCOME CRITERIA

The person will:

1. Express willingness to participate in prevention of pressure ulcers
2. Describe causes and prevention measures
3. Demonstrate skin integrity free of pressure ulcers

⊞ GENERIC INTERVENTIONS

1. Maintain sufficient fluid intake for adequate hydration (approximately 2500 mL daily, unless contraindicated); check mucous membranes in mouth for moisture, and check urine-specific gravity.
2. Establish a schedule for emptying bladder (begin with every 2 hours). If person is confused, determine what incontinence pattern is, and intervene before incontinence occurs. Explain problem to individual, and secure cooperation for plan.
3. When incontinent, wash perineum with a liquid soap that will not alter skin pH, and apply a protective barrier to the perineal region (incontinence film barrier spray or wipes).
4. Encourage ROM exercises and weight-bearing mobility, when possible.
5. Turn or instruct person to turn or shift weight every 30 minutes to 2 hours, depending on other causative factors present and the ability of the skin to recover from pressure.
6. Frequency of turning schedule should be increased if any reddened areas that appear do not disappear within 1 hour after turning.
7. Keep bed as flat as possible to reduce shearing forces; limit Fowler's position to only 30 minutes at a time.
8. Use enough personnel to lift person up in bed or chair rather than pull or slide skin surfaces.
9. Instruct person to lift self using chair arms every 10 minutes if possible or assist person in rising up off the chair every 10 to 20 minutes, depending on risk factors present.
10. Observe for erythema and blanching, and palpate for warmth and tissue sponginess with each position change.
11. Do not rub reddened areas or over bony prominences.
12. Increase protein and carbohydrate intake to maintain a positive nitrogen balance; weigh the person daily, and determine serum albumin level weekly to monitor status.
13. Instruct person and family in specific techniques to use at home to prevent pressure ulcers.

🏛 OLDER ADULT FOCUS INTERVENTIONS

1. Explain high-risk age-related factors.
   a. Decreased subcutaneous fat
   b. Drier skin, decreased elasticity
   c. Slowed rate of dermal healing
   d. Decreased skin strength (loss of collagen)
   e. Proteins, vitamins, and mineral deficiencies
   f. Immobility
   g. Urinary or bowel incontinence

Oral Mucous Membrane, Altered

DEFINITION

Altered Oral Mucous Membrane: The state in which an individual experiences or is at risk of experiencing disruptions in the oral cavity.

DEFINING CHARACTERISTICS

Major (Must Be Present)

Disrupted oral mucous membranes

Minor (May Be Present)

Coated tongue	Leukoplakia
Xerostomia (dry mouth)	Edema
Stomatitis	Hemorrhagic gingivitis
Oral tumors	Purulent drainage
Oral lesions	

RELATED FACTORS

Pathophysiological

Related to inflammation secondary to:
Diabetes mellitus	Periodontal disease
Oral cancer	Infection

Treatment-Related

Related to drying effects of:
    NPO status for 24 hours
    Radiation to head or neck
    Prolonged use of steroids or other immunosuppressives
    Use of antineoplastic drugs
Related to mechanical irritation secondary to: endotracheal or nasogastric intubation

Situational (Personal, Environmental)

Related to chemical irritants secondary to: acidic foods, drugs, noxious agents, alcohol, or tobacco
Related to mechanical trauma secondary to: broken or jagged teeth, ill-fitting dentures, braces
Related to malnutrition
Related to dehydration
Related to mouth breathing
Related to inadequate oral hygiene
Related to lack of knowledge of oral hygiene
Related to decreased salivation

OUTCOME CRITERIA

The person will:

1. Demonstrate integrity of the oral cavity
2. Be free of oral discomfort during food and fluid intake
3. Demonstrate knowledge of optional oral hygiene

⊞ GENERIC INTERVENTIONS

1. Discuss the importance of daily oral hygiene and periodic dental examinations.
2. Evaluate the person's ability to perform oral hygiene.
3. Teach correct oral care.
   a. Remove and clean dentures and bridges daily.
   b. Floss teeth (every 24 hours).
   c. Brush teeth (after meals and before sleep).
   d. Inspect mouth for lesions, sores, or excessive bleeding.
4. Perform oral hygiene on person who is unconscious or at risk for aspiration as often as needed.

5. Teach preventive oral hygiene to individuals at risk of developing stomatitis.
    a. Perform the regimen after meals and before sleep (if there is excessive exudate, also perform regimen before breakfast).
    b. Floss teeth only once in 24 hours.
    c. Omit flossing if excessive bleeding occurs, and use extreme caution with persons with platelet counts of less than 50,000.
    d. Avoid mouthwashes with high alcohol content, lemon/glycerine swabs, or prolonged use of hydrogen peroxide.
    e. Use an oxidizing agent to loosen thick, tenacious mucus (gargle and expectorate), for example, hydrogen peroxide and water quarter strength (avoid prolonged use) or sodium bicarbonate 1 teaspoon in 8 oz warm water (can flavor these with mouthwash or one drop of oil of wintergreen).
    f. Rinse mouth with saline solution after gargling.
    g. Apply lubricant to lips every 2 hours and as needed (*e.g.*, lanolin, A&D ointment, petroleum jelly).

6. For person who is unable to tolerate brushing or swabbing, teach to irrigate mouth (every 2 hours and as needed).
    a. With baking soda solution (4 teaspoons in 1 L warm water) using an enema bag (labeled for oral use only) with a soft irrigation catheter tip
    b. By placing catheter tip in mouth and slowly increasing flow while standing over a basin or having a basin held under chin
    c. Removing dentures before irrigation and not replacing in person with severe stomatitis

7. Inspect oral cavity three times daily with tongue blade and light; if stomatitis is severe, inspect mouth every 4 hours. Teach client to inspect mouth.

8. Ensure that oral hygiene regimen is done every 2 hours while awake and every 6 hours (4 if severe) during the night.

9. Instruct individual to:
    a. Avoid commercial mouthwashes, citrus fruit juices, spicy foods, extremes in food temperature (hot, cold), crusty or rough foods, alcohol, mouthwashes with alcohol.

      b. Eat bland, cool foods (sherbets).

      c. Drink cool liquids every 2 hours and as needed.

10. Consult with physician or advanced practice nurse for an oral pain-relief solution.

      a. Use lidocaine (Xylocaine Viscous) 2% oral swish and expectorant every 2 hours and before meals (if throat is sore, the solution can be swallowed; if swallowed, lidocaine produces local anesthesia and may affect the gag reflex).

      b. Mix equal parts of lidocaine, 0.5 aqueous diphenhydramine (Benadryl) solution, and magnesium hydroxide; swish and swallow 1 oz of mixture every 2 to 4 hours as needed.

      c. Mix equal parts of 0.5 aqueous diphenhydramine solution and kaolin (Kaopectate); swish and swallow every 2 to 4 hours as needed.

11. Teach person and family the factors that contribute to the development and progression of stomatitis.

12. Have individual describe or demonstrate home care regimen.

🌀 CHILD FOCUS INTERVENTIONS

1. If thrush (oral candidiasis) is present:

      a. Rinse mouth with plain water after each feeding.

      b. Boil nipples and bottles for at least 20 minutes.

      c. Boil pacifiers once a day.

      d. Apply topical medication as prescribed.

2. Explain the need to teach 2 year olds how to brush their teeth after meals and before bedtime.

3. Encourage parent to have toddler accompany him or her to dentist office to meet personnel.

4. Discuss the importance of routine dental examinations every 6 months beginning at 3 to 4 years old.

🌀 MATERNAL FOCUS INTERVENTIONS

1. Stress the importance good oral hygiene and continuance of dental examinations.

2. Remind to advise dentist of pregnancy.

3. Explain that gum hypertrophy and tenderness are normal during pregnancy.

OLDER ADULT FOCUS INTERVENTIONS

1. Explain high-risk age-related factors (Miller, 1999):
    a. Degenerative bone disease
    b. Diminished oral blood supply
    c. Dry mouth
    d. Vitamin deficiencies
2. Explain that some medications cause dry mouth.
    a. Laxatives
    b. Antibiotics
    c. Antidepressants
    d. Analgesics
    e. Iron sulfate
    f. Cardiovascular
    g. Anticholinergics
3. Determine the presence of barriers to dental care.
    a. Financial
    b. Mobility
    c. Dexterity
    d. Lack of knowledge

Relocation Stress (Syndrome)

DEFINITION

Relocation Stress (Syndrome): A state in which an individual experiences physiological and/or psychological disturbances as a result of transfer from one environment to another.

Author's Note:

Relocation represents a disruption for all individuals involved. It can occur with a transfer from one unit to another or from one facility to another. It can involve a permanent move to a long-term care facility or to a new home. All age groups involved are disturbed by the relocation. When physiological and psychological disturbances compromise functioning, the nursing diagnosis Relocation Stress (Syndrome) is appropriate.

(Continued)

Author's Note (Continued):

The most optimal nursing approach to relocation stress is to initiate preventive measures, using Risk for Relocation Stress as the diagnosis.

This diagnosis has been accepted by NANDA as a syndrome diagnosis. Relocation Stress as a syndrome diagnosis does not fit the criteria for a syndrome diagnosis, which is a cluster of actual or high-risk nursing diagnoses as defining characteristics. The defining characteristics associated with Relocation Stress are observable or reportable cues consistent with Relocation Stress, not Relocation Stress Syndrome. The author recommends deleting syndrome from the label.

Other terms found in the literature that describe relocation stress include: admission stress, postrelocation crisis, relocation crisis, relocation shock, relocation trauma, transfer stress, transfer trauma, translocation syndrome, and transplantation shock.

DEFINING CHARACTERISTICS
(Harkulich & Brugler, 1988)

Major (80%–100%)

Responds to transfer or relocation with:
Loneliness
Apprehension
Depression
Anxiety
Increased confusion (older adult population)

Minor (50%–79%)

Change in former eating habits
Change in former sleep patterns
Demonstration of dependency
Demonstration of insecurity
Demonstration of lack of trust
Gastrointestinal disturbances
Increased verbalization of needs
Need for excessive reassurance
Restlessness
Sad affect
Unfavorable comparison of post-transfer to pretransfer staff

Verbalization of being concerned/upset about transfer
Verbalization of insecurity in new living situation
Vigilance
Weight change
Withdrawal

RELATED FACTORS

Pathophysiological

Related to compromised ability to adapt to changes secondary to:
    (Decreased physical health status)
        Physical difficulties
    (Decreased psychosocial health status)
        Increased/perceived stress before relocation
        Depression
        Decreased self-esteem

Situational (Personal, Environmental)

Related to moderate to high degree of environmental change secondary to:
    Decreased control of individual care
    Decrease and/or change in available caregivers
    Decrease/increase in patient monitoring equipment
    Physical differences between the two environments
    Increased noise/activities in post-transfer environment
    Inconsistencies in care
    Decreased privacy changes in lifestyle
    Loss of privacy
Related to negative history with previous transfers secondary to:
    Involuntary move(s)
    Frequent moves within short time spans
    Transfers occurring at evening/nights
Related to concurrent, recent, and past interpersonal losses secondary to:
    Negative experiences dealing with earlier separation(s) (for adults as well as children)
    Loss of social and familial ties
    Abandonment
    Perceived/actual rejection by caregivers
    Anticipation of lengthy and/or permanent stay in new environment
    Threat to financial security
    Change in relationship with family members

Related to little or no preparation for the impending move
Lack of predictability in new environment
Little or no time between when an individual is notified of an impending move and the actual move
Unrealistic expectations of individual/family members regarding facility and staff
Lack of decision making and control on behalf of the person who is moving

Maturational

School-age and adolescents
Related to losses associated with moving secondary to fear of rejection, loss of peer group, or school-related problems
Decreased security in new adolescent peer group and school

OUTCOME CRITERIA

The person will:

1. Voice concerns about the move to a new environment
2. Participate in decision-making activities concerning the new environment
3. Become involved in activities in the new environment

⮂ GENERIC INTERVENTIONS

1. Reduce environmental differences between old and new settings; promote continuity of care in new environment.
   a. Maintain person on same activity level and diet through pretransfer and post-transfer units.
   b. Transfer person to similar, proximal area when possible.
   c. Wean any monitoring equipment gradually before transfer.
   d. Transfer all personal items (*e.g.*, mobility aids, eyeglasses, hearing aids, dentures, prostheses, and belongings) with the person.
   e. Transfer person during daytime hours.
2. Offer person decision-making opportunities throughout relocation experience.
3. Promote person's input about new environment when possible, such as use of decorations and arrangement of furniture.
4. Encourage family members to share their perceptions of relocation with each other.

5. Offer the person help in maintaining contact with significant others by telephone calls, writing letters, and visits with previous roommates when applicable.
6. Provide follow-up visit with nurse from pretransfer unit to person on post-transfer unit.
7. Retain highly anxious person in pretransfer unit until anxiety decreases, when possible.
8. Identify individuals at high risk for selected physiological responses.
   a. Musculoskeletal/neurological deficits
   b. Advanced age
   c. Infections
   d. Changes in orientation
   e. Cardiovascular deficits
9. Assess vital signs and level of orientation prior to relocation.

🐟 CHILD FOCUS INTERVENTIONS

1. Teach parents technique to assist their child(ren) with the move.
   a. Remain positive about the move before, during, and after with the acceptance that the child may not be optimistic.
   b. Instruct parents to explore various options with their children on how to communicate with friends/families in previous environment.
   c. Keep regular routines in the new environment.
   d. Acknowledge the difficulty of peer losses with the adolescent.
   e. Access the organizations to which the child previously belonged (*e.g.*, Girl Scouts, sports).
   f. Plan a trip to school during a class and lunch period to reduce fear of unknown.
   g. Ask teacher or counselor at new school to introduce child to a student who recently relocated to that school.

🏛 OLDER ADULT FOCUS INTERVENTIONS

1. Promote integration after transfer into a long-term care nursing facility.
   a. Allow as many choices as possible.
   b. Encourage person to bring familiar objects from home.
   c. Encourage person to interact with other individuals in new facility.

317

d. Assist person to maintain previous interpersonal relationships.

Respiratory Function, Risk for Altered*

Dysfunctional Ventilatory Weaning Response

Dysfunctional Ventilatory Weaning Response, Risk for

Ineffective Airway Clearance

Ineffective Breathing Patterns

Impaired Gas Exchange

Inability to Sustain Spontaneous Ventilation

Respiratory Function, Risk for Altered

DEFINITION

Risk for Altered Respiratory Function (ARF): The state in which an individual is at risk of experiencing a threat to the passage of air through the respiratory tract and to the exchange of gases (O_2–CO_2) between the lungs and vascular system.

*This diagnosis is not currently on the NANDA list but has been included for clarity or usefulness.

Author's Note:

This diagnosis has been added by the author to describe a state in which the entire respiratory system may be affected, not just isolated areas, such as airway clearance or gas exchange. Smoking, allergy, and immobility are examples of factors that affect the entire system and thus make it incorrect to use Impaired Gas Exchange related to immobility, because immobility also affects airway clearance and breathing patterns. It is advised that Risk for Altered Respiratory Function not be used to describe an actual problem, which is a collaborative problem—not a nursing diagnosis.

The diagnoses Ineffective Airway Clearance and Ineffective Breathing Patterns can be used when the nurse can definitively alter the contributing factors that are influencing respiratory function, for example, ineffective cough, immobility, or stress. The nurse is cautioned not to use this diagnosis to describe acute respiratory disorders, which are the primary responsibility of physicians and nurses together (*i.e.*, a collaborative problem). This can be labeled Potential Complication: Hypoxemia or Potential Complication: Pulmonary edema.

RISK FACTORS

Presence of risk factors that can change respiratory function (see Related Factors)

RELATED FACTORS

Pathophysiological

Related to excessive or thick secretions secondary to: infection, cystic fibrosis, or influenza

Related to immobility, stasis of secretions, and ineffective cough secondary to:

Diseases of the nervous system (*e.g.*, Guillain-Barré syndrome, multiple sclerosis, myasthenia gravis)

CNS depression/head trauma

Cerebrovascular accident (stroke)

Quadriplegia

Treatment-Related

Related to immobility secondary to: sedating effects of medications (specify): anesthesia, general or spinal

319

Related to suppressed cough reflex secondary to (specify):
Related to decreased oxygen in the inspired air

Situational (Personal, Environmental)

Related to immobility secondary to: surgery or trauma, pain,
fear, anxiety, fatigue, or perception/cognitive impairment
Related to extreme high or low humidity
Related to diminished ciliary cleansing mechanisms, inflammatory response, and increased production of mucus secondary to smoking, mouth breathing

OUTCOME CRITERIA

The person will:

1. Perform hourly deep-breathing exercises (sigh) and cough sessions as needed
2. Achieve maximum pulmonary function
3. Relate importance of daily pulmonary exercises

⬛ GENERIC INTERVENTIONS

1. Assess for optimal pain relief with minimal period of fatigue or respiratory depression.
2. Encourage ambulation as soon as consistent with plan of care.
3. If unable to walk, establish a regimen for being out of bed in a chair several times a day (*e.g.*, 1 hour after meals and 1 hour before bedtime).
4. Increase activity gradually, explaining that respiratory function will improve and dyspnea will decrease with practice.
5. Assist to reposition, turning frequently from side to side (hourly if possible).
6. Encourage deep-breathing and controlled-coughing exercises five times every hour.
7. Teach individual to use blow bottle or incentive spirometer every hour while awake (with severe neuromuscular impairment, the person may have to be awakened during the night as well).
8. Auscultate lung field every 8 hours; increase frequency if altered breath sounds are present.

🐞 CHILD FOCUS INTERVENTIONS

1. Observe for nasal flaring, retractions, or cyanosis.
2. Allow child to select the color of water in blow bottles.
3. Monitor intake, output, and urine-specific gravity.
4. Provide age-appropriate explanation for deep-breathing exercises.

Dysfunctional Ventilatory Weaning Response

DEFINITION

Dysfunctional Ventilatory Weaning Response (DVWR): A state in which an individual cannot adjust to lowered levels of mechanical ventilator support, which interrupts and prolongs the weaning process.

Author's Note:

DVWR is a specific diagnosis within the category of Risk for Altered Respiratory Function. Ineffective Airway Clearance, Ineffective Breathing Patterns, and Impaired Gas Exchange can also be encountered in the weaning situation, either as indicators of lack of weaning readiness or as factors related to the onset of DVWR. DVWR is a separate client state. Its distinctive etiologies and treatments arise from the process of separating the client from the mechanical ventilator.

DEFINING CHARACTERISTICS

DVWR is a progressive state, and experienced nurses have identified three levels of defining characteristics that can occur in response to weaning (Logan & Jenny, 1991).

Mild

Major (Must Be Present, One or More)

Restlessness
Slight increase in respiratory rate from baseline

Minor (May Be Present)

Expressed feelings of increased oxygen need, breathing discomfort, fatigue, warmth

Queries about possible machine dysfunction

Increased concentration on breathing

Moderate

Major (Must Be Present, One or More)

Slight increase in blood pressure <20 mm Hg or less from baseline

Slight increase in heart rate <20 beats/min or less from baseline

Increase in respiratory rate <5 breaths per minute or less from baseline

Minor (May Be Present)

Hypervigilance to activities

Inability to respond to coaching

Inability to cooperate

Apprehension

Diaphoresis

Eye-widening (wide-eyed look)

Decreased air entry heard on auscultation

Skin color changes: pale, slight cyanosis

Slight respiratory accessory muscle use

Severe

Major (Must Be Present, One or More)

Agitation

Significant deterioration in arterial blood gases from baseline

Increase in blood pressure >20 mm Hg from baseline

Increase in heart rate >20 beats/min from baseline

Rapid, shallow breathing >25 breaths per minute

Minor (May Be Present)

Full respiratory accessory muscle use

Shallow, gasping breaths

Paradoxical abdominal breathing

Adventitious breath sounds

Cyanosis
Profuse diaphoresis
Discoordinated breathing with the ventilator
Decreased level of consciousness

RELATED FACTORS

Pathophysiological

Related to muscle weakness and fatigue secondary to:
  Unstable hemodynamic status
  Decreased level of consciousness
  Anemia
  Infection
  Metabolic abnormalities or acid–base imbalance
  Fluid or electrolyte imbalance
  Severe disease process
  Chronic respiratory disease
  Chronic neuromuscular disability
  Multisystem disease
  Chronic nutritional deficit
  Debilitated condition
Related to ineffective airway clearance

Treatment-Related

Related to obstructed airway
Related to muscle weakness and fatigue secondary to:
  Excess sedation, analgesia
  Uncontrolled pain
Related to inadequate nutrition (deficit in calories, excess carbohydrates, inadequate fat and protein intake)
Related to prolonged ventilator dependence (>1 week)
Related to previous unsuccessful ventilator weaning attempt(s)
Related to too-rapid pacing of the weaning process

Situational (Personal, Environmental)

Related to insufficient knowledge of the weaning process
Related to excessive energy demands (self-care activities, diagnostic and treatment procedures, visitors)
Related to inadequate social support
Related to insecure environment (noisy, upsetting events, busy room)

Related to fatigue secondary to interrupted sleep patterns
Related to inadequate self-efficacy
Related to moderate to high anxiety related to breathing efforts
Related to fear of separation from ventilator
Related to feelings of powerlessness
Related to feelings of hopelessness

OUTCOME CRITERIA

The person will:

1. Achieve progressive weaning goals
2. Remain extubated *or*
3. Demonstrate a positive attitude toward the next weaning trial: collaborate willingly with the weaning plan, communicate comfort status during the weaning process, attempt to control the breathing pattern, and try to control emotional responses
4. Be tired from the work of weaning but not exhausted

⬧ GENERIC INTERVENTIONS

1. If applicable, assess causative factors for previous unsuccessful weaning attempts.
   a. Inadequate energy substrates: oxygen, nutrition, and rest
   b. Inadequate comfort status
   c. Excessive activity demands
   d. Decreased self-esteem, confidence, feelings of control
   e. Lack of knowledge of their role in weaning
   f. Lack of trust relationship with staff
   g. Negative emotional state
   h. Adverse weaning environment
2. Determine readiness for weaning (Geisman, 1989).
   a. Oxygen concentration of 50% or less on the ventilator
   b. Positive end-expiratory pressure less than 5 cm of water pressure
   c. Respiratory rate less than 30 breaths per minute
   d. Minute ventilation of less than 10 L/min
   e. Low dynamic and static pressures, with compliance of at least 35 cm of water pressure
   f. Adequate respiratory muscle strength

      g. Rested, controlled discomfort

      h. Willingness to try weaning

3. If readiness for weaning is determined to be present, engage client in establishing the plan.

      a. Explain the weaning process.

      b. Jointly negotiate progressive weaning goals.

      c. Explain that these goals will be reexamined daily with the individual.

4. Refer to unit protocols for specific weaning procedures.

5. Explain client's role in the weaning process.

6. Strengthen feelings of self-esteem, self-efficacy, and control.

7. Demonstrate confidence in client's ability to wean.

8. Maintain client's confidence by adopting a weaning pace (may require a doctor's order) that will ensure success and minimize setbacks.

9. Promote trust in the staff and environment.

10. Reduce negative effects of anxiety and fatigue.

      a. Monitor status frequently to avoid undue fatigue and anxiety.

      b. Provide regular periods of rest before fatigue is advanced.

      c. If the individual is starting to get agitated, talk him or her down while remaining at the bedside.

      d. If weaning trial is discontinued, address person's perceptions of weaning failure. Reassure him or her that the trial was good exercise and a useful form of training.

11. Create a positive weaning environment, which increases the person's feelings of security.

12. Provide sufficient rest periods to prevent undue fatigue.

13. Coordinate necessary activities to promote adequate time for rest or relaxation.

14. Coordinate analgesia schedule with the weaning schedule.

15. Start weaning trial when the person is rested, usually in the morning after a night's sleep.

16. Discuss elements of the weaning process with other clinicians to maximize the probability of weaning success.

      a. Starting time

      b. Pace of the weaning

      c. Adherence to the care plan

      d. Diversional activities (*e.g.*, trips outside the unit)

      e. Scheduling of activities and rest periods

🌀 CHILD FOCUS INTERVENTIONS

1. Withhold oral feedings 2 hours before weaning attempts and after extubation.

Dysfunctional Ventilatory Weaning Response, Risk for

DEFINITION

Risk for Dysfunctional Ventilatory Weaning Response: The state in which an individual is at risk for experiencing an inability to adjust to lowered levels of mechanical ventilator support during the weaning process, related to physical or psychological unreadiness to wean.

RISK FACTORS

Pathophysiological

Related to airway obstruction
Related to muscle weakness and fatigue secondary to:
  Impaired respiratory functioning
  Unstable hemodynamic status
  Anemia
  Dysrhythmia
  Decreased level of consciousness
  Mental confusion
  Infection
  Fever
  Metabolic abnormalities
  Acid–base abnormalities
  Fluid or electrolyte imbalance
  Severe disease process
  Multisystem disease

Treatment-Related

Related to ineffective airway clearance
Related to excess sedation, analgesia
Related to uncontrolled pain
Related to fatigue

Related to inadequate nutrition (deficit in calories, excess carbohydrates, inadequate fat and protein intake)

Related to prolonged ventilator dependence of more than 1 week

Related to previous unsuccessful ventilator weaning attempt(s)

Related to too-rapid pacing of the weaning process

Situational (Personal, Environmental)

Related to muscle weakness and fatigue secondary to:
    Chronic nutritional deficit
    Obesity
    Ineffective sleep patterns

Related to knowledge deficit related to the weaning process

Related to inadequate self-efficacy related to weaning

Related to moderate to high anxiety related to breathing efforts

Related to fear of separation from ventilator

Related to feelings of powerlessness

Related to depressed mood

Related to feelings of hopelessness

Related to uncontrolled energy demands (self-care activities, diagnostic and treatment procedures, visitors)

Related to inadequate social support

Related to insecure environment (noisy, upsetting events, busy room)

OUTCOME CRITERIA

The person will:

1. Demonstrate a willingness to start weaning
2. Demonstrate a positive attitude about ability to succeed
3. Maintain emotional control
4. Collaborate with planning of the weaning

⊞ GENERIC INTERVENTIONS

1. Assess for causative and contributory factors of inadequate self-efficacy about weaning readiness.
   a. Verbalizes continued need for ventilator support
   b. Uses excuses for delaying the start of weaning
   c. Displays concern about ability to adjust to lowered level of ventilator support or about the probability of success of weaning
   d. Is agitated when weaning is mentioned
   e. Has elevated blood pressure, pulse, and respirations when weaning is discussed

2. Reduce risk factors.
   a. Negotiate with the medical staff for a delayed start and a weaning plan with a slow pace that ensures success at each stage.
   b. See *Dysfunctional Ventilatory Weaning Response.*

Ineffective Airway Clearance

DEFINITION

Ineffective Airway Clearance: The state in which an individual experiences a threat to respiratory status related to inability to cough effectively.

DEFINING CHARACTERISTICS

Major (Must Be Present, One or More)

Ineffective or absent cough
Inability to remove airway secretions

Minor (May Be Present)

Abnormal breath sounds
Abnormal respiratory rate, rhythm, depth

RELATED FACTORS

See *Risk for Altered Respiratory Function.*

OUTCOME CRITERIA

The person will:

1. Not experience aspiration
2. Demonstrate effective coughing and increased air exchange in the lungs

⬔ GENERIC INTERVENTIONS

1. Instruct person on the proper method of controlled coughing.
   a. Breathe deeply and slowly while sitting up as high as possible.

b. Use diaphragmatic breathing.
c. Hold breath for 3 to 5 seconds and then slowly exhale as much of this breath as possible through the mouth (lower rib cage and abdomen should sink down).
d. Take a second breath, hold, and cough forcefully from the chest (not from the back of the mouth or throat), using two short forceful coughs.

2. Assess present analgesic regimen.
   a. Assess its effectiveness: Is the individual too lethargic? Is the individual still in pain?

3. Initiate coughing when person appears to have best pain relief with optimal level of alertness and physical performance.

4. Splint abdominal or chest incisions with hand, pillow, or both.

5. Maintain adequate hydration (increase fluid intake to 2 to 3 quarts a day if not contraindicated by decreased cardiac output or renal disease).

6. Maintain adequate humidity of inspired air.

7. Plan for rest periods (after coughing, before meals).

8. Vigorously coach and encourage coughing, using positive reinforcement.

9. Proceed with health teaching with constant reinforcement in principles of care. Acknowledge and encourage good individual effort and progress.

❦ CHILD FOCUS INTERVENTIONS

1. Position to prevent aspiration.
2. Suction secretions from airway as needed.
3. Provide humidified atmosphere.

Ineffective Breathing Patterns

DEFINITION

Ineffective Breathing Patterns: The state in which an individual experiences an actual or potential loss of adequate ventilation related to an altered breathing pattern.

Author's Note:
This diagnosis has limited clinical utility except to describe situations that nurses definitively treat, such as hyperventilation. For individuals with chronic pulmonary disease with Ineffective Breathing Patterns, refer to Activity Intolerance. Individuals with periodic apnea and hypoventilation have a collaborative problem that can be labeled Potential Complication: Hypoxemia to indicate that the person is to be monitored for a variety of respiratory dysfunctions. If the person is more vulnerable to a specific respiratory complication, the collaborative problem can then be written as Potential Complication: Pneumonia or Potential Complication: Pulmonary embolism. Hyperventilation is a manifestation of anxiety or fear. The nurse can use Anxiety or Fear related to (specify event) as manifested by hyperventilation as a more descriptive diagnosis.

DEFINING CHARACTERISTICS

Major (Must Be Present, One or More)

Changes in respiratory rate or pattern (from baseline)
Changes in pulse (rate, rhythm, quality)

Minor (May Be Present)

Orthopnea
Tachypnea, hyperpnea, hyperventilation
Dysrhythmic respirations
Splinted/guarded respirations

RELATED FACTORS

See *Risk for Altered Respiratory Function.*

OUTCOME CRITERIA

The person will:

1. Demonstrate an effective respiratory rate and experience improved gas exchange in the lungs
2. Relate the causative factors, if known, and relate adaptive ways of coping with them

⬢ GENERIC INTERVENTIONS

For hyperventilation:

1. Reassure person that measures are being taken to ensure safety.
2. Distract person from thinking about anxious state by having person maintain eye contact with you. Say, "Now look at me and breathe slowly with me like this."
3. Consider use of paper bag as means of rebreathing expired air.
4. Stay with person, and coach in taking slower, more effective breaths.
5. Explain that one can learn to overcome hyperventilation through conscious control of breathing even when the cause is unknown.
6. Discuss possible causes, physical and emotional, and methods of coping effectively (see *Anxiety*).

⬢ CHILD FOCUS INTERVENTIONS

1. If child is prone to bronchospasm, medication may be indicated.

Impaired Gas Exchange

DEFINITION

Impaired Gas Exchange: The state in which an individual experiences an actual or potential decreased passage of gases (oxygen and carbon dioxide) between the alveoli of the lungs and the vascular system.

Author's Note:

This diagnosis does not represent a situation for which nurses prescribe definitive treatment. Nurses do not treat Impaired Gas Exchange, but nurses can treat the functional health patterns that decreased oxygenation can affect, such as activity, sleep, nutrition,

(Continued)

Author's Note (Continued):

and sexual function. Thus, Activity Intolerance related to insufficient oxygenation for activities of daily living better describes the nursing focus. If an individual is at risk or has experienced respiratory dysfunction, the nurse can describe the situation as Potential Complication: Respiratory or be even more specific with Potential Complication: Embolism.

DEFINING CHARACTERISTICS

Major (Must Be Present)

Dyspnea on exertion

Minor (May Be Present)

Confusion/agitation
Tendency to assume a three-point position (sitting, one hand on each knee, bending forward)
Pursed-lip breathing with prolonged expiratory phase
Lethargy and fatigue
Increased pulmonary vascular resistance (increased pulmonary artery/right ventricular pressure)
Decreased gastric motility, prolonged gastric emptying
Decreased oxygen content, decreased oxygen saturation, increased PCO_2, as measured by blood gas studies
Cyanosis

RELATED FACTORS

See *Risk for Altered Respiratory Function.*

Inability to Sustain Spontaneous Ventilation

DEFINITION

Inability to Sustain Spontaneous Ventilation: A state in which an individual is unable to maintain adequate breathing to support life. This is measured by deterioration of arterial blood gases, increased work of breathing, and decreasing energy.

Author's Note:
This diagnosis represents respiratory insufficiency with corresponding metabolic changes that are incompatible with life. This situation requires rapid nursing and medical management, specifically resuscitation and mechanical ventilation. Inability to sustain spontaneous ventilation is not appropriate as a nursing diagnosis—it is hypoxemia, a collaborative problem. Hypoxemia is insufficient plasma oxygen saturation due to alveolar hypoventilation, pulmonary shunting, or ventilation–perfusion inequality. As a collaborative problem, the definitive treatments are prescribed by physicians; however, both nursing and medical-prescribed interventions are required for management. The nursing accountability is to monitor status continuously and to manage changes in status with the appropriate interventions using protocols. (For interventions refer to Potential Complication: Hypoxemia in Section III in Carpenito, L.S. (1999). *Nursing Diagnosis: Application to Clinical Practice, 8th Edition*, Philadelphia, Lippincott-Raven.)

DEFINING CHARACTERISTICS

Major

Dyspnea

Increased metabolic rate

Minor

Increased restlessness
Apprehension
Increased use of accessory
  muscles
Decreased tidal volume

Increased heart rate
Decreased PO_2
Increased PCO_2
Decreased cooperation
Decreased SaO_2

Role Performance, Altered

DEFINITION

Altered Role Performance: The state in which an individual experiences or is at risk of experiencing a disruption in the way he or she perceives that his or her role performance matches norms or expectations.

Author's Note:

This nursing diagnosis had previously been a subcategory under Self-Concept Disturbance. The use of this diagnosis in its present state may prove problematic. If a woman were unable to continue her household responsibilities because of illness and these responsibilities were assumed by other family members, the situations that might arise would better be described as Risk for Self-Concept Disturbance related to recent loss of role responsibility secondary to illness and Risk for Impaired Home Maintenance Management related to lack of knowledge of family members. Until clinical research defines this diagnosis more definitively, use Altered Role Performance as a cause of Self-Concept Disturbance or Risk for Impaired Home Maintenance Management. If the role disturbance relates to parenting, Parental Role Conflict should be considered.

DEFINING CHARACTERISTICS

Major (Must Be Present)

Conflict related to role perception or performance

Minor (May Be Present)

Change in self-perception of role
Denial of role
Change in others' perception of role
Change in physical capacity to resume role
Lack of knowledge of role
Change in usual patterns of responsibility

Self-Care Deficit Syndrome*

Feeding Self-Care Deficit

Bathing/Hygiene Self-Care Deficit

Dressing/Grooming Self-Care Deficit

Toileting Self-Care Deficit

Instrumental Self-Care Deficit†

Self-Care Deficit Syndrome

DEFINITION

Self-Care Deficit Syndrome: The state in which the individual experiences an impaired motor function or cognitive function, causing a decreased ability to perform each of the five self-care activities.

> **Author's Note:**
> Self-care encompasses the activities needed to meet daily needs, usually called *activities of daily living.* Activities of daily living are learned and become life-long habits. Enmeshed in the
> *(Continued)*

---

*Hoskins, L. M. (1989). Self-care deficit. In G. McFarland & E. McFarlane (Eds.), *Nursing diagnosis and interventions.* St. Louis: C.V. Mosby.

†This diagnosis is not currently on the NANDA list but has been included for clarity or usefulness.

broad category of self-care activities are tasks that *are* to be done (hygiene, bathing, dressing, toileting, feeding), *how* these tasks are done, and *when, here, with whom* they are to be done. Self-Care Deficit Syndrome, not currently on the NANDA list, has been added to describe an individual with compromised ability in all five self-care activities. The nurse will assess functioning in each of the five areas and identify the level of participation of which the individual is capable. The goal will be to maintain that functioning or to increase participation and independence. The syndrome distinction will cluster all five self-care deficits together to provide clustering of interventions when indicated (*e.g.*, to ensure that the individual is wearing the corrective lenses required). It will also permit specialized interventions for one of the five activities (*e.g.*, to lay out clothes in the order in which they will be put on by the person).

The danger of Self-Care Deficit diagnoses is that the nurse could prematurely label an individual as unable to participate at any level. This would eliminate a rehabilitation focus. The nurse must classify the functional level of the client to promote independence.

DEFINING CHARACTERISTICS*

Major (One deficit must be present in each activity):

1. Self-feeding deficits
   a. Unable to cut food or open packages
   b. Unable to bring food to mouth
2. Self-bathing deficits (includes washing entire body, combing hair, brushing teeth, attending to skin and nail care, and applying makeup)
   a. Unable or unwilling to wash body or body parts
   b. Unable to obtain a water source

*Evaluate each of the activities of daily living using the following coding scale:

0 = Completely independent
1 = Requires use of assistive device
2 = Needs minimal help
3 = Needs assistance or some supervision
4 = Needs total supervision
5 = Needs total assistance or unable to assist

    c. Unable to regulate temperature or water flow

    d. Inability to perceive need for hygienic measures

3. Self-dressing deficits (including donning regular or special clothing, not nightclothes)

    a. Impaired ability to put on or take off clothing

    b. Unable to fasten clothing

    c. Unable to groom self satisfactorily

    d. Unable to obtain or replace articles of clothing

4. Self-toileting deficits

    a. Unable or unwilling to get to toilet or commode

    b. Unable or unwilling to carry out proper hygiene

    c. Unable to transfer to and from toilet or commode

    d. Unable to handle clothing to accommodate toileting

    e. Unable to flush toilet or empty commode

5. Instrumental self-care deficits

    a. Difficulty using telephone

    b. Difficulty accessing transportation

    c. Difficulty laundering, ironing

    d. Difficulty preparing meals

    e. Difficulty shopping

    f. Difficulty managing money

    g. Difficulty with medication administration

RELATED FACTORS

Pathophysiological

Related to lack of coordination secondary to (specify)
Related to spasticity or flaccidity secondary to (specify)
Related to muscular weakness secondary to (specify)
Related to partial or total paralysis secondary to (specify)
Related to atrophy secondary to (specify)
Related to muscle contractures secondary to (specify)
Related to comatose state
Related to visual disorders secondary to (specify)
Related to nonfunctioning or missing limb(s)
Related to regression to an earlier level of development
Related to excessive ritualistic behaviors
Related to somatoform deficits (specify)

Treatment-Related

Related to external devices (specify), *e.g.*, cast, splints, braces, IV equipment
Related to postoperative fatigue and pain

Situational (Personal, Environmental)

Related to cognitive deficits
Related to pain
Related to decreased motivation
Related to fatigue
Related to confusion
Related to disabling anxiety

Maturational

Older adult
Related to decreased visual and motor ability, muscle
weakness

ASSESSMENT

Subjective/Objective Data

Observed or reported inability or difficulty in performing
some activity in each of the five areas of self-care

OUTCOME CRITERIA

The person will:

1. Identify preferences in self-care activities (*e.g.*, time, products, location)
2. Demonstrate optimal hygiene after assistance with care
3. Participate physically or verbally in feeding, dressing, toileting, bathing, and instrumental activities.

GENERIC INTERVENTIONS

1. Assess causative or contributing factors:
   a. Visual deficits
   b. Impaired cognition
   c. Decreased motivation
   d. Impaired mobility
   e. Lack of knowledge
   f. Inadequate social support
   g. Regression
   h. Excessive ritualistic behavior
2. Promote optimal participation.
3. Promote self-esteem and self-determination:
   a. During self-care activities, provide choices and request preferences.

4. Evaluate ability to participate in each self-care activity.
5. Encourage to express feelings about self-care deficits.
6. For self-care deficits associated with mental disorders:
   a. Encourage independence and involvement. Praise involvement.
   b. Provide assistance with self-care activities. Remain nonjudgmental.
   c. Avoid increasing person's dependency by doing for the person when he or she has demonstrated the ability.
   d. Explore person's feelings about his or her disability and the need for help. Gently explore the disability and its purpose.
7. Refer to interventions under each diagnosis, *Feeding, Bathing/Hygiene, Dressing/Grooming, Toileting, and Instrumental Self-Care Deficit*, as indicated.

Feeding Self-Care Deficit

DEFINITION

Feeding Self-Care Deficit: A state in which the individual experiences an impaired ability to perform or complete feeding activities for oneself.

DEFINING CHARACTERISTICS

Unable to cut food or open packages
Unable to bring food to mouth

RELATED FACTORS

See *Self-Care Deficit Syndrome.*

OUTCOME CRITERIA

The person will:

1. Demonstrate increased ability to feed self *or*
2. Report that he or she is unable to feed self
3. Demonstrate ability to make use of adaptive devices, if indicated
4. Demonstrate increased interest and desire to eat

5. Describe rationale and procedure for treatment
6. Describe causative factors for feeding deficit

⊕ GENERIC INTERVENTIONS

1. Ascertain from person or family members what foods the person likes or dislikes.
2. Have meals taken in the same setting: pleasant surroundings that are not too distracting.
3. Maintain correct food temperatures (hot foods hot, cold foods cold).
4. Provide pain relief, because pain can affect appetite and ability to feed self.
5. Provide good oral hygiene before and after meals.
6. Encourage person to wear dentures and eyeglasses.
7. Place person in the most normal eating position suited to his or her physical disability (best is sitting in a chair at a table).
8. Provide social contact during eating.
9. For perceptual deficits:
   a. Choose different-colored dishes to help distinguish items (*e.g.*, red tray, white plates).
   b. Ascertain person's usual eating patterns, and provide food items according to preference (or arrange food items in clock like pattern); record on care plan the arrangement used (*e.g.*, meat, 6 o'clock; potatoes, 9 o'clock; vegetables, 12 o'clock).
   c. Encourage eating of "finger foods" (*e.g.*, bread, bacon, fruit, hot dogs) to promote independence.
10. To enhance maximum amount of independence, provide necessary adaptive devices:
    a. Plate guard to avoid pushing food off plate
    b. Suction device under plate or bowl for stabilization
    c. Padded handles on utensils for a more secure grip
    d. Wrist or hand splints with clamp to hold eating utensils
    e. Special drinking cup
    f. Rocker knife for cutting
11. Assist with setup if needed, opening containers, napkins, condiment packages; cutting meat; buttering bread.
12. For people with cognitive deficits:
    a. Provide isolated, quiet atmosphere until person is able to attend to eating and is not easily distracted from the task.

b. Orient person to location and purpose of feeding equipment.

c. Place person in the most normal eating position he or she is physically able to assume.

d. Encourage person to attend to the task, but be alert for fatigue, frustration, or agitation.

13. For people who are fearful of being poisoned:

a. Allow person to open canned foods.

b. Eat one cookie first.

c. Have family-style meals.

14. Assess to ensure that both person and family understand the reason and purpose of all interventions.

Bathing/Hygiene Self-Care Deficit

DEFINITION

Bathing/Hygiene Self-Care Deficit: A state in which the individual experiences an impaired ability to perform or complete bathing/hygiene activities for oneself.

DEFINING CHARACTERISTICS

Self-bathing deficits (including washing entire body, combing hair, brushing teeth, attending to skin and nail care, and applying makeup)

Unable or unwilling to wash body or body parts

Unable to obtain a water source

Unable to regulate temperature or water flow

Inability to perceive need for hygienic measures

RELATED FACTORS

See *Self-Care Deficit Syndrome.*

OUTCOME CRITERIA

The person will:

1. Perform bathing activity at expected optimal level *or*

2. Report satisfaction with accomplishments despite limitations
3. Relate feeling of comfort and satisfaction with body cleanliness
4. Demonstrate ability to use adaptive devices
5. Describe causative factors of bathing deficit
6. Relate rationale and procedures for treatment

⬥ GENERIC INTERVENTIONS

1. Encourage person to wear prescribed corrective lenses or hearing aid.
2. Keep bathroom temperature warm; ascertain individual's preferred water temperature.
3. Provide for privacy during bathing routine.
4. Provide all bathing equipment within easy reach.
5. Provide for safety in the bathroom (nonslip mats, grab bars).
6. When person is physically able, encourage use of either tub or shower stall, depending on which facility is at home (the person should practice in the hospital in preparation for going home).
7. Provide for adaptive equipment as needed:
   a. Chair or stool in bathtub or shower
   b. Long-handled sponge to reach back or lower extremities
   c. Grab bars on bathroom walls where needed to assist in mobility
   d. Bath board for transferring to tub chair or stool
   e. Safety treads or nonslip mat on floor of bathroom, tub, and shower
   f. Washing mitts with pocket for soap
   g. Adapted toothbrushes
   h. Shaver holders
   i. Hand-held shower spray
8. For people with visual deficits:
   a. Place bathing equipment in location most suitable to individual.
   b. Keep call bell within reach if person is to bathe alone.
   c. Give the visually impaired individual the same degree of privacy and dignity as any other person.
   d. Verbally announce yourself before entering or leaving the bathing area.

    e. Observe the person's ability to locate all bathing utensils.

    f. Observe the person's ability to perform mouth care, hair combing, and shaving tasks.

    g. Provide place for clean clothing within easy reach.

9. For people with affected or missing limbs:

    a. Bathe early in morning or before bed at night to avoid unnecessary dressing and undressing.

    b. Encourage person to use a mirror during bathing to inspect the skin of paralyzed areas.

    c. Encourage the person with amputation to inspect remaining foot or stump for good skin integrity.

    d. Provide only the amount of supervision or assistance necessary for relearning the use of extremity or adaptation to the handicap.

10. For people with cognitive deficits:

    a. Provide a consistent time for the bathing routine as part of a structured program to help decrease confusion.

    b. Keep instructions simple, and avoid distractions; orient to purpose of bathing equipment.

    c. If person is unable to bathe the entire body, have the individual bathe one part until it is done correctly; give positive reinforcement for success.

    d. Supervise activity until person can safely perform the task unassisted.

    e. Encourage attention to the task, but be alert for fatigue that may increase confusion.

11. Evaluate bathing facilities at home, and assist in determining if there is any need to make adaptations; refer to occupational therapy or social service for help in obtaining needed home equipment.

Dressing/Grooming Self-Care Deficit

DEFINITION

Dressing/Grooming Self-Care Deficit: A state in which the individual experiences an impaired ability to perform or complete dressing and grooming activities for oneself.

DEFINING CHARACTERISTICS

Self-dressing deficits (including donning regular or special clothing, not nightclothes)

Impaired ability to put on or take off clothing

Unable to fasten clothing

Unable to groom self satisfactorily

Unable to obtain or replace articles of clothing

RELATED FACTORS

See *Self-Care Deficit Syndrome.*

OUTCOME CRITERIA

The person will:

1. Demonstrate increased ability to dress self *or*
2. Report the need of having someone else assist him or her in performing the task
3. Demonstrate ability to learn how to use adaptive devices to facilitate optimal independence in the task of dressing
4. Demonstrate increased interest in wearing street clothes
5. Describe causative factors for dressing deficit
6. Relate rationale and procedures for treatments

⮆ GENERIC INTERVENTIONS

1. Encourage person to wear prescribed corrective lenses or hearing aid.
2. Promote independence in dressing through continual and unaided practice.
3. Choose clothing that is loose fitting, with wide sleeves and pant legs and front fasteners.
4. Allow sufficient time for dressing and undressing, because the task may be tiring, painful, or difficult.
5. Plan for person to learn and demonstrate one part of an activity before progressing further.
6. Lay clothes out in the order in which they will be needed to dress.
7. Provide dressing aids as necessary (some commonly used aids include dressing stick, Swedish reacher, zipper pull, buttonhook, long-handled shoehorn, and shoe fasteners adapted with elastic laces, Velcro closures, or flip-back

tongues; all garments with fasteners may be adapted with Velcro closures).

8. Encourage person to wear ordinary or special clothing rather than nightclothes.

9. Provide for privacy during dressing routine.

10. For people with visual deficits:
    a. Allow person to ascertain the most convenient location for clothing, and adapt the environment to accomplish the task (*e.g.*, remove unnecessary barriers).
    b. Verbally announce yourself before entering or leaving the dressing area.

11. For people with cognitive deficits:
    a. Establish a consistent dressing routine to provide a structured program to decrease confusion.
    b. Keep instructions simple, and repeat them frequently; avoid distractions.
    c. Introduce one article of clothing at a time.
    d. Encourage attention to the task; be alert for fatigue, which may increase confusion.

12. Assess understanding and knowledge of individual and family for above instructions and rationale.

Toileting Self-Care Deficit

DEFINITION

Toileting Self-Care Deficit: A state in which the individual experiences an impaired ability to perform or complete toileting activities.

DEFINING CHARACTERISTICS

Unable or unwilling to get to toilet or commode
Unable or unwilling to carry out proper hygiene
Unable to transfer to and from toilet or commode
Unable to handle clothing to accommodate toileting
Unable to flush toilet or empty commode

RELATED FACTORS

See *Self-Care Deficit Syndrome.*

OUTCOME CRITERIA

The person will:

1. Demonstrate increased ability to toilet self *or*
2. Report that he or she is unable to toilet self
3. Demonstrate ability to make use of adaptive devices to facilitate toileting
4. Describe causative factors for toileting deficit
5. Relate rationale and procedures for treatment

✚ GENERIC INTERVENTIONS

1. Encourage person to wear prescribed corrective lenses or hearing aid.
2. Obtain bladder and bowel history from individual or significant other (see *Constipation* or *Altered Patterns of Urinary Elimination*).
3. Ascertain communication system person uses to express the need to toilet.
4. Maintain bladder and bowel record to determine toileting patterns.
5. Avoid development of "bowel fixation" by less frequent discussion and inquiries about bowel movements.
6. Be alert to possibility of falls when toileting person (be prepared to ease him or her to floor without causing injury to either of you).
7. Achieve independence in toileting by continual and unaided practice.
8. Allow sufficient time for the task of toileting to avoid fatigue (lack of sufficient time to toilet may cause incontinence or constipation).
9. Avoid use of indwelling catheters and condom catheters to expedite bladder continence (if possible).
10. For people with visual deficits:
    a. Keep call bell easily accessible so person can quickly obtain help to toilet; answer call bell promptly to decrease anxiety.
    b. If bedpan or urinal is necessary for toileting, be sure it is within person's reach.
    c. Verbally announce yourself before entering or leaving toileting area.

    d. Observe person's ability to obtain equipment or get to the toilet unassisted.

    e. Provide for a safe and clear pathway to toilet area.

11. For people with affected or missing limbs:

    a. Provide only the amount of supervision and assistance necessary for relearning or adapting to the prosthesis.

    b. Encourage person to look at affected area or limb and use it during toileting tasks.

    c. Encourage useful transfer techniques taught by occupational or physical therapy (the nurse should familiarize himself or herself with planned mode of transfer).

    d. Provide the necessary adaptive devices to enhance the maximum amount of independence and safety (commode chairs, spill-proof urinals, fracture bedpans, raised toilet seats, support side rails for toilets).

    e. Provide for a safe and clear pathway to toilet area.

12. For people with cognitive deficits:

    a. Offer toileting reminders every 2 hours, after meals, and before bedtime.

    b. When person is able to indicate the need to toilet, begin toileting at 2-hour intervals, after meals, and before bedtime.

    c. Answer call bell immediately to avoid frustration and failure to be continent.

    d. Encourage wearing ordinary clothes (many confused individuals are continent while wearing regular clothing).

    e. Avoid the use of bedpans and urinals; if physically possible, provide a normal atmosphere of elimination in bathroom (the toilet used should remain constant to promote familiarity).

    f. Give verbal cues as to what is expected of the individual, and give positive reinforcement for success.

    g. See *Altered Patterns of Urinary Elimination* for additional information on incontinence.

13. Ascertain home toileting needs, and refer to occupational therapy or social services for help in obtaining necessary equipment.

Instrumental Self-Care Deficit

DEFINITION

Instrumental Self-Care Deficit: A state in which the individual experiences an impaired ability to perform certain activities or access certain services essential for managing a household.

> **Author's Note:**
> Instrumental Self-Care Deficit is not currently on the NANDA list but has been added for clarity and usefulness. Instrumental Self-Care Deficit describes problems in performing certain activities or accessing certain services needed to live in the community (*e.g.*, phone use, shopping, money management). This diagnosis is important to consider in discharge planning and during assessment by the community nurse.

DEFINING CHARACTERISTICS

Major (Must Be Present, One or More)

Observed or reported difficulty in:
Using a telephone
Accessing transportation
Laundering, ironing
Preparing meals
Shopping (food, clothes)
Managing money
Medication administration

RELATED FACTORS

See *Self-Care Deficit.*

OUTCOME CRITERIA

The person/family will:

1. Demonstrate use of adaptive devices (*e.g.*, phone, cooking aids)
2. Describe a method to ensure adherence to medication schedule

3. Report ability to call and answer telephone
4. Report regular laundering by self or others
5. Report daily intake of two nutritious meals
6. Identify transportation options to stores, health care, house of worship, social activities
7. Demonstrate management of simple money transactions
8. Identify individual(s) who will assist with money matters

⊞ GENERIC INTERVENTIONS

1. Assess for causative and contributing factors:
   a. Visual, hearing deficits
   b. Impaired cognition
   c. Impaired mobility
   d. Lack of knowledge
   e. Inadequate social support
2. Assist to identify self-help devices.
3. Promote self-care and safety with individuals with cognitive deficits:
   a. Evaluate activities that are achievable.
   b. Evaluate ability to procure, select, and prepare nutritious food daily.
   c. Teach hints for adherence to medicine schedule (*e.g.*, 7-day pill holder, separate pill for each time to be taken).
   d. Evaluate ability to understand money, budget money, and pay bills.
4. Determine sources of transportation (*e.g.*, church groups, neighbors).
5. Determine sources of social support (transportation, laundry, money matters).
6. Discuss the importance of identifying need for assistance (*e.g.*, Department of Social Services, agency on aging).

Self-Concept Disturbance*

Body Image Disturbance

Personal Identity Disturbance

Self-Esteem Disturbance

Chronic Low Self-Esteem

Situational Low Self-Esteem

Self-Concept Disturbance

DEFINITION

Self-Concept Disturbance: The state in which an individual experiences or is at risk of experiencing a negative state of change about the way he or she feels, thinks, or views himself or herself. It may include a change in body image, self-ideal, self-esteem, role performance, or personal identity.

> **Author's Note:**
> Self-Concept Disturbance represents a broad category under which more specific categories fall. Initially the nurse may not have sufficient clinical data to validate a more specific diagnosis as Chronic Low Self-Esteem or Body Image Disturbance; thus, Self-Concept Disturbance can be used until more specific diagnoses can be supported with data.

*This diagnosis is not currently on the NANDA list but has been included for clarity or usefulness.

DEFINING CHARACTERISTICS

Since a self-concept disturbance may include a change in any one or a combination of its five component parts (body image, self-ideal, self-esteem, role performance, personal identity) and the nature of the change causing the alteration can be so varied, there is no "typical" response for this diagnosis. Reactions may include the following:

Refusal to touch or look at a body part

Refusal to look into a mirror

Unwillingness to discuss a limitation, deformity, or disfigurement

Refusal to accept rehabilitation efforts

Inappropriate attempts to direct own treatment

Denial of the existence of a deformity or disfigurement

Increasing dependence on others

Signs of grieving: weeping, despair, anger

Refusal to participate in own care or take responsibility for self-care (self-neglect)

Self-destructive behavior (alcohol, drug abuse)

Displaying hostility toward the healthy

Withdrawal from social contacts

Changing usual patterns of responsibility

Showing change in ability to estimate relationship of body to environment

RELATED FACTORS

A self-concept disturbance can occur as a response to a variety of health problems, situations, and conflicts. Some common sources include the following.

Pathophysiological

Related to change in appearance, lifestyle, role, and response of others secondary to:

Loss of body part(s)   Chronic disease

Loss of body function(s)   Pain

Severe trauma

Situational (Personal, Environmental)

Related to feelings of abandonment or failure secondary to: divorce, separation from, or death of a significant other or loss of job or ability to work

Related to immobility or loss of function

Related to unsatisfactory relationships (parental, spousal)

Maturational

Refer to *Self-Concept Disturbance*.

OUTCOME CRITERIA

The person will:

1. Appraise self in situations in a realistic manner without distortions
2. Verbalize and demonstrate increased feelings of self-concept
3. Demonstrate a healthy adaptation, coping skills

GENERIC INTERVENTIONS

1. Encourage person to express feelings, especially about the way person feels, thinks, or views self.
2. Encourage person to ask questions about health problem, treatment, progress, prognosis.
3. Provide reliable information, and reinforce information already given.
4. Elicit areas that he or she would like to change. Encourage to problem solve options.
5. Clarify any misconceptions the person has about self, care, or caregivers.
6. Avoid negative criticism.
7. Provide privacy and a safe environment.
8. If indicated, refer to *Self-Esteem Disturbance* or *Body Image Disturbance* for interventions under the category.
9. Teach person what community resources are available, if needed (*e.g.*, mental health centers, self-help groups such as Reach for Recovery, Make Today Count).

CHILD FOCUS INTERVENTIONS

1. Allow the child to bring his or her own experiences into the situation (Johnson & Saunders, 1995; *e.g.*, some children say that an injection feels like a insect sting, and some say they don't feel anything). "After we do this, you can tell me how it felt."

2. Avoid using good or bad to describe behavior. Be specific and descriptive (*e.g.*, "You really helped me by holding still. Thank you for helping"; Johnson & Saunders, 1995).

3. Connect a previous experience with the present one (*e.g.*, "The x-ray camera will look different from the last time. You will have to hold real still again. The table will move too"; Johnson & Saunders, 1995).

4. Convey optimism with positive self-talk (*e.g.*, "I am so busy today. I wonder if I will get all my work done? I bet I can." "When you come back from surgery, you will need to stay in bed. What would you like to do when you come back?").

5. Help the child plan playtime with choices. Encourage crafts that produce a product.

6. Encourage interaction with peers and supportive adults.

7. Encourage to decorate room with crafts and personal items.

Body Image Disturbance

DEFINITION

Body Image Disturbance: The state in which an individual experiences or is at risk of experiencing confusion in the way one perceives one's physical self.

DEFINING CHARACTERISTICS

Major (Must Be Present)

Verbal or nonverbal negative response to actual or perceived change in structure or function (*e.g.*, shame, embarrassment, guilt, revulsion)

Minor (May Be Present)

Not looking at body part
Not touching body part
Hiding or overexposing body part
Change in social involvement
Negative feelings about body, feelings of helplessness, hopelessness, powerlessness, vulnerability

Preoccupation with change or loss
Refusal to verify actual change
Depersonalization of part or loss
Self-destructive behaviors (*e.g.*, mutilation, suicide attempts, overeating, undereating)

RELATED FACTORS

Pathophysiological

Related to changes in appearance secondary to: chronic disease, loss of body part, loss of body function, or severe trauma
Related to unrealistic perceptions of appearance secondary to: psychoses, anorexia nervosa, or bulimia

Treatment-Related

Related to changes in appearance secondary to: hospitalization, surgery, chemotherapy, or radiation

Situational

Related to physical trauma secondary to: sexual abuse or rape (perpetrator known or unknown)
Related to effects of (specify) on appearance (*e.g.*, obesity, pregnancy, immobility)

Maturational

Related to developmental change

OUTCOME CRITERIA

The person will:

1. Implement new coping patterns
2. Verbalize and demonstrate acceptance of appearance (grooming, dress, posture, eating patterns, presentation of self)
3. Demonstrate a willingness and ability to resume self-care/role responsibilities
4. Initiate new or reestablish existing support systems

⊡ GENERIC INTERVENTIONS

1. Encourage person to express feelings, especially about the way he or she feels, thinks, or views self.

2. Encourage person to ask questions about health problem, treatment, progress, prognosis.
3. Provide reliable information, and reinforce information already given.
4. Clarify any misconceptions the person has about self, care, or caregivers.
5. Prepare significant others for physical and emotional changes. Support family as they adapt.
6. Encourage visits from peers and significant others. Advise to share with the person their value and importance to them.
7. Encourage contact (letters, telephone) with peers and family.
8. Provide opportunity to share with people going through similar experiences.
9. For loss of body part or function:
   a. Assess the meaning of the loss for the individual and significant others, as related to visibility of loss, function of loss, and emotional investment.
   b. Expect the individual to respond to the loss with denial, shock, anger, and depression.
   c. Be aware of the effect of the responses of others to the loss; encourage sharing of feelings between significant others.
   d. Allow individual to ventilate feelings and grieve.
   e. Use role-playing to assist with sharing.
   f. Explore realistic alternatives, and provide encouragement.
   g. Explore strengths and resources with person.
10. Assist with the resolution of a surgically created alteration of body image.
    a. Replace the lost body part with prosthesis as soon as possible.
    b. Encourage viewing of site.
    c. Encourage touching of site.
11. For changes associated with chemotherapy (Cooley et al., 1986):
    a. Discuss the possibility of hair loss, absence of menses, temporary or permanent sterility, decreased estrogen levels, vaginal dryness, mucositis.
    b. Encourage person to share concerns, fears, and perception of the impact of these changes on the person's life.
    c. Explain where hair loss may occur (head, eyelashes, eyebrows, and axillary, pubic, and leg hair).

    d. Explain that hair will grow back after treatment but may change in color and texture.

    e. Have person select a wig and wear it before hair loss. Consult a beautician for tips on how to vary the look of the wig (*e.g.*, combs, clips).

    f. Encourage the wearing of scarves, turbans when wig is not on.

    g. Teach to minimize the amount of hair loss by:

        • Avoiding excessive shampooing, using a conditioner twice weekly

        • Patting hair dry gently

        • Avoiding electric curlers, dryers, and curling irons

        • Avoiding pulling hair with bands, clips, or bobby pins

        • Avoiding hair spray and hair dye

        • Using wide-tooth comb, avoiding vigorous brushing

    h. Refer to American Cancer Society for information regarding new or used wigs. Inform that the wig is a tax-deductible item.

12. Discuss the difficulty that others (spouse, friends, co-workers) may have with visible changes.

13. Allow significant others opportunities to share feelings and fears.

14. Assist significant others to identify positive aspects of the client and ways this can be shared.

15. Teach person what community resources are available if needed (*e.g.*, mental health centers, such self-help groups as Reach for Recovery, Make Today Count).

✿ CHILD FOCUS INTERVENTIONS

1. Discuss with parents how body image develops and what interactions contribute to their child's self-perceptions.

    a. Teach the names and functions of body parts

    b. Acknowledge changes (*e.g.*, height)

    c. Allow some choices of what to wear

2. Ask child to draw a picture of his or her body just after a bath (naked). Ask to describe picture.

3. Focus child on body changes (*e.g.*, "What can you do now that you couldn't do when you were little?").

For Adolescents

1. Discuss with parents the adolescent's need to "fit in."
   a. Do not dismiss adolescent's concerns too quickly.
   b. Be flexible and compromise when possible (*e.g.,* clothes are temporary, tattoos are not).
   c. Negotiate a time to think about it (*e.g.,* 4–6 weeks).
   d. Provide reasons for denying a request. Elicit adolescent's reasons. Compromise if possible (*e.g.,* curfew parents want, 11:00; adolescent, 12:00; compromise 11:30).
2. Provide opportunities to discuss concerns when parents are not present.
3. Ask to describe best features and those they dislike.
4. Prepare for impending development changes.

MATERNAL FOCUS INTERVENTIONS

1. Teach couples about anticipated physiological changes and possible changes in sexual response.
2. Allow woman opportunities to discuss her feelings regarding body changes.

Personal Identity Disturbance

DEFINITION

Personal Identity Disturbance: The state in which an individual experiences or is at risk of experiencing an inability to distinguish between self and nonself.

Author's Note:

This diagnosis is a subcategory under Self-Concept Disturbance. Until clinical research defines and differentiates this diagnosis from others, refer to Self-Concept Disturbance or Altered Growth and Development for assessment criteria and interventions.

DEFINING CHARACTERISTICS

See Defining Characteristics for *Self-Concept Disturbance* or *Altered Growth and Development*.

Self-Esteem Disturbance

DEFINITION

Self-Esteem Disturbance: The state in which an individual experiences or is at risk of experiencing negative self-evaluation about self or capabilities.

> **Author's Note:**
> Self-esteem is one of the four components of Self-Concept. Self-Esteem Disturbance is the general diagnostic category. Chronic Low Self-Esteem and Situational Low Self-Esteem represent specific types of Self-Esteem Disturbances, thus involving more specific interventions. Initially, the nurse may not have sufficient clinical data to validate a more specific diagnosis, such as Chronic Low Self-Esteem or Situational Low Self-Esteem. Refer to the major Defining Characteristics under these diagnoses for validation.

DEFINING CHARACTERISTICS

Overt or covert:
   Self-negating verbalization*
   Expressions of shame or guilt*
   Evaluation of self as unable to deal with events*
   Rationalizing away/rejecting positive feedback and
      exaggerates negative feedback about self*
   Inability to set goals
   Indecisiveness
   Lack of/poor problem solving

*Norris, J., & Kunes-Connell, M. (1987). Self-esteem disturbance: A clinical validation study. In A. McLane (Ed.), *Classification of nursing diagnoses: Proceedings of the seventh conference.* St. Louis: C.V. Mosby.

Signs of depression (sleeping, eating)
Seeking approval/reassurance excessively
Poor body presentation (posture, eye contact, movements)
Self-abusive behavior (mutilation, suicide attempts, nail
  biting, substance abuse, becoming a victim)
Hesitation to try new things/situations*
Denial of problems obvious to others
Projection of blame/responsibility for problems*
Rationalization of personal failures*
Hypersensitivity to slight criticism*
Grandiosity*

RELATED FACTORS

Self-Esteem Disturbance can be either an episodic event or a
chronic problem. Failure to resolve a problem or multiple se-
quential stresses can result in Chronic Low Self-Esteem. Factors
that occur with time and are associated with Chronic Low Self-
Esteem are indicated by CLSE.

Pathophysiological

Related to change in appearance secondary to:
  Loss of body part(s)
  Loss of body function(s)
  Disfigurement (trauma, surgery, birth defects)

Situational (Personal, Environmental)

Related to unmet dependency needs
Related to lack of positive feedback
Related to feelings of abandonment secondary to: death of
  significant other, child abduction/murder, separation from
  significant other
Related to feelings of failure secondary to:
  Unemployment
  Financial problems
  Loss of job or ability to work
  Relationship problems
    Marital discord
    Separation
    Step-parents
    In-laws
  Increase/decrease in weight

*Norris, J., & Kunes-Connell, M. (1987). Self-esteem disturbance: A
clinical validation study. In A. McLane (Ed.), *Classification of nursing
diagnoses: Proceedings of the seventh conference.* St. Louis: C.V. Mosby.

Premenstrual syndrome

Related to failure in school

Related to history of ineffective relationship with own parents (CLSE)

Related to history of abusive relationships (CLSE)

Related to unrealistic expectations of child by parent (CLSE)

Related to unrealistic expectations of self (CLSE)

Related to unrealistic expectations of parent by child (CLSE)

Related to parental rejection (CLSE)

Related to inconsistent punishment (CLSE)

Related to feelings of helplessness or failure secondary to: institutionalization (*e.g.*, mental health facility, jail, orphanage, halfway house)

Related to history of numerous failures (CLSE)

Maturational

Infant/toddler/preschool

Related to lack of stimulation or closeness (CLSE)

Related to separation from parents/significant others (CLSE)

Related to continual negative evaluation by parents

Related to inadequate parental support (CLSE)

Related to inability to trust significant other (CLSE)

School age

Related to failure to achieve grade-level objectives

Related to loss of peer group

Related to repeated negative feedback (CLSE)

Adolescent

Related to loss of independence and autonomy secondary to (specify)

Related to disruption of peer relationships

Related to scholastic problems

Related to loss of significant others

Middle age

Related to changes associated with aging

Older adult

Related to losses (people, function, financial, retirement)

OUTCOME CRITERIA

The person will:

1. Verbalize feelings and thinking about self
2. Identify two positive attributes about self

▶ GENERIC INTERVENTIONS

1. Establish a trusting nurse–client relationship.
   a. Encourage person to express feelings, especially about the way he or she thinks or views self.
   b. Encourage person to ask questions about health problem, treatment, progress, prognosis.
   c. Provide reliable information, and reinforce information already given.
   d. Clarify any misconceptions the person has about self, care, or caregivers.
   e. Avoid negative criticism.
   f. Provide privacy and a safe environment.
2. Promote social interaction.
   a. Assist person to accept help from others.
   b. Avoid overprotection while still limiting the demands made on the individual.
   c. Encourage movement.
   d. Support family as they adapt.
3. Explore strengths and resources with person.
4. Discuss expectations.
   a. Discuss if realistic.
   b. Explore realistic alternatives.
5. Refer to community resources as indicated (*e.g.*, counseling, assertiveness courses).

Chronic Low Self-Esteem

DEFINITION

Chronic Low Self-Esteem: The state in which an individual experiences a long-standing negative self-evaluation about self or capabilities.

DEFINING CHARACTERISTICS
(Norris & Kunes-Connell, 1987)

Major (80%–100%)

Long-standing or chronic:
  Self-negating verbalization
  Expressions of shame/guilt

Evaluation of self as unable to deal with events
Rationalization away/rejection of positive feedback and
    exaggeration negative feedback about self
Hesitation to try new things/situations

Minor (50%–79%)

Frequent lack of success in work or other life events
Overly conforming, dependent on opinions of others
Poor body presentation (eye contact, posture, movements)
Nonassertive/passive
Indecisive
Excessively seeking reassurance

RELATED FACTORS

See *Self-Esteem Disturbance*.

OUTCOME CRITERIA

The individual will:

1. Modify excessive and unrealistic self-expectations
2. Verbalize acceptance of limitations
3. Verbalize nonjudgmental perceptions of self
4. Identify positive aspects of self
5. Cease self-abusive behavior
6. Report freedom from symptoms of depression
7. Begin to take verbal and behavioral risks

⏩ GENERIC INTERVENTIONS

1. Assist the person to reduce present anxiety level.
2. Enhance the person's sense of self.
    a. Be attentive.
    b. Respect individual's personal space.
    c. Validate your interpretation of what person is say-
       ing or experiencing ("Is this what you mean?").
3. Provide encouragement as a task or skill is attempted.
   Allow person to perform as independently as possible.
4. Assist person in expressing thoughts and feelings.
5. Encourage visits/contact with peers and significant others
   (letters, telephone).
6. Be a role model in one-to-one interactions.
7. Involve in activities, especially when strengths can be used.

8. Do not allow person to isolate self (refer to *Social Isolation* for further interventions).
9. Set limits on problematic behavior, such as aggression, poor hygiene, ruminations, and suicidal preoccupation. Refer to *Risk for Suicide* or *Risk for Violence* if these are assessed as problems.
10. Encourage activities that exercise large muscles (*e.g.*, walking, biking, swimming). Avoid competitive activities.
11. Provide for development of social and vocational skills.
12. Refer for vocational counseling, if indicated.

♀ CHILD FOCUS INTERVENTIONS

1. Provide opportunities for child to be successful and needed.
2. Personalize the child's environment with pictures, possessions, and crafts made.
3. Provide structured and unstructured playtime.
4. Ensure continuance of academic experiences in the hospital or home. Provide uninterrupted time for school work.

🏛 OLDER ADULT FOCUS INTERVENTIONS
(Miller, 1999)

1. Acknowledge person by name.
2. Use a tone of voice that you use for your peer group.
3. Avoid words associated with babies (*e.g.*, diapers).
4. Ask about family pictures, personal items, and past experiences.
5. Avoid attributing disabilities to "old age."
6. Knock on door of bedrooms and bathrooms.
7. Allow person enough time to accomplish tasks at own pace.

Situational Low Self-Esteem

DEFINITION

Situational Low Self-Esteem: The state in which an individual who previously had positive self-esteem experiences negative feelings about self in response to an event (loss, change).

DEFINING CHARACTERISTICS
(Norris & Kunes-Connell, 1987)

Major (80%–100%)

Episodic occurrence of negative self-appraisal in response to life events in a person with a previously positive self-evaluation

Verbalization of negative feelings about self (helplessness, uselessness)

Minor (50%–79%)

Self-negating verbalizations
Expressions of shame/guilt
Evaluation of self as unable to handle situations/events
Difficulty making decisions
Self-neglect
Social isolation

RELATED FACTORS

See *Self-Esteem Disturbance*.

OUTCOME CRITERIA

The person will:

1. Identify source of threat to self-esteem and work through that issue
2. Identify positive aspects of self
3. Express a positive outlook for the future
4. Analyze own behavior and its consequences

5. Identify ways of exerting control and influencing outcomes
6. Resume previous level of functioning

⬈ GENERIC INTERVENTIONS

1. Assist the individual in identifying and expressing feelings.
2. Assist in identifying positive self-evaluations.
3. Examine and reinforce positive abilities and traits (*e.g.*, hobbies, skills, school, relationships, appearance, loyalty, industriousness).
4. Encourage an activity that exercises large muscles (*e.g.*, walking, swimming, biking). Avoid competitive situations.
5. Help individual accept positive and negative feelings.
6. Encourage examination of current behavior and its consequences (*e.g.*, dependency, procrastination, isolation).
7. Help to identify negative automatic thoughts and overgeneralizing.
8. Assist in identifying own responsibility and control in a situation (*e.g.*, when continually blaming others for problems).
9. Assess and mobilize current support system.
10. Refer to community resources as indicated (*e.g.*, Reach for Recovery).

Risk for Self-Harm*

Risk for Self-Abuse*

Risk for Self-Mutilation

Risk for Suicide*

Risk for Self-Harm*

DEFINITION

Risk for Self-Harm: A state in which an individual is at risk for inflicting direct harm on himself or herself. This may include one or more of the following: self-abuse, self-mutilation, suicide.

Author's Note:

Risk for Self-Harm represents a broad diagnosis that can encompass self-abuse, self-mutilation, or risk for suicide. Although initially they may appear the same, the distinction lies in the intent. "Self-mutilation and self-abuse are pathological attempts to relieve stress (temporary reprieve), whereas suicide is an attempt to die (to relieve stress permanently)" (Casscaden, 1992; personal communication). Risk for Self-Harm can also be a useful early diagnosis when insufficient data are present to differentiate one from the other.

DEFINING CHARACTERISTICS

Major

Expresses desire or intent to harm self
Expresses desire to die or commit suicide
Has history of attempts to harm self

*This diagnosis is not currently on the NANDA list but has been included for clarity or usefulness.

Minor

Reports or observed
- Depression
- Poor self-concept
- Hallucinations/delusion
- Substance abuse
- Poor impulse control
- Agitation
- Hopelessness
- Helplessness
- Lack of support system
- Emotional pain
- Hostility

RELATED FACTORS

Risk for Self-Harm can occur as a response to a variety of health problems, situations, and conflicts. Some sources are listed:

Pathophysiological

Related to feelings of helplessness, loneliness, or hopelessness secondary to:
- Disabilities
- Terminal illness
- Chronic illness
- Chronic pain
- Psychiatric disorder
  - Schizophrenia
  - Bipolar disorder
  - Post-traumatic syndrome
- Chemical dependency
- Substance abuse
- Mental impairment (organic or traumatic)
  - Personality disorder
  - Adolescent adjustment disorder
  - Somatoform disorders

Treatment-Related

Related to unsatisfactory outcome of treatment (medical, surgical, psychological)

Related to prolonged dependence on, for example, dialysis, insulin injections, chemotherapy/radiation, ventilator

Situational (Personal, Environmental)

Related to:
- Depression
- Ineffective individual coping skills
- Parental/marital conflict
- Substance abuse in family
- Child abuse (present, past)

Related to real or perceived loss secondary to:
- Finances/job
- Status/prestige
- Threat of abandonment

Separation/divorce
Death of significant others
Someone leaving home
Related to wish for revenge on real or perceived injury (body or self-esteem)

Maturational

Adolescent
Related to feelings of abandonment
Related to unrealistic expectations of child by parents
Related to peer pressure or rejection
Related to depression
Related to relocation
Related to significant loss
Older adult
Related to multiple losses secondary to retirement, social isolation, significant loss, or illness

OUTCOME CRITERIA

The person will:

1. Acknowledge self-harm thoughts
2. Admit to use of self-harm behavior if it occurs
3. Make a commitment to control behaviors
4. Be able to identify personal triggers
5. Learn to identify and tolerate uncomfortable feelings properly
6. Choose alternatives that are not harmful

⚡ GENERIC INTERVENTIONS

1. Demonstrate an acceptance of the individual as a worthwhile person through the use of nonjudgmental statements and behavior.
   a. Actively listen or provide support by just being there if the person is silent.
   b. Label the behavior, not the person.
2. Assist in recognizing the presence of hope and the element of alternatives.
3. Orient individual as required. Point out sensory or environmental misperceptions without belittling fears or indicating disapproval of verbal expressions.

4. Help reframe old thinking/feeling patterns
   a. Assist in identifying thought–feeling–behavior concept.
   b. Help assess payoffs and drawbacks to self-harm.
   c. Encourage identification of personal triggers.
   d. Facilitate the development of new behaviors.
5. Validate good coping skills already in existence.
6. Encourage the use of positive affirmations, meditation and relaxation techniques, and other esteem-building exercises.
7. Encourage journaling, keeping a diary of triggers, thoughts, and feelings, and alternatives that do or do not work.
8. Assist in developing body awareness as a method of ascertaining triggers and determining levels of impending self-harm.
9. Introduce "contracting" to individual.
10. Assist in role playing to problem solve situations/relationships.
11. Reduce excessive stimuli.
12. Intervene at earliest stages to assist person to regain control, prevent escalation, and allow treatment in the least restrictive manner.
13. Promote the use of alternatives:
    a. Stress that there are always alternatives.
    b. Stress that self-harm is a choice, not something uncontrollable.
    c. Allow opportunities for verbal expression of thoughts and feelings.
    d. Provide acceptable physical outlets.
14. Initiate support systems to community when indicated.
    a. Teach family:
       • Constructive expression of feelings
       • How to recognize levels of impending self-harm
       • How to assist with appropriate interventions
       • How to deal with self-harm behavior/results
    b. Supply phone number of 24-hour emergency hotlines.
    c. Counseling:
       • Leisure/vocational counseling
       • Halfway houses
       • Other community resources

Risk for Self-Abuse

DEFINITION

Risk for Self-Abuse: A state in which an individual is at risk to perform a deliberate act upon the self, without the intent to kill, which may or may not cause harm to the body.

DEFINING CHARACTERISTICS

Major (Must Be Present, One or More)

Expresses a desire or intent to harm self
Evidence of self-abuse: *e.g.,*
  Head banging
  Slapping
  Picking
  Scratching
  Nonlethal use of drugs/poison
  Anorexic/bulimic behaviors
  Swallowing foreign objects (glass, needles, safety pins, straight pins, various hardware [*e.g.,* nails, screws])

RELATED FACTORS

See *Risk for Self-Harm.*

OUTCOME CRITERIA

See *Risk for Self-Harm.*

⏎ GENERIC INTERVENTIONS

See *Risk for Self-Harm.*

☻ CHILD FOCUS INTERVENTIONS

1. Redirect child back to the activity or task.
2. Praise his or her attention to the activity.
3. If applicable, look away from the child; make no eye contact.
4. If quiet room is used, limit as much as possible.

Risk for Self-Mutilation

DEFINITION

Risk for Self-Mutilation: A state in which an individual is at risk to perform a deliberate act upon the self with the intent to injure, not kill, which produces immediate tissue damage to the body.

DEFINING CHARACTERISTICS

Major (Must Be Present, One or More)

Expresses desire or intent to harm self
History of attempts to harm self: *e.g.*,
Cutting
Slashing
Stabbing
Scratching
Picking
Gouging

RELATED FACTORS

See *Risk for Self-Harm.*

OUTCOME CRITERIA

See *Risk for Self-Harm.*

GENERIC INTERVENTIONS

See *Risk for Self-Harm.*

Risk for Suicide

DEFINITION

Risk for Suicide: The state in which an individual is at risk for killing himself or herself.

Author's Note:
Risk for Suicide is not currently on the NANDA list but has been added for clarity. Risk for Violence: Self-directed Medications is included under Risk for Violence. The term *violence* is described as a swift and intense force or a rough or injurious physical force. Suicide can be violent, but it can also be nonviolent (overdose of barbiturates). Using the term violence can unfortunately cause the risk for suicide to be undetected because of the belief that an individual is not capable of violence.

Risk for Suicide clearly denotes an individual at high risk for suicide and the need for protection. The treatment of the diagnosis comprises validation, contracting, and protection. The treatment of the underlying depression and hopelessness should be addressed with other nursing diagnoses (*e.g.*, Ineffective Individual Coping, Hopelessness).

RISK FACTORS

Major (Must Be Present, One or More)

Suicidal ideation
Previous suicidal attempts

Minor (May Be Present)

See *Risk for Self-Harm.*

RELATED FACTORS

See *Risk for Self-Harm.*

OUTCOME CRITERIA

The person will:

1. Not harm self
2. Accept help from significant others and community
3. Use effective coping mechanisms to handle stress

✚ GENERIC INTERVENTIONS

1. Assess level of risk status (Table I-3):
   a. High, moderate, low

2. Assess level of long-term risk:
   a. Lifestyle, lethality of plan, usual coping mechanisms
3. Provide closely supervised environment for high-risk person.
   a. Restrict glass, nail files, scissors, nail polish remover, mirrors, needles, razors, soda cans, plastic bags, lighters, electric equipment, belts, hangers, knives, tweezers, alcohol, guns.
   b. Meals should be provided in a closely supervised area.
   c. When administering oral medications, check to ensure that all medications are swallowed.
   d. Provide checks on the person as designated by institution's policy.
   e. Restrict the individual to the unit unless specifically ordered by physician. When off unit, provide a staff member to accompany the person.
   f. Instruct visitors on restricted items.
   g. The acutely suicidal person may be required to wear a hospital gown to prevent unauthorized leaving.
   h. Room searches should be done periodically according to institution policy.
   i. Use seclusion and restraint if necessary (refer to *Risk for Violence* for discussion).
   j. Notify police if the person leaves and is at risk for suicide.
4. Notify all staff that this person is at risk for suicide.
5. Make a no-suicide contract with the individual (include family if person is at home).
   a. Written contract
   b. Mutual agreement
6. Encourage appropriate expression of anger and hostility.
7. Set limits on ruminations about suicide or previous attempts.
8. Assist in recognizing predisposing factors: "What was happening before you started having these thoughts?"
9. Facilitate examination of life stresses and past coping mechanisms.
10. Explore alternative behaviors.
11. Anticipate future stresses, and assist in planning alternatives.

(Text continues on p. 376)

TABLE I-3.
Assessing the Degree of Suicidal Risk

Behavior or Symptom	Intensity of Risk		
	LOW	**MODERATE**	**HIGH**
Anxiety	Mild	Moderate	High or panic state
Depression	Mild	Moderate	Severe
Isolation/withdrawal	Some feelings of isolation; no withdrawal	Some feelings of hopelessness, and withdrawal	Hopeless, withdrawn, and self-deprecating, isolation
Daily functioning	Effective	Moody	Depressed
	⚔ Good grades in school	⚔ Variable grades	Poor grades
	Close friends	Some friends	⚔ Few or no close friends
	No prior suicide attempt	Prior suicidal thoughts	Prior suicide attempts
	Stable job		Erratic or poor work history
Lifestyle	Stable	Moderately stable	Unstable
Alcohol/drug use	Infrequently to excess	Frequently to excess	Continual abuse
Previous suicide attempts	None or of low lethality (few pills)	One or more (pills, super-ficial wrist slash)	One or more (entire bottle of pills, gun, hanging)

Associated events	None or an argument	⚹ Disciplinary action ⚹ Failing grades Work problems Family illness	Relationship breakup Death of a loved one Loss of job Pregnancy
Purpose of act	None or not clear	Relief of shame or guilt To punish others To get attention	⚹ Wants to die Escape to join deceased Debilitating disease
Family's reaction and structure	Supportive Intact family Good coping and mental health No history of suicide	Mixed reaction Divorced/separated Usually copes and understands	Angry and unsupportive Disorganized Rigid/abusive History of suicide in family
Suicide plan (method, location, time)	No plan	Frequent thoughts, occasional ideas about a plan	Specific plan

⚹ Applies only to children and adolescents.
(Adapted from Hatton, C. L., & McBride, S. [1984]. *Suicide: Assessment and intervention.* Norwalk, CT: Appleton-Century-Crofts and Jackson, D. B., & Saunders, R. B. [1993]. *Child health nursing.* Philadelphia: J. B. Lippincott.)

12. Involve person in planning the treatment goals and evaluating progress.
13. Instruct significant others in how to recognize an increase in risk: change in behavior, verbal, nonverbal communication, withdrawal, signs of depression.
14. Supply phone numbers of 24-hour emergency hotlines.
15. Refer to community agency or ongoing therapy.

CHILD FOCUS INTERVENTIONS

1. Take all suicide threats seriously.
2. Engage parents, friends, school personnel, and the individual in behavior contracts to "keep safe."
3. Explore feelings and reason for suicidal feelings.
4. Consult with a psychiatric expert regarding the most appropriate environment for treatment.
5. Participate in programs in schools to teach about the symptoms of depression and signs of suicidal behavior.

OLDER ADULT FOCUS INTERVENTIONS
(Miller, 1999)

1. Be direct (*e.g.*, "Are you thinking of hurting yourself?").
2. Acknowledge the intent with concern; remain nonjudgmental.
3. Help to identify other options.
4. Accept the person's feelings of helplessness and hopelessness.
5. Discuss the problem with family.

Sensory–Perceptual Alterations

DEFINITION

Sensory–Perceptual Alterations: The state in which an individual/group experiences or is at risk of experiencing a change in the amount, pattern, or interpretation of incoming stimuli.

Author's Note:

The diagnosis Sensory–Perceptual Alterations describes an individual with altered perception and cognition influenced by physiological factors (*e.g.*, pain, sleep deprivation, immobility, and excessive or decreased meaningful stimuli from the environment). Altered Thought Processes can also manifest with altered perception and cognition. Sensory–Perceptual Alterations result when barriers or factors interfere with a person's ability to interpret stimuli accurately. When personality or mental disorders interfere with one's ability to interpret stimuli accurately, Altered Thought Processes is more accurate than Sensory–Perceptual Alterations.

The diagnosis Sensory–Perceptual Alterations has six subcategories: visual, auditory, kinesthetic, gustatory, tactile, and olfactory. When an individual has a visual or hearing deficit, how does the nurse intervene with the diagnosis Sensory–Perceptual Alterations: visual related to effects of glaucoma? What would the outcome criteria be? The nurse should assess for the individual's response to the visual loss and specifically label the response, not the deficit.

The diagnosis Sensory–Perceptual Alterations is more clinically useful without the addition of the specific sense. Examples of responses to sensory deficits may be:

Visual
    Risk for Injury   Self-Care Deficit
Auditory
    Impaired Communication   Social Isolation
Kinesthetic
    Risk for Injury
Olfactory
    Altered Nutrition
Tactile
    Risk for Injury
Gustatory
    Altered Nutrition

DEFINING CHARACTERISTICS

Major (Must Be Present)

Inaccurate interpretation of environmental stimuli *and/or*
Negative change in amount or pattern of incoming stimuli

377

Minor (May Be Present)

Disorientation about time
 or place
Disorientation about people
Altered problem-solving
 ability
Altered behavior or
 communication pattern

Restlessness
Auditory or visual
 hallucinations
Irritability
Poor concentration

RELATED FACTORS

Many factors in an individual's life can contribute to Sensory–
Perceptual Alterations. Some common factors are listed below.

Pathophysiological

Related to misinterpretations secondary to:
   (Sensory organ alterations)
      Visual, gustatory, auditory, olfactory, and tactile deficits
   (Neurological alterations)
      Cerebrovascular accident   Neuropathies
      Encephalitis/meningitis
   (Metabolic alterations)
      Fluid and electrolyte   Acidosis
         imbalance   Alkalosis
      Elevated blood urea
         nitrogen
   (Impaired oxygen transport)
      Cerebral   Respiratory
      Cardiac   Anemia
Related to mobility restrictions secondary: to paraplegia or
   quadriplegia

Treatment-Related

Related to misinterpretations secondary to:
   Medications (sedatives, tranquilizers)
   Surgery (glaucoma, cataract, detached retina)
Related to physical isolation (reverse isolation, communicable
   disease, prison)
Related to immobility
Related to mobility restrictions (bed rest, traction, casts,
   Stryker frame, CircOlectric bed)

Situational (Personal, Environmental)

Related to misinterpretations secondary to: pain or stress
Related to socially restricted environment
Related to excessive noise
Related to complex environment (noise, lights, constant
  changes, excess activity, frequent demands)
Related to monotonous environment
Related to loss of socialization

OUTCOME CRITERIA

The person will:

1. Demonstrate decreased symptoms of sensory overload as evident by (specify)
2. Identify and eliminate the potential risk factors if possible
3. Describe the rationale for the treatment modality

◆ GENERIC INTERVENTIONS

1. Reduce excess noise or light.
2. Share with person the source of the noise.
3. Discuss the use of a radio with earplugs to provide soft, relaxing music.
4. Share with personnel the need to reduce noise and provide individuals with uninterrupted sleep for at least 2 to 4 hours.
5. Attempt to reduce fears and concerns by explaining equipment, its purpose, and noises.
6. Encourage person to share perceptions of noises.
7. Orient to all three spheres (person, place, time).
8. Offer simple explanations of each task.
9. Allow person to participate in task, such as washing own face.
10. Promote movement in and out of bed.
11. Avoid isolation of the person; change environment daily (*e.g.*, move into hall).
12. Provide at least four undisturbed sleep and rest periods for 100 minutes every 24 hours.
13. Use a variety of methods to stimulate senses (*e.g.*, perfume, pet therapy, ambulate to window).
14. Ask family to bring in familiar possessions.
15. Limit use of sedation.
16. If at risk for injury, refer to *Risk for Injury*.

Sexuality Patterns, Altered

Sexual Dysfunction

Sexuality Patterns, Altered

DEFINITION

Altered Sexuality Patterns: The state in which an individual experiences or is at risk of experiencing a change in sexual health. Sexual health is the integration of somatic, emotional, intellectual, and social aspects of sexual being in ways that are enriching and that enhance personality, communication, and love.

> **Author's Note:**
> The diagnoses Altered Sexuality Patterns and Sexual Dysfunction are difficult to differentiate. Altered Sexuality Patterns is a broad diagnosis of which sexual dysfunction can be one part. Sexual health is the integration of somatic, emotional, intellectual, and social aspects of sexual being in ways that are enriching and that enhance personality communication and love (World Health Organization).
> Sexual Dysfunction may be more appropriately used by a nurse with advanced preparation in sex therapy. Until Sexual Dysfunction is differentiated from Altered Sexuality Patterns, it is unnecessary for most nurses to use this diagnosis.

DEFINING CHARACTERISTICS

Major (Must Be Present)

Actual or anticipated negative changes in sexual functioning or sexual identity

Minor (May Be Present)

Expression of concern about sexual functioning or sexual identity

Inappropriate sexual verbal or nonverbal behavior
Changes in primary and/or secondary sexual characteristics

RELATED FACTORS

Altered sexuality patterns can occur as a response to a variety of
health problems, situations, and conflicts. Some common sources
are listed:

Pathophysiological

Related to biochemical effects on energy and libido secondary
to:
(Endocrine)
Diabetes mellitus
Decreased hormone
production
Myxedema
(Genitourinary)
Chronic renal failure
(Neuromuscular and
skeletal)
Arthritis
Multiple sclerosis
Amyotrophic lateral
sclerosis
(Cardiorespiratory)
Myocardial infarction
Congestive heart failure
Peripheral vascular disorders
Chronic respiratory disorders
(Cancer)

Hyperthyroidism
Addison's disease
Acromegaly

Disturbances of the
nerve supply to the
brain, spinal cord,
sensory nerves, and
autonomic nerves

Related to fears associated with (specify)(sexually transmitted
diseases [STDs])
HIV/AIDS
Herpes
Syphilis

Human papilloma virus
Chlamydia
Gonorrhea

Related to the effects of alcohol on performance
Related to decreased vaginal lubrication secondary to
(specify)
Related to fear of premature ejaculation
Related to (specify) phobia, *e.g.*, pregnancy, cancer, venereal
disease

381

Treatment-Related

Related to the effects of medications or radiation treatment
Related to altered self-concept from change in appearance
(trauma, radical surgery)

Situational (Personal, Environmental)

Related to partner problem (specify), for example, unwilling,
uninformed, abusive, not available, separated, divorced
Related to no privacy
Related to stressors secondary to: job problems, financial
worries, conflicting values, or religious conflict
Related to misinformation or lack of knowledge
Related to fatigue
Related to fear of rejection secondary to obesity
Related to pain
Related to fear of sexual failure
Related to fear of pregnancy
Related to depression
Related to anxiety
Related to guilt
Related to fear of sexually transmitted disease
Related to history of unsatisfactory sexual experiences

Maturational

Adolescent
  Related to ineffective role models
  Related to negative sexual teaching
  Related to absence of sexual teaching
Adult
  Related to adjustment to parenthood
  Related to effects of pregnancy on energy levels and body
    image
  Related to values conflict
  Related to menopause

OUTCOME CRITERIA

The person will:

1. Share concerns regarding sexual functioning
2. Express increased satisfaction with sexual patterns
3. Identify stressors in life
4. Resume previous sexual activity
5. Report a desire to resume sexual activity

⊞ GENERIC INTERVENTIONS

1. Acquire a sexual history.
    a. Usual sexual pattern
    b. Satisfaction (individual, partner)
    c. Sexual knowledge
    d. Problems (sexual, health)
    e. Expectations
    f. Mood, energy level
2. Encourage to ask questions about sexuality or sexual functioning that may be disturbing him or her.
3. Explore his or her relationship with partner.
4. If stressors or a stressful lifestyle have negatively impacted functioning:
    a. Assist person in modifying lifestyle to reduce stress.
    b. Encourage identification of present stressors in life; group as those person can control and those person cannot.
        • *Can control*
            ○ Personal lateness
            ○ Involvement in community activities
        • *Cannot control*
            ○ Report due
            ○ Daughter's illness
    c. Initiate a regular exercise program for stress reduction. See *Health Seeking Behaviors* for interventions.
5. Identify alternative methods for dispersing sexual energy when partner is unavailable or unwilling.
    a. Use masturbation, if acceptable to individual.
    b. Teach the physical and psychological benefits of regular physical activity (at least three times a week for 30 minutes).
    c. If partner is deceased, explore opportunities to meet and socialize with others (night school, singles club, community work).
6. If a change or loss of body part has negatively impacted functioning:
    a. Assess the stage of adaptation of the individual and partner to the loss (denial, depression, anger, resolution; see *Grieving*).
    b. Explain the normalcy of the foregoing responses to loss.

    c. Explain the need to share concerns with partner.
- Imagined response of partner
- Fear of rejection
- Fear of future losses
- Fear of physically hurting partner

    d. Encourage the partner to discuss the strengths of their relationship and to assess the influence of the loss on their strengths.

    e. Encourage person to resume sexual activity as close to previous pattern as possible.

7. Identify barriers to satisfying sexual functioning (*e.g.*, hypoxia, pain, impaired mobility, pregnancy, side effects of medications).

8. Teach techniques to:

    a. Reduce oxygen consumption
- Use oxygen during sexual activity if indicated.
- Engage in sexual activity after intermittent positive-pressure breathing treatment or postural drainage.
- Plan sexual activities for time of day person is most rested.
- Use positions for intercourse that are comfortable and permit unrestricted breathing.

    b. Reduce cardiac workload
- Cardiac patients should avoid sexual activity:
  - In extremes of temperature
  - Directly after eating or drinking
  - When intoxicated
  - When tired
  - With unfamiliar partner
- Rest before engaging in sexual activity (mornings are best).
- Cardiac patients should terminate sexual activity if chest discomfort or dyspnea occurs.

    c. Reduce or eliminate pain
- If vaginal lubrication is decreased, use a water-soluble lubricant.
- Take medication for pain before beginning sexual activity.
- Use whatever relaxes individual before beginning sexual activity (hot packs, hot showers).

9. Initiate health teaching and referrals as indicated; discuss with individuals or couples the availability of self-help groups (*e.g.*, Reach for Recovery, United Ostomy Association).

♋ CHILD FOCUS INTERVENTIONS

1. Clarify the confidentiality of the discussion.
2. Strive to be open, warm, objective, unembarrassed, and reassuring.
3. Explore feelings and sexual experiences. Encourage questions. Clarify myths.
4. Discuss how bacteria are transferred (vaginally, anally, orally).
5. For young women, explain the relationship of sexually transmitted diseases and pelvic inflammatory disease, infertility, and atopic pregnancies.
6. Show a diagram of reproductive structures.
7. Emphasize that most sexually transmitted diseases have no symptoms initially.
8. Discuss abstinence from sexual perspective (*e.g.*, right to say no, commitment, unwanted pregnancies, sexually transmitted diseases).
9. Differentiate contraceptive methods available (*e.g.*, pill, Depo-Provera, intrauterine device, condoms, foam, diaphragm, spermicides). Discuss:
   a. How it works
   b. Effectiveness
   c. Cost
   d. Prevention of sexually transmitted diseases
10. Explain and provide written instructions for method chosen.

♊ MATERNAL FOCUS INTERVENTIONS

1. Discuss body changes during pregnancy. Encourage couple to share their feelings.
2. Reassure that unless problems exist (preterm labor, previous early loss, bleeding or rupture of membrane) intercourse is allowed until labor begins.
3. Orgasms from intercourse or masturbation should be discouraged if spotting or bleeding occurs, fetal membranes rupture prematurely, or there is a repeated history of miscarriage.

385

4. Suggest alternative sexual positions for later pregnancy to prevent abdominal pressure (*e.g.*, side-lying, woman kneeling, woman on top). Give reassurance about post-partum changes. Reassure that this is a temporary state and will resolve in 2 to 3 months.

5. Reassure that sexual attitudes change throughout pregnancy from feeling very desirous of sex to wanting only to be cuddled.

6. Encourage honest communication with partner concerning desires or changes in interest.

7. Acknowledge fatigue, especially during first trimester, last month, and postpartum.

8. Encourage person to make time for her relationship, in sexual and other contexts.

9. Teach couples to abstain from any sex play or intercourse and seek the advice of their health care provider if any of the following situations are present (May & Mahlmeister, 1994).
    a. Vaginal bleeding
    b. Premature dilation
    c. Multiple pregnancy
    d. Engaged fetal head or lightening
    e. Placenta previa
    f. Rupture of membranes
    g. History of premature delivery
    h. History of miscarriage

OLDER ADULT FOCUS INTERVENTIONS

1. Explain that normal aging affects reproductive abilities but has little effect on sexual functioning.

2. Explore interest, activity, attitude, and knowledge regarding sexual functioning.

3. If pertinent, discuss the effects of chronic diseases on functioning.

4. Explain the effects of certain medications on sexual functioning (*e.g.*, cardiovascular, antidepressants, antihistamine, gastrointestinal, sedatives, alcohol).

5. If sexual dysfunction is related to medications, explore alternatives (*e.g.*, medication change, dose reduction).

6. With women, discuss the quality of vaginal lubrication and available water-soluble lubricants.

7. Encourage questions. If needed, refer to urologist or other specialist.

Sexual Dysfunction

DEFINITION

Sexual Dysfunction: The state in which an individual experiences or is at risk of experiencing a change in sexual function that is viewed as unrewarding or inadequate.

> **Author's Note:**
> Refer to Altered Sexuality Patterns.

DEFINING CHARACTERISTICS

Major (Must Be Present, One or More)

Verbalization of problem with sexual function
Reports limitations on sexual performance imposed by
  disease or therapy

Minor (May Be Present)

Fears future limitations on sexual performance
Is misinformed about sexuality
Lacks knowledge about sexuality and sexual function
Has value conflicts involving sexual expression (cultural,
  religious)
Experiencing altered relationship with significant other
Is dissatisfied with sex role (perceived or actual)

Sleep Pattern Disturbance

Sleep Deprivation

Sleep Pattern Disturbance

DEFINITION

Sleep Pattern Disturbance: The state in which an individual experiences or is at risk of experiencing a change in the quantity or quality of his or her rest pattern that causes discomfort or interferes with desired lifestyle.

DEFINING CHARACTERISTICS

Adults

Major (Must Be Present)

Difficulty falling or remaining asleep

Minor (May Be Present)

Fatigue on awakening or
   during the day
Dozing during the day

Agitation
Mood alterations

Children

Sleep disturbances in children are frequently related to fear, enuresis, or inconsistent responses of parents to the child's requests for changes in sleep rules, such as requests to stay up late.

Reluctance to retire
Frequent awakening during the night
Desire to sleep with parents

RELATED FACTORS

Many factors in life can contribute to Sleep Pattern Disturbances. Some common factors are listed below.

Pathophysiological

Related to frequent awakenings secondary to:

Angina	Retention
Peripheral arteriosclerosis	Dysuria
Respiratory disorders	Frequency
Circulatory disorders	Hyperthyroidism
Diarrhea	Gastric ulcers
Constipation	Hepatic disorders
Incontinence	

Treatment-Related

Related to difficulty assuming usual position secondary to: casts, traction, pain, or intravenous therapy

Related to excessive daytime sleeping secondary to medications (*e.g.*):

Tranquilizers	Corticosteroids
Sedatives	Soporifics
Hypnotics	Monoamine oxidase
Antidepressants	inhibitors
Antihypertensives	Barbiturates
Amphetamines	

Situational (Personal, Environmental)

Related to excessive hyperactivity secondary to: bipolar disorder, panic anxiety, or attention-deficit disorder

Related to excessive daytime sleeping

Related to inadequate daytime activities

Related to depression

Related to pain

Related to anxiety response

Related to discomforts secondary to pregnancy

Related to lifestyle disruptions (*e.g.*, occupational, emotional, social, sexual, financial)

Related to environmental changes (*e.g.*, hospitalization [noise, disturbing roommate, fear] or travel)

Related to circadian rhythm changes

Related to fears

Maturational

Child
  Related to fear of the dark

Adult women
Related to hormonal changes (*e.g.*, perimenopausal)

OUTCOME CRITERIA

The person will:

1. Describe factors that prevent or inhibit sleep
2. Identify techniques to induce sleep
3. Report an optimal balance of rest and activity

▶ GENERIC INTERVENTIONS

1. Reduce noise.
2. Organize procedures to provide the fewest number of disturbances during sleep period (*e.g.*, when individual awakens for medication, also administer treatments and obtain vital signs).
3. If voiding during the night is disruptive, have person limit nighttime fluids and void before retiring.
4. Establish with person a schedule for a daytime program of activity (walking, physical therapy).
5. Limit amount and length of daytime sleeping if excessive (*i.e.*, more than 1 hour).
6. Assess with person, family, or parents the usual bedtime routine—time, hygiene practices, rituals (reading, toy)—and adhere to it as closely as possible.
7. Limit intake of caffeinated drinks after midafternoon.
8. Explain to person and significant others the causes of sleep/rest disturbance and possible ways to avoid it (Boyd & Nihart, 1998).
   a. Avoid alcohol.
   b. Keep regular bedtimes and rising times.
   c. Set a relaxing routine to prepare for sleep (*e.g.*, herbal tea, warm bath).
   d. Keep bedroom slightly cool.
   e. Wear ear plugs if noise is a problem.
   f. Do not exercise within 3 hours of bedtime.

♥ CHILD FOCUS INTERVENTIONS

1. Explain night to the child (stars and moon).
2. Discuss how some persons (nurses, factory workers) work at night.

3. Compare the contrast that when night comes for them, day is coming for other persons in another country.
4. If a nightmare occurs, encourage the child to talk about it if possible. Reassure child that it is a dream, even if it seems so real. Share with child that you have dreams too.
5. Provide child with a night light or a flashlight to use to give child control over the dark.
6. Reassure child that you will be nearby all night.
7. Explain the possible problems of sleeping with child.

MATERNAL FOCUS INTERVENTIONS

1. Explain some reasons for sleeping difficulties during pregnancy (*e.g.*, leg cramps, backache).
2. Teach how to position pillows in side-lying position (one between legs, one under abdomen, one under top arm, one under head).
3. Teach to avoid caffeine and large meal within 2 to 3 hours of bedtime.
4. Teach to exercise daily and take a warm bath at bedtime.

OLDER ADULT FOCUS INTERVENTIONS

1. Explain the effects of alcohol on sleep (*e.g.*, nightmares, frequent awakenings).
2. Explain that sleeping pills (prescribed or over the counter) are not effective after 1 month and that they interfere with the quality of sleep and daytime functioning.
3. Instruct to avoid over-the-counter sleeping pills because of their antihistamine effects.
4. If sleeping pills are needed for a few days, advise to consult primary care provider for a type with a short half-life.

Sleep Deprivation

DEFINITION

Sleep Deprivation: The state in which an individual experiences prolonged periods of time without sustained, natural, periodic states of relative unconsciousness.

Author's Note:

This diagnostic label represents a situation in which insufficient sleep is achieved. It is the most common type of sleep pattern disturbance and will probably be used for most clinical situations.

DEFINING CHARACTERISTICS

Refer to *Sleep Pattern Disturbance.*

RELATED FACTORS

Refer to *Sleep Pattern Disturbance.*

OUTCOME CRITERIA

Refer to *Sleep Pattern Disturbance.*

INTERVENTIONS

Refer to *Sleep Pattern Disturbance.*

Social Interaction, Impaired

DEFINITION

Impaired Social Interaction: The state in which an individual experiences or is at risk of experiencing negative, insufficient, or unsatisfactory responses from interactions.

DEFINING CHARACTERISTICS

Major (Must Be Present, One or More)

Reports inability to establish and/or maintain stable supportive relationships
Is dissatisfied with social network

Minor (May Be Present)

Social isolation
Superficial relationships
Blaming others for
  interpersonal problems
Avoidance of others
Interpersonal difficulties at
  work

Others reporting problematic
  patterns of interaction
Feelings of being
  misunderstood .
Feelings of rejection

RELATED FACTORS

Impaired Social Interactions can result from a variety of situations and health problems that are related to the inability to establish and maintain rewarding relationships. Some common sources are as follows:

Pathophysiological

Related to embarrassment or limited physical mobility or energy secondary to: loss of body function, terminal illness, or loss of body part
Related to communication barriers secondary to hearing deficits, mental retardation, visual deficits, speech impediments, or chronic mental illness

Treatment-Related

Related to surgical disfigurement
Related to therapeutic isolation

Situational (Personal, Environmental)

Related to alienation from others secondary to:
  Constant complaining
  Rumination
  Overt hostility
  Manipulative behaviors
  Mistrust or suspicions
  Illogical ideas
  Egocentric behavior
  Emotional immaturity
  Aggressive responses

  High anxiety
  Impulsive behavior
  Delusions
  Hallucinations
  Disorganized thinking
  Dependent behavior
  Strong unpopular beliefs
  Depressive behavior

Related to language/cultural barriers
Related to lack of social skills
Related to change in usual social patterns secondary to divorce, relocation, or death

Maturational

Child/adolescent
   Related to impulse control
   Related to altered appearance
   Related to speech impediments
Adult
   Related to loss of ability to practice vocation
Older adult
   Related to change in usual social patterns secondary to
      Death of spouse   Functional deficits
      Retirement

OUTCOME CRITERIA

The person will:

1. Acknowledge problems with socialization
2. Identify new behaviors to promote effective socialization
3. Report or role play the use of a constructive substitute behavior

⬢ GENERIC INTERVENTIONS

1. Provide an individual, supportive relationship.
2. Help to identify how stress precipitates problems.
3. Support healthy defenses.
4. Help to identify alternative courses of action.
5. Assist in analyzing approaches that work best.
6. Role play situations that are problematic. Discuss feelings.
7. If in group therapy:
   a. Focus on here and now.
   b. Establish group norms that discourage inappropriate behavior.
   c. Encourage testing of new social behavior.
   d. Use snacks or coffee to decrease anxiety during sessions.
   e. Role model certain accepted social behaviors (*e.g.*, responding to a friendly greeting versus ignoring it).
   f. Foster development of relationships among members through self-disclosure and genuineness.
   g. Use questions and observations to encourage persons with limited interaction skills.

  h. Encourage members to validate their perception with others.

  i. Identify strengths among members, and ignore selected weaknesses.

8. For family members of persons with chronic mental illness:

  a. Assist family members in understanding and providing support.

  b. Provide factual information concerning illness, treatment, and progress to family members.

  c. Validate family members' feelings of frustration when dealing with daily problems.

  d. Provide guidance on overstimulating or understimulating environments.

  e. Allow families to discuss their feelings of guilt and how their behavior affects the person.

  f. Develop an alliance with family.

  g. Arrange for periodic respite care.

9. For individuals with chronic mental illness, teach (McFarland, 1993):

  a. Responsibilities of his or her role as a client (making requests clearly known, participating in therapies)

  b. To outline activities of the day and focus on accomplishing them

  c. How to approach others to communicate

  d. To identify which interactions encourage others to give him or her consideration and respect

  e. To identify how he or she can participate in formulating family roles and responsibility to comply

  f. To recognize signs of anxiety and methods to relieve them

  g. To identify his or her positive behavior and experience satisfaction with self in selecting constructive choices

10. As indicated, refer to community agencies (*e.g.*, social service, occupational counseling, family therapy, crisis intervention).

✌ CHILD FOCUS INTERVENTIONS

1. If impulse control is a problem (Johnson & Saunders, 1995):

  a. Set firm, responsible limits.

  b. Do not lecture.

  c. State them simply, and back them up.

d. Maintain routines.
e. Limit play to one playmate to learn appropriate play skills (*e.g.*, relative, adult, quiet child).
f. Gradually increase number of playmates.
g. Provide immediate and constant feedback.

2. Teach parents to:
   a. Avoid harsh criticism
   b. Do not disagree in front of child
   c. Establish eye contact before giving instructions and ask child to repeat what was said

3. Teach older child to self-monitor target behaviors and to develop self-reliance.

4. If antisocial behavior is present, help to (Johnson & Saunders, 1995):
   a. Describe behaviors that interfere with socialization
   b. Role play alternate responses
   c. Limit social circle to a manageable size
   d. Elicit peer feedback for positive and negative behavior

Social Isolation

DEFINITION

Social Isolation: The state in which an individual or group experiences or perceives a need or desire for increased involvement with others but is unable to make that contact.

Author's Note:

In 1994, NANDA added a new diagnosis, Risk for Loneliness. Although this diagnosis is only in stage 1 of a four-stage developmental process, it more accurately adheres to the NANDA definition of "response to." Social isolation is not a response but a cause or contributing factor to loneliness. In addition, one can experience loneliness even with many persons around. I recommend deleting Social Isolation from clinical use and using Loneliness or Risk for Loneliness.

DEFINING CHARACTERISTICS

Because Social Isolation is a subjective state, all inferences made about a person's feelings of aloneness must be validated because the causes vary, and people show their aloneness in different ways.

Major (Must Be Present, One or More)

Expresses feelings of aloneness, rejection
Desire for more contact with people
Reports insecurity in social situations*
Describes a lack of meaningful relationships*

Minor (May Be Present)

Time passing slowly ("Mondays are so long for me.")
Inability to concentrate and make decisions
Feelings of uselessness
Feelings of rejection
Underactivity (physical or verbal)
Appearing depressed, anxious, or angry
Failure to interact with others nearby
Sad, dull affect*
Uncommunicative*
Withdrawn*
Poor eye contact*
Preoccupied with own thoughts and memories

RELATED FACTORS

A state of social isolation can result from a variety of situations and health problems that are related to a loss of established relationships or to a failure to generate these relationships. Some common sources follow.

Pathophysiological

Related to fear of rejection secondary to:
Obesity
Cancer (disfiguring surgery of head or neck, superstitions of others)
Physical handicaps (paraplegia, amputation, arthritis, hemiplegia)

*Elsen, J., & Blegen, M. (1991). Social isolation. In M. Maas, K. Buckwalter, & M. Hardy (Eds.), *Nursing diagnoses and interventions for the elderly.* Redwood City, CA: Addison-Wesley Nursing.

Emotional handicaps (extreme anxiety, depression, paranoia, phobias)

Incontinence (embarrassment, odor)

Communicable diseases (AIDS, hepatitis)

Psychiatric illness (schizophrenia, bipolar affective disorder, personality disorders)

Treatment-Related

Therapeutic isolation

Situational (Personal, Environmental)

Related to death of a significant other

Related to divorce

Related to disfiguring appearance

Related to fear of rejection secondary to: obesity, extreme poverty, hospitalization or terminal illness (dying process), or unemployment

Related to moving to another culture (*e.g.*, unfamiliar language)

Related to history of unsatisfying relationships secondary to: drug abuse, alcohol abuse, immature behavior, unacceptable social behavior, or delusional thinking

Related to loss of usual means of transportation

Maturational

Child

Related to protective isolation or a communicable disease

Older adult

Related to loss of usual social contacts

Sorrow, Chronic

DEFINITION

Chronic Sorrow: The state in which a person experiences or is at risk to experience permanent sadness, variable in intensity in response to a loved one forever changed by an event or condition, and the ongoing losses of normality (Teel, 1991).

Author's Note:
Chronic Sorrow was identified in 1962 by Olchansky. Chronic sorrow is different from grieving. Grieving is time-limited and ends in adaptation to the loss. Chronic sorrow will vary in intensity, but it persists as long as the person with the disability or chronic sorrow condition lives (Eakes, 1995).

DEFINING CHARACTERISTICS

Life-long episodic sadness due to the loss of normality in a loved one who is disabled
Variable in intensity

RELATED FACTORS

Situational (Personal, Environmental)

Related to the chronic loss of normality secondary to child's condition. Examples:

Autism	Mental retardation
Down syndrome	Psychiatric condition
Severe scoliosis	Spina bifida

Related to lifetime losses associated with infertility
Related to ongoing losses associated with a degenerative condition. Examples:
Multiple sclerosis
Alzheimer's disease

OUTCOME CRITERIA

The person will:

1. Express his or her sadness
2. Discuss the losses periodically
3. Be assisted to anticipate developmental events that can trigger heightened sadness

⊞ GENERIC INTERVENTIONS

1. Explain the difference between chronic sorrow and chronic grieving:
   a. Normal response

  b. Focused on loss of normality
  c. Not time-limited
  d. Persists throughout life
2. Encourage to share his or her feelings since the change, *e.g.*, birth of child, accident.
3. Gently encourage to share lost dreams or hopes.
4. Assist to identify developmental milestones that will exacerbate the loss of normality, *e.g.*, school play, sports, prom, dating.
5. Encourage to participate in support groups with others experiencing chronic sorrow.
6. Link the family with appropriate services, *e.g.*, home health, respite counselor.
7. Clarify that his or her feelings will fluctuate (intensify, diminish) through the years, but the sorrow will not disappear.

Spiritual Distress

Spiritual Distress, Risk for

Spiritual Distress

DEFINITION

Spiritual Distress: The state in which an individual or group experiences or is at risk of experiencing a disturbance in the belief or value system that provides strength, hope, and meaning to life.

DEFINING CHARACTERISTICS

Major (Must Be Present)

Experiences a disturbance in belief system

Minor (May Be Present)

Questions meaning of life, death, and suffering
Questions credibility of belief system

Demonstrates discouragement or despair
Chooses not to practice usual religious rituals
Has ambivalent feelings (doubts) about beliefs
Expresses that he or she has no reason for living
Feels a sense of spiritual emptiness
Shows emotional detachment from self and others
Expresses concern—anger, resentment, fear—about the
meaning of life, suffering, death
Requests spiritual assistance for a disturbance in belief system

RELATED FACTORS

Pathophysiological

Related to challenges to belief system or separation from spiritual ties secondary to:

Loss of body part or function	Pain
	Trauma
Terminal illness	Miscarriage, stillbirth
Debilitating disease	

Treatment-Related

Related to conflict between (specify prescribed regimen) and beliefs
Abortion
Surgery
Blood transfusion
Dietary restrictions
Isolation
Amputation
Medications
Medical procedures

Situational (Personal, Environmental)

Related to death or illness of significant other
Related to embarrassment at practicing spiritual rituals
Related to barriers to practicing spiritual rituals
Intensive care restrictions
Confinement to bed or room
Lack of privacy
Lack of availability of special foods/diet
Related to beliefs opposed by family, peers, health care providers
Related to divorce, separation from loved ones

OUTCOME CRITERIA

The person will:

1. Continue spiritual practices not detrimental to health
2. Express decreasing feelings of guilt and anxiety
3. Express satisfaction with spiritual condition

⊕ GENERIC INTERVENTIONS

1. Communicate acceptance of various spiritual beliefs and practices.
2. Convey nonjudgmental attitude.
3. Acknowledge importance of spiritual needs.
4. Express willingness of health care team to help in meeting spiritual needs.
5. Provide privacy and quiet as needed for daily prayer, visit of spiritual leader, and spiritual reading and contemplation.
6. Contact spiritual leader to clarify practices and perform religious rites or services if desired.
7. Maintain diet with spiritual restrictions when not detrimental to health.
8. Encourage spiritual rituals not detrimental to health.
9. Provide opportunity for individual to pray with others or be read to by members of own religious group or a member of the health care team who feels comfortable with these activities.
10. Give "permission" to discuss spiritual matters with nurse by bringing up subject of spiritual welfare if necessary.
11. Use questions about past beliefs and spiritual experiences to assist person in putting this life event into wider perspective.
12. Offer to pray/meditate/read with client if you are comfortable with this, or arrange for another member of health care team if more appropriate.
13. Be available and willing to listen when client expresses self-doubt, guilt, or other negative feelings.
14. Offer to contact other spiritual support person (*e.g.*, pastoral care, hospital chaplain) if person cannot share feelings with usual spiritual leader.

⊗ CHILD FOCUS INTERVENTIONS

1. Provide child with opportunity to engage in usual spiritual practices (*e.g.*, bedtime prayers, visit to chapel).

2. Discuss if being sick has changed their beliefs (*e.g.,* prayer requests).
3. Clarify that accidents or illnesses are not punishments for "bad acts."
4. Support an adolescent who may be struggling for understanding of spiritual teachings.
5. For parent conflict about treatment of child:
    a. If parents refuse treatment of child, encourage consideration of alternative methods of therapy (*e.g.,* use of Christian Science nurses and practitioners; special surgeons and techniques for surgery without blood transfusions); support individual making informed decision even if decision conflicts with own values.
    b. If treatment is still refused, physician or hospital administrator may obtain court order appointing temporary guardian to consent to treatment.
    c. Call spiritual leader to support parents (and possibly child).
    d. Encourage expression of negative feelings.

Spiritual Distress, Risk for

DEFINITION

Risk for Spiritual Distress: The state in which the individual or group is at risk of experiencing a disturbance in the belief or value system that provides strength, hope, and meaning to life.

RISK FACTORS

Refer to *Spiritual Distress* for related factors.

OUTCOME CRITERIA

The person will:

1. Continue to practice useful spiritual rituals
2. Express increased comfort after assistance

◆ GENERIC INTERVENTIONS

Refer to *Spiritual Distress* for interventions.

Spiritual Well-Being, Potential for Enhanced

DEFINITION

Potential for Enhanced Spiritual Well-Being: An individual who experiences affirmation of life in a relationship with a higher power (as defined by the person), self, community, and environment that nurtures and celebrates wholeness (The National Interfaith Coalition on Aging, 1980, as cited in Carson, 1989).

> **Author's Note:**
> Refer to Spiritual Distress.

DEFINING CHARACTERISTICS (Carson, 1989)

Inner strengths that nurture

Sense of awareness	Sacred source
Trust relationships	Inner peace
Unifying force	

Intangible motivation and commitment directing toward ultimate values of love, meaning, hope, beauty, and truth

Trust relations with or in the transcendent that provide bases for meaning and hope in life's experiences and love in one's relationships

Has meaning and purpose to one's existence

RISK FACTORS

Refer to Related Factors.

RELATED FACTORS

Because this is a diagnosis of positive functioning, the use of related factors is not warranted.

OUTCOME CRITERIA

The person will:

1. Maintain previous relationship with his or her higher being or source of peace

2. Continue spiritual practices not detrimental to health
3. Express continued spiritual harmony and wholeness

🔁 GENERIC INTERVENTIONS

1. Support the person's spiritual practices.
   a. Refer to Interventions to reduce barriers for spiritual practices under *Spiritual Distress.*

Surgical Recovery, Delayed

DEFINITION

Delayed Surgical Recovery: The state in which an individual experiences, or is at risk to experience, an extension of the number of postoperative days required to initiate and perform self-care activities.

> **Author's Note:**
> This newly accepted diagnosis represents an individual who has not achieved recovery from a surgical procedure during the expected time period. As one reviews the defining characteristics from NANDA, there is some confusion regarding the difference between defining characteristics (signs and symptoms) and related factors. Those with an * are not defining characteristics but are factors that can cause or contribute to Delayed Surgical Recovery. Currently the diagnosis has not been developed sufficiently for clinical use. This author recommends utilizing other nursing diagnoses, such as Self-Care Deficit, Acute Pain, or Altered Nutrition.

DEFINING CHARACTERISTICS (NANDA, 1998)

Postpones resumption of activities (home, work)
Perception that more time is needed to recover
Requires help to complete self-care
*Evidence of interrupted healing of surgical area
*Loss of appetite with or without nausea
*Difficulty in moving about
*Reports pain or discomfort

*Refer to Author's Note for explanation of *.

Thought Processes, Altered

Memory, Impaired

Thought Processes, Altered

DEFINITION

Altered Thought Processes: The state in which an individual experiences a disruption in such mental activities as conscious thought, reality orientation, problem solving, judgment, and comprehension related to coping, personality, and/or mental disorder.

Author's Note:

The diagnosis Altered Thought Processes describes an individual with altered perception and cognition that interferes with daily living. Causes are biochemical or psychological disturbances (*e.g.*, depression, personality disorders). The focus of nursing is to reduce disturbed thinking and promote reality orientation.

The nurse should be cautioned when using this diagnosis as a "waste-basket" diagnosis for all clients with disturbed thinking or confusion. Frequently, confusion in older adults is erroneously attributed to aging. Confusion in the older adult can be caused by a single factor or multiple factors (*e.g.*, dementia, medication side effects, depression, or metabolic disorder). Depression causes impaired thinking in older adults more frequently than dementia (Miller, 1990). Refer to Confusion for additional information.

DEFINING CHARACTERISTICS

Major (Must Be Present)

Inaccurate interpretation of stimuli, internal or external

Minor (May Be Present)

Cognitive deficits, including abstraction, problem solving, memory deficits

Suspiciousness
Delusions
Hallucinations
Phobias
Obsessions
Distractibility
Lack of consensual
  validation

Confusion/disorientation
Ritualistic behavior
Impulsivity
Inappropriate social behavior

RELATED FACTORS

Pathophysiological

Related to physiological changes secondary to:
  Drug or alcohol withdrawal
Related to biochemical alterations

Situational (Personal, Environmental)

Related to emotional trauma
Related to abuse [physical, sexual, mental]
Related to torture
Related to childhood trauma
Related to repressed fears
Related to panic level of anxiety
Related to continued low levels of stimulation
Related to decreased attention span and ability to process information secondary to:
  Depression   Anxiety
  Fear   Grieving

Maturational

Older adult
  Isolation, late-life depression

OUTCOME CRITERIA

The person will:

1. Identify situations that evoke anxiety
2. Express delusional material less frequently
3. Describe problems in relating with others
4. Differentiate between reality and fantasy
5. Demonstrate an increase in self-care activities

⊕ GENERIC INTERVENTIONS

1. Approach in a calm, nurturing manner.
2. Recognize when person is testing the trustworthiness of others.
3. Avoid making promises that cannot be fulfilled.
4. Initial staff contact should be minimal and brief with suspicious person; increase time as suspicion decreases.
5. Verify your interpretation of what person is experiencing ("I understand you are fearful of others.").
6. Use communication that helps person maintain own individuality (*e.g.*, "I" instead of "we").
7. For hallucinations:
   a. Observe for verbal and nonverbal hallucinations—inappropriate laughter, delayed verbal response, eye movements, moving lips without sound, increased motor movements, grinning.
   b. Direct the focus from delusional expression to discussion of reality-centered situations.
   c. Encourage differentiation of stimuli arising from inner sources from those from outside (*e.g.*, in response to "I hear voices," say, "Those are the voices of persons on television" or "I hear no one speaking now; they are your own thoughts.").
   d. Avoid the impression that you confirm or approve reality distortions; tactfully express doubt.
   e. Set limits for discussing repetitive delusional material ("You've already told me about that; let's talk about something realistic.").
   f. Identify the underlying needs being met by the delusions/hallucinations.
   g. Help connect false beliefs with increased levels of anxiety.
8. Assist in communicating more effectively.
   a. Ask for the meaning of what is said; do not assume that you understand.
   b. Validate your interpretation of what is being said ("Is this what you mean?").
   c. Clarify all global pronouns—we, they ("Who is *they*?").
   d. Refocus when person changes the subject in the middle of an explanation or thought.
   e. Tell the person when you are not following his or her train of thought.

    f. Do not mimic or restate words or phrases that you do not understand.

    g. Teach the person to validate consensually with others.

9. Assist person to set limits on own behavior.

    a. Discuss alternative methods of coping (*e.g.*, taking a walk instead of crying).

    b. Confront person with the attitude that regression is not acceptable behavior.

    c. Help delay gratification (*e.g.*, "I want you to wait 5 minutes before you repeat your request for help in making your bed.").

    d. Encourage person to achieve realistic expectations.

    e. Pace expectations to avoid frustration.

10. Encourage and support person in the decision-making process.

    a. Compliment the person who assumes more responsibility.

    b. Provide opportunity for person to contribute to own treatment plan.

    c. Help establish future goals that are realistic; examine problems in achieving a goal, and suggest various alternatives.

11. Assist person to differentiate between needs and demands.

    a. Explain the difference between needs and demands (*e.g.*, food and clothing are needs; expectations that others dress and feed person, if he or she can do it, are demands).

    b. Assist person to examine the effects of behavior on others; encourage a change in behavior if it evokes negative responses.

12. Help person recognize behaviors that stimulate rejection.

    a. Identify activities that reduce interpersonal anxiety (*e.g.*, exercise, controlled-breathing exercises).

    b. Set limits firmly and kindly on destructive behavior.

    c. Allow expression of negative emotions, verbally or in constructive activity.

    d. Help person accept responsibility for responses he or she elicits from others.

    e. Encourage discussion of problems in relating after visits with family members.

      f. Help person test new skills in relating to others in role-playing situations.

13. Anticipate difficulties in adjusting to community living; discuss concerns about returning to community, and elicit family reaction to individual's discharge.

14. Provide health teaching that will prepare person to deal with life stresses (methods of relaxation, problem-solving skills, how to negotiate with others, how to express feelings constructively).

15. Inform individual of social agencies that offer help in adjusting to community living.

16. Provide sensory input that is sufficient and meaningful.
    a. Keep person oriented to time and place.
       • Refer to time of day and place each morning.
       • Provide person with a clock and calendar large enough to see.
       • Provide person with opportunity to see daylight and dark through a window, or take person outdoors.
       • Single out holidays with cards or pins (*e.g.*, wear a red heart for Valentine's day).
    b. Encourage family to bring in familiar objects from home (photographs, afghan).
    c. Discuss current events, seasonal events (snow, water activities); share your interests (travel, crafts).
    d. Assess if person can perform an activity with own hands (*e.g.*, latch rugs, wood crafts).
       • Provide reading materials, audio tapes, puzzles (manual, computer, crossword).
       • Encourage person to keep own records if possible (*e.g.*, intake and output).
       • Provide tasks to perform (addressing envelopes, occupational therapy).

17. Refer to *Risk for Injury* for strategies for assessing and manipulating the environment for hazards.

🌀 CHILD FOCUS INTERVENTIONS

1. For children with thought disturbance, assess for signs of dissociative disorder (Johnson & Saunders, 1995).
    a. Abusive history (physical, sexual)
    b. Amnestic periods

c. Switching between alter personalities
d. Affect disturbances
e. Abrupt behavioral changes
2. Refer for multidiscipline evaluation.

Memory, Impaired

DEFINITION

Impaired Memory: The state in which an individual experiences a temporary or permanent inability to remember or recall bits of information or behavioral skills.

Author's Note:

This diagnosis is useful when the person can be helped to function better because of improved memory. If the person's memory cannot be improved because of cerebral degeneration, this diagnosis is not appropriate. Instead the nurse should evaluate the effects of impaired memory on functioning as Self-Care Deficits or Risk for Injury. The focus of interventions would be on improving self-care or protection, not on improving memory.

DEFINING CHARACTERISTICS

Major (Must Be Present, One or More)

Observed or reported experiences of forgetting
Inability to determine if a behavior was performed
Inability to learn or retain new skills or information
Inability to perform a previously learned skill
Inability to recall factual information
Inability to recall recent or past events

RELATED FACTORS

Pathophysiological

Related to central nervous system changes secondary to:
degenerative brain disease, lesion, head injury, or cerebrovascular accident

Related to reduced quantity and quality of information processed secondary to visual deficits, poor physical fitness, learning habits, educational level, hearing deficits, fatigue, or intellectual skills

Related to nutritional deficiencies (*e.g.*, vitamins C, B$_{12}$, folate, niacin, thiamin)

Treatment-Related

Related to effects of medication (specify) on memory storage

Situational (Personal, Environmental)

Related to self-fulfilling expectations

Related to excessive self-focusing and worrying secondary to grieving, depression, or anxiety

Related to alcohol consumption

Related to lack of motivation

Related to lack of stimulation

Related to difficulty concentrating secondary to: stress, distractions, lack of intellectual stimulation, pain, or sleep disturbances

OUTCOME CRITERIA

The individual will:

1. Identify three techniques to improve memory

GENERIC INTERVENTIONS

1. Discuss the person's beliefs about memory deficits.
   a. Correct misinformation.
   b. Explain that negative expectations can result in memory deficits.
   c. If a person is older, provide accurate information about age-related changes.
2. Explain that if one wants to improve memory, the intent to remember and the knowledge about techniques for remembering are needed (Miller, 1999).
3. If the person has difficulty concentrating, explain the favorable effects of relaxation and imagery.

4. Teach the person two or three methods for improving memory skills (Miller, 1999).
    a. Write things down (*e.g.*, use lists, calendars, and notebooks).
    b. Use auditory cues (*e.g.*, timers, alarm clocks) in conjunction with written cues.
    c. Have specific places for specific items, and keep the items in their proper place (*e.g.*, keep keys on a hook near the door).
    d. Put reminders in appropriate places (*e.g.*, place shoes to be repaired near the door).
    e. Use active observation—pay attention to details of what's going on around you, and be alert to the environment.
    f. Make associations between names and mental images (*e.g.*, Carol and Christmas carol).
    g. Rehearse items you want to remember by repeating them aloud or writing the information on paper.
    h. Divide information into small "chunks" that can be remembered easily (*e.g.*, to remember an address or a zip code, divide it into groups ["seven hundred sixty, fifty five"]).
    i. Search the alphabet while focusing on what you are trying to remember (*e.g.*, to remember that someone's name is Martin, start with names that begin with "A" and continue naming names through the alphabet until your memory is jogged for the correct one).
5. Explain that when one is trying to learn or remember something:
    a. Minimize distractions.
    b. Do not rush.
    c. Maintain some form of organization of routine tasks.
    d. Carry a note pad or calendar or use written cues.
6. When teaching (Miller, 1999; Stanley & Beare, 1995):
    a. Eliminate distractions.
    b. Present information as concretely as possible.
    c. Use practical examples.
    d. Allow learner to pace the learning.
    e. Use visual, auditory aids.
    f. Provide advance organizers: outlines, written cues.
    g. Encourage use of aids.

　　h. Make sure glasses are clean and lights are soft-white.
　　i. Correct wrong answers immediately.
　　j. Encourage verbal responses.

🏛 OLDER ADULT FOCUS INTERVENTIONS

1. Encourage to share concerns about memory problems.
2. Explain that short-term memory may decline with aging.
3. Explain that memory aides can improve memory. Refer to Generic Interventions.

Tissue Perfusion, Altered: (Specify)

Altered Peripheral Tissue Perfusion

Tissue Perfusion, Altered

DEFINITION

Altered Tissue Perfusion: The state in which an individual experiences or is at risk of experiencing a decrease at the capillary level in oxygenation.

Author's Note:

This nursing diagnosis is restricted to represent only diminished peripheral tissue perfusion situations in which nurses prescribe definitive treatment to reduce, eliminate, or prevent the problem.

In the other situations of diminished cardiopulmonary, cerebral, renal, or gastrointestinal tissue perfusion, the nurse should focus

(Continued)

Author's Note (Continued)

on the functional abilities of the individual that are or may be compromised because of the decreased tissue perfusion. The nurse should also monitor to detect physiological complications of decreased tissue perfusion and label these situations as collaborative problems. The following illustrates examples of a compromised functional health problem (nursing diagnosis) and a potential complication (collaborative problem) for an individual with compromised cerebral tissue perfusion:

> *Risk for Injury* related to vertigo secondary to recent head injury (nursing diagnosis)
> *Potential Complication: Increased intracranial pressure* (collaborative problem)

Refer to Chapter 2 of Carpenito, L.J.: *Nursing Diagnosis: Application to Clinical Practice* (7th ed.), Philadelphia, Lippincott, 1997, for additional information on collaborative problems. For additional examples of nursing diagnoses and collaborative problems grouped under medical conditions, refer to Section II of this handbook.

Altered Peripheral Tissue Perfusion

DEFINITION

Altered Peripheral Tissue Perfusion: The state in which an individual experiences or is at risk of experiencing a decrease in nutrition and respiration at the peripheral cellular level because of a decrease in capillary blood supply.

DEFINING CHARACTERISTICS

Major (Must Be Present, One or More)

Presence of one of the following types
    Claudication (arterial)   Aching pain (arterial)
    Rest pain (arterial)
Diminished or absent arterial pulses
Skin color changes
    Pallor (arterial)   Reactive hyperemia (arterial)
    Cyanosis (venous)

Skin temperature changes
    Cooler (arterial)
    Warmer (venous)
Decreased blood pressure (arterial)
Capillary refill greater than 3 seconds (arterial)

Minor (May Be Present)

Edema (venous)
Change in sensory function (arterial)
Change in motor function (arterial)
Trophic tissue changes (arterial)
    Hard, thick nails
    Loss of hair
    Nonhealing wound

RELATED FACTORS

Pathophysiological

Related to compromised blood flow secondary to:
    (Vascular disorders)

Arteriosclerosis	Raynaud's disease/
Hypertension	syndrome
Aneurysm	Varicosities
Arterial thrombosis	Buerger's disease
Deep vein thrombosis	Sickle cell crisis
Collagen vascular disease	Cirrhosis
Rheumatoid arthritis	Alcoholism
Leriche's syndrome	

Diabetes mellitus
Hyptension
Blood dyscrasias (platelet disorders)
Renal failure
Cancer/tumor

Treatment-Related

Related to immobilization
Related to presence of invasive lines
Related to pressure sites/constriction (Ace bandages, stockings)
Related to blood vessel trauma or compression

3. For a person in a wheelchair, obtain a lapboard (preferably Plexiglas), and position affected arm on lapboard with fingertips at midline; encourage person to look for arm on board.

4. For an ambulatory person, obtain an arm sling to prevent the arm from dangling and causing shoulder subluxation.

5. Constantly cue person to the environment.

6. Encourage person to wear prescribed corrective lenses or hearing aids.

7. For bathing, dressing, and toileting:
   a. Instruct person to attend to affected extremity/side first when performing activities of daily living.
   b. Instruct person always to look for affected extremity when performing activities of daily living, to know where it is at all times.
   c. Encourage person to integrate affected extremity during bathing; encourage person to feel extremity by rubbing and massage.

8. For eating:
   a. Instruct person to eat in small amounts; place food on unaffected side of mouth.
   b. Instruct person to use tongue to sweep out "pockets" of food from affected side after every bite.
   c. After meals/medications, check oral cavity for pocketed food/medication.
   d. Provide oral care t.i.d. and as needed.
   e. Initially place food in visual field; gradually move food out of field, and teach person to scan entire visual field.

9. Retrain person to scan entire environment.

10. Have person stroke involved side with uninvolved hand; the person should watch arm or leg as he or she strokes it.

11. Evaluate that both person and family understand the purpose and rationale of all interventions.

Urinary Elimination, Altered Patterns of

Maturational Enuresis*

Functional Incontinence

Reflex Incontinence

Stress Incontinence

Total Incontinence

Urge Incontinence

Urge Incontinence, Risk for

Urinary Retention

Author's Note:

All of these diagnoses pertain to urine elimination, not urine formulation. Anuria, oliguria, and renal failure should be labeled collaborative problems, such as Potential Complication: Anuria. Altered Patterns of Urinary Elimination represents a broad diagnosis, probably too broad for clinical use. It is recommended that a more specific diagnosis, such as Stress Incontinence be used instead. When the etiological or contributing factors have not been identified for incontinence, the diagnosis can temporarily be written Incontinence related to unknown etiology.

*This diagnosis is not currently on the NANDA list but has been included for clarity or usefulness.

Urinary Elimination, Altered Patterns of

DEFINITION

Altered Patterns of Urinary Elimination: The state in which an individual experiences or is at risk of experiencing urinary elimination dysfunction.

DEFINING CHARACTERISTICS

Major (Must Be Present, One or More)

Reports or experiences a urinary elimination problem, such as

Urgency	Dribbling
Frequency	Bladder distention
Hesitancy	Incontinence
Nocturia	Large residual urine
Enuresis	volumes

RELATED FACTORS

Pathophysiological

Related to incompetent bladder outlet secondary to congenital urinary tract anomalies

Related to decreased bladder capacity or irritation to bladder secondary to infection, trauma, urethritis, glucosuria, or carcinoma

Related to diminished bladder cues or impaired ability to recognize bladder cues secondary to:

Cord injury/tumor/infection	Diabetic neuropathy
Brain injury/tumor/infection	Alcoholic neuropathy
Cerebrovascular accident	Tabes dorsalis
Demyelinating diseases	Parkinsonism
Multiple sclerosis	

Treatment-Related

Related to effects of surgery on bladder sphincter secondary to: postprostatectomy or extensive pelvic dissection

Related to diagnostic instrumentation

Related to decreased bladder muscle tone secondary to:
General or spinal anesthesia

423

Drug therapy (iatrogenic)
 Antihistamines
 Epinephrine
 Anticholinergics
 Sedatives
Postindwelling catheters

Immunosuppressant therapy
Diuretics
Tranquilizers
Muscle relaxants

Situational (Personal, Environmental)

Related to weak pelvic floor muscles secondary to: obesity, aging, recent substantial weight loss, or childbirth

Related to inability to communicate needs

Related to bladder outlet obstruction secondary to fecal impaction or chronic constipation

Related to decreased bladder muscle tone secondary to dehydration

Related to decreased attention to bladder cues secondary to: depression, confusion, intentional suppression, or delirium

Related to environmental barriers to bathroom secondary to: distant toilets, poor lighting, unfamiliar surroundings, bed too high, or side rails

Related to inability to access bathroom on time secondary to: impaired mobility or caffeine/alcohol use

Maturational

Child
 Related to small bladder capacity
 Related to lack of motivation

OUTCOME CRITERIA

The person will:

1. Be continent (specify during day, night, 24 hours)
2. Be able to identify the cause of incontinence and rationale for treatment

⊟ GENERIC INTERVENTIONS

1. Determine if there is acute cause of problem.
   a. Infection (*e.g.*, urinary tract, sexually transmitted disease, gonorrhea)
   b. Renal disease

3. Assess for motor/mobility deficits.
4. Reduce environmental barriers.
   a. Obstacles, lighting, and distance
   b. Adequacy of toilet height and need for grab bars
5. Provide a commode between bathroom and bed, if needed.
6. For an individual with cognitive deficits, offer toileting reminders every 2 hours, after meals, and before bedtime.
7. For persons with limited hand function:
   a. Assess person's ability to remove and replace clothing.
   b. Clothing that is loose is easier to manipulate.
   c. Provide dressing aids as necessary: Velcro closures in seams for wheelchair patients, zipper pulls; all garments with fasteners may be adapted with Velcro closures.
8. Initiate referral to visiting nurse (occupational therapy department) for assessment of bathroom facilities at home.

OLDER ADULT FOCUS INTERVENTIONS

1. Emphasize that incontinence is not an inevitable age-related event.
2. Explain not to restrict fluid intake for fear of incontinence.
3. Explain not to rely on thirst as a signal to drink fluids.
4. Teach the need to have easy access to bathroom at night. If needed, consider commode chair or urinal.

Reflex Incontinence

DEFINITION

Reflex Incontinence: The state in which an individual experiences predictable, involuntary loss of urine with no sensation of urge, voiding, or bladder fullness.

DEFINING CHARACTERISTICS

Major (Must Be Present, One or More)

Uninhibited bladder contractions
Involuntary reflexes that produce spontaneous voiding

Partial or complete loss of sensation of bladder fullness or urge to void

RELATED FACTORS

Pathophysiological

Related to impaired conduction of impulses above the reflex arc level secondary to: cord injury, tumor, or infection

OUTCOME CRITERIA

The person will:

1. Report a state of dryness that is personally satisfactory
2. Have a residual urine volume of less than 50 mL
3. Use triggering mechanisms to initiate reflex voiding

◀ GENERIC INTERVENTIONS

1. Explain to person rationale for treatment.
2. Teach cutaneous triggering mechanisms:
   a. Repeated deep, sharp suprapubic tapping (most effective)
   b. Instruct individual to:
      - Position self in a half-sitting position
      - Tapping is aimed directly at bladder wall
      - Rate is seven to eight times for 5 seconds (50 single blows)
      - Use only one hand
      - Shift site of stimulation over bladder to find most successful site
      - Continue stimulation until a good stream starts
      - Wait approximately 1 minute, repeat stimulation until bladder is empty
      - One or two series of stimulations without response signifies that nothing more will be expelled
   c. If the above is ineffective, perform each of the following for 2 to 3 minutes each.
   d. Wait 1 minute between facilitation attempts.
      - Stroking glans penis
      - Punching abdomen above inguinal ligaments (lightly)
      - Stroking inner thigh

3. Encourage person to void or trigger at least every 3 hours.
4. Persons with abdominal muscle control should use the Valsalva maneuver during triggered voiding.
5. Indicate on intake and output sheet which mechanism was used to induce voiding.
6. Teach person that if fluid intake is increased, he or she also needs to increase the frequency of triggering to prevent overdistention.
7. If needed, schedule intermittent catheterization program.
8. Instruct person in signs and symptoms of dysreflexia:
   a. Elevated blood pressure, decreasing pulse
   b. Flushing and sweating above the level of the lesion
   c. Cool and clammy below the level of the lesion
   d. Pounding headache
   e. Nasal stuffiness
   f. Anxiety, "feeling of impending doom"
   g. Goose pimples
   h. Blurred vision
9. Instruct person in measures to reduce or eliminate symptoms:
   a. Elevate head
   b. Check blood pressure
   c. Rule out bladder distention; empty bladder by catheter (do not trigger); use lidocaine lubricant for catheter.
10. If condition persists after emptying bladder, check for bowel distention. If stool is present in the rectum, use a dibucaine (Nupercainal) suppository to desensitize the area before removing stool.
11. If condition persists or person has not been able to identify cause, notify physician immediately, or seek help in an emergency room.
12. Instruct person to carry an identification card that states signs, symptoms, and management in the event that the person would not be able to direct others.

Stress Incontinence

DEFINITION

Stress Incontinence: The state in which an individual experiences an immediate involuntary loss of urine during an increase in intra-abdominal pressure.

DEFINING CHARACTERISTICS

Major (Must Be Present, One or More)

The individual reports loss of urine (usually less than 50 mL) occurring with increased abdominal pressure from standing, sneezing, coughing, running, or lifting heavy objects

RELATED FACTORS

Pathophysiological

Related to incompetent bladder outlet secondary to congenital urinary tract anomalies

Related to degenerative changes in pelvic muscles and structural supports secondary to estrogen deficiency

Situational (Personal, Environmental)

Related to high intra-abdominal pressure and weak pelvic muscles secondary to: obesity, pregnancy, sex, poor personal hygiene

Related to weak pelvic muscles and sphincter incompetence secondary to: recent substantial weight loss, childbirth

Maturational

Older adult
  Related to loss of muscle tone

OUTCOME CRITERIA

The person will:

1. Report a reduction or elimination of stress incontinence
2. Be able to explain the cause of incontinence and rationale for treatment

◤ GENERIC INTERVENTIONS

1. Assess pattern of voiding/incontinence and fluid intake.
2. Explain to the person the effect of incompetent floor muscles on continence.
3. Teach person to identify pelvic floor muscles, and strengthen them with exercise (Kegel exercises).
   a. "For posterior pelvic floor muscles, imagine you are trying to stop the passage of stool and tighten your anal muscles without tightening your legs or your abdominal muscles."

b. "For anterior pelvic floor muscles, imagine you are trying to stop the passage of urine, tighten the muscles (back and front) for 4 seconds and then release them; repeat 10 times, 6 to 10 times a day." (Can be increased to four times an hour if indicated.)

c. Instruct person to stop and start the urine stream several times during voiding.

4. Explain the relationship of obesity and stress incontinence and teach:
   a. Kegel exercises
   b. person to refer to community programs if weight loss is desired
   c. Void every 2 hours
   d. Avoid prolonged periods of standing

5. Explain the relationship of decreased estrogen production and stress incontinence. Suggest vaginal estrogen cream.

6. For individuals who do not improve, refer to a urologist for evaluation of possible detrusor instability or atony, mechanical obstruction, or neuron injury.

MATERNAL FOCUS INTERVENTIONS

1. Teach to decrease abdominal pressure with pregnancy
   a. Teach to avoid prolonged periods of standing.
   b. Teach the benefit of frequent voiding at least every 2 hours.
   c. Teach Kegel exercises. (Refer to Generic Interventions.)

Total Incontinence

DEFINITION

Total Incontinence: The state in which an individual experiences continuous unpredictable loss of urine without distention or awareness of bladder fullness.

Author's Note:
This diagnosis is used only after the other types of incontinence have been ruled out.

DEFINING CHARACTERISTICS

Major (Must Be Present)

Constant flow of urine without distention
Nocturia more than two times during sleep
Incontinence refractory to other treatments

Minor (May Be Present)

Unaware of bladder cues to void
Unaware of incontinence

RELATED FACTORS

Pathophysiological

Refer to *Altered Patterns of Urinary Elimination.*

OUTCOME CRITERIA

The person will:

1. Be continent (specify during day, night, 24 hours)
2. Be able to identify the cause of incontinence and rationale for treatment

⬕ GENERIC INTERVENTIONS

1. Maintain optimal hydration.
   a. Increase fluid intake to 2000 to 3000 mL/day, unless contraindicated.
   b. Space fluids every 2 hours.
   c. Decrease fluid intake after 7 PM, and provide only minimal fluids during the night.
   d. Reduce intake of coffee, tea, dark colas, alcohol, and grapefruit juice because of their diuretic effect.
   e. Avoid large amounts of tomato and orange juice because they tend to make the urine more alkaline.
2. Maintain adequate nutrition to ensure bowel elimination at least once every 3 days.
3. Promote micturition.
   a. Ensure privacy and comfort.
   b. Use toilet facilities, if possible, instead of bedpans.
   c. Provide male with opportunity to stand, if possible.

d. Assist person on bedpan to flex knees and support back.

e. Teach postural evacuation (bend forward while sitting on toilet).

4. Promote personal integrity, and provide motivation to increase bladder control.

5. Convey to person that incontinence can be cured or at least controlled to maintain dignity.

6. Expect person to be continent, not incontinent (*e.g.*, encourage street clothes, discourage use of bedpans, protective pads).

7. Promote skin integrity.

a. Identify individuals at risk for developing pressure ulcers.

b. Wash area, rinse, and dry well after incontinent episode.

c. Use a protective ointment if needed (for area burns, use hydrocortisone cream; for fungal irritations, use antifungal ointment).

8. Assess the person's potential for participation in a bladder-retraining program (cognition, willingness to participate, desire to change behavior).

9. Provide individual with rationale for plan, and acquire informed consent.

10. Encourage individual to continue program by providing accurate information concerning reasons for success or failure.

11. Assess voiding pattern.

a. Time and amount of fluid intake

b. Type of fluid

c. Amount of incontinence

d. Amount of void, whether it was voluntary or involuntary

e. Presence of sensation of need to void

f. Amount of retention

g. Amount of residual urine

h. Amount of triggered urine

i. Identify certain activities that precede voiding (*e.g.*, restlessness, yelling, exercise)

12. Schedule fluid intake and voiding times.

13. Schedule intermittent catheterization program, if indicated.

14. Teach intermittent catheterization to person and family for long-term management of bladder.

a. Explain the reasons for the catheterization program.

     b. Explain the relationship of fluid intake and the frequency of catheterization.

     c. Explain the importance of emptying the bladder at the prescribed time regardless of circumstances because of the hazards of an overdistended bladder (*e.g.*, circulation contributes to infection, and stasis of urine contributes to bacterial growth).

15. Teach prevention of urinary tract infections.

     a. Encourage regular, complete emptying of the bladder.

     b. Ensure adequate fluid intake.

     c. Keep urine acidic; avoid citrus juices, dark colas, and coffee.

     d. Monitor urine pH.

16. Teach individual to monitor for signs and symptoms of urinary tract infections.

     a. Increase in mucus and sediment

     b. Blood in urine (hematuria)

     c. Change in color (from normal straw-colored) or odor

     d. Elevated temperature, chills, and shaking

     e. Changes in urine properties

     f. Suprapubic pain

     g. Painful urination

     h. Urgency

     i. Frequent, small voids or frequent, small incontinences

     j. Increased spasticity in spinal cord-injured individuals

     k. Increase in urine pH

     l. Nausea/vomiting

     m. Lower back or flank pain

17. Refer to community nurses for assistance in bladder reconditioning if indicated.

Urge Incontinence

DEFINITION

Urge Incontinence: The state in which an individual experiences an involuntary loss of urine associated with a strong sudden desire to void.

DEFINING CHARACTERISTICS

Major (Must Be Present)

Urgency followed by incontinence

RELATED FACTORS

Pathophysiological

Related to decreased bladder capacity secondary to:

Infection
Trauma
Urethritis
Neurogenic disorders or
  injury
Brain injury/tumor/infection

Cerebrovascular accident
Demyelinating diseases
Diabetic neuropathy
Alcoholic neuropathy
Parkinsonism

Treatment-Related

Related to decreased bladder capacity secondary to:
Abdominal surgery
Post–indwelling catheters

Situational (Personal, Environmental)

Related to irritation of bladder stretch receptors secondary to:
Alcohol
Caffeine
Excess fluid intake

Related to decreased bladder capacity secondary to frequent
voiding

Maturational

Child
Related to small bladder capacity
Older adult
Related to decreased bladder capacity

OUTCOME CRITERIA

The person will:

1. Report an absence or decreased episodes of incontinence
   (specify)
2. Explain causes of incontinence

⮕ GENERIC INTERVENTIONS

1. Explain the causative or contributing factors.
   a. Bladder irritants
      - Infection
      - Inflammation
      - Alcohol, caffeine, or dark cola ingestion
      - Concentrated urine
   b. Diminished bladder capacity
      - Self-induced deconditioning (frequent, small voids)
      - Post–indwelling catheter
   c. Overdistended bladder
      - Increased urine production (diabetes mellitus, diuretics)
      - Intake of alcohol or large quantities of fluids
   d. Uninhibited bladder contractions
      - Neurological disorders
         ○ Cerebrovascular accident
         ○ Brain tumor/trauma/infection
         ○ Parkinson's disease
2. Explain the risk of insufficient fluid intake and its relation to infection and concentrated urine.
3. Explain the relationship between incontinence and intake of alcohol, caffeine, and dark colas (irritants).
4. Determine amount of time between urge to void and need to void (record how long person can hold off urination).
5. For a person with difficulty prolonging waiting time, communicate to personnel the need to respond rapidly to request for assistance for toileting (note on care plan).
6. Teach person to increase waiting time by increasing bladder capacity.
   a. Determine volume of each void.
   b. Ask person to "hold off" urinating as long as possible.
   c. Give positive reinforcement.
   d. Discourage frequent voiding that is result of habit, not need.
   e. Develop bladder reconditioning program.
7. For uninhibited bladder contractions, provide an opportunity to void on awakening; after meals, physical exercise, bathing, and drinking coffee or tea; and before going to sleep.

Urge Incontinence, Risk for

DEFINITION

Risk for Urge Incontinence: The state in which an individual is at risk to experience an involuntary loss of urine associated with a strong, sudden desire to void.

RISK FACTORS

Refer to Related Factors in *Urge Incontinence.*

OUTCOME CRITERIA

The person will:

1. Continue to report satisfactory voiding patterns

INTERVENTIONS

Refer to *Urge Incontinence* for interventions.

Urinary Retention

DEFINITION

Urinary Retention: The state in which an individual experiences a chronic inability to void followed by involuntary voiding (overflow incontinence).

Author's Note:

This diagnosis is not recommended for use with individuals with acute episodes of urinary retention (*e.g.*, fecal impaction, postanesthesia, postdelivery), in which cases catheterization, treatment of the cause, or surgery (prostatic hypertrophy) cure urinary retention. These situations are collaborative problems: Potential Complication: Acute urinary retention.

DEFINING CHARACTERISTICS

Major (Must Be Present, One or More)

Bladder distention (not related to acute, reversible etiology) *or*
Bladder distention with small, frequent voids or dribbling
  (overflow incontinence)
100 mL or more residual urine

Minor (May Be Present)

The individual states that it feels as though the bladder is not
  empty after voiding.

RELATED FACTORS

Pathophysiological

Related to sphincter blockage secondary to:
  Strictures   Ureterocele
  Prostate enlargement   Bladder neck contractures
  Perineal swelling
Related to impaired afferent pathways or inadequacy sec-
  ondary to:
  Cord injury/tumor/infection   Multiple sclerosis
  Brain injury/tumor/infection   Diabetic neuropathy
  Cerebrovascular accident   Alcoholic neuropathy
  Demyelinating diseases   Tabes dorsalis

Treatment-Related

Related to bladder outlet obstruction or impaired afferent
  pathways secondary to drug therapy (iatrogenic)
  Antihistamines   Theophylline
  Epinephrine   Isoproterenol
  Anticholinergics

Situational (Personal, Environmental)

Related to bladder outlet obstruction secondary to fecal impaction
Related to detrusor inadequacy secondary to deconditioned
  voiding associated with stress or discomfort

OUTCOME CRITERIA

The person will:

1. Empty the bladder using Credé's or Valsalva maneuvers with residual urine of less than 50 mL if indicated
2. Void voluntarily
3. Achieve a state of dryness that is personally satisfactory

⮔ GENERIC INTERVENTIONS

1. Develop a bladder retraining or reconditioning program (see *Total Incontinence* for general interventions).
2. Teach person abdominal strain and Valsalva maneuver, if indicated.
    a. Lean forward on thighs.
    b. Contract abdominal muscles if possible, and strain or "bear down;" hold breath while straining (Valsalva maneuver).
    c. Hold strain or breath until urine flow stops; wait 1 minute, and strain again as long as possible.
    d. Continue until no more urine is expelled.
3. Teach person Credé's maneuver if indicated.
    a. Place hands flat (or place fist) just below umbilical area.
    b. Place one hand on top of the other.
    c. Press firmly down and in toward the pelvic arch.
    d. Repeat six or seven times until no more urine can be expelled.
    e. Wait a few minutes and repeat to ensure complete emptying.
4. Teach person anal stretch maneuver, if indicated.
    a. Sit on commode or toilet.
    b. Lean forward on thighs.
    c. Place one gloved hand behind buttocks.
    d. Insert one to two lubricated fingers into the anus to the anal sphincter.
    e. Spread fingers apart, or pull to posterior direction.
    f. Gently stretch the anal sphincter and hold it distended.
    g. Bear down and void.
    h. Take a deep breath and hold it while straining (Valsalva).
    i. Relax and repeat the procedure until the bladder is empty.

5. Instruct individual to try all three techniques or a combination of techniques to determine which is most effective in emptying the bladder.
6. Indicate on the intake and output record which technique was used to induce voiding.
7. Obtain postvoid residuals after attempts at emptying bladder; if residual urine volumes are greater than 100 ml, schedule intermittent catheterization program.

Violence, Risk for

DEFINITION

Risk for Violence: The state in which an individual has been or is at risk to be assaultive toward others or the environment.

> **Author's Note:**
> This diagnosis can be made more specific by adding Risk for Violence: Self-directed or directed at others. The author has added Risk for Suicide to describe individuals at risk for self-inflicted injuries; thus, the descriptor *self-directed* is not needed. Therefore, the content for Risk for Violence will focus exclusively on violence directed at others.

RISK FACTORS

Presence of risk factors (see also Related Factors)

RELATED FACTORS

Pathophysiological

Related to history of aggressive acts and perception of environment as threatening secondary to: *or*

Related to history of aggressive acts and delusional thinking secondary to: *or*

Related to history of aggressive acts and manic excitement secondary to: *or*

Related to history of aggressive acts and inability to verbalize feelings secondary to: *or*

Related to history of aggressive acts and psychic overload
   secondary to:

Temporal lobe epilepsy	Hormonal imbalance
Progressive CNS deter-	Viral encephalopathy
ioration (brain tumor)	Mental retardation
Head injury	Minimal brain dysfunction

Related to toxic response to alcohol or drugs
Related to organic brain syndrome

Treatment-Related

Related to toxic reaction to medication

Situational (Personal, Environmental)

Related to history of overt aggressive acts
Related to increase in stressors within a short period
Related to acute agitation
Related to suspiciousness
Related to persecutory delusions
Related to verbal threats of physical assault
Related to low frustration tolerance
Related to poor impulse control
Related to fear of the unknown
Related to response to catastrophic event
Related to response to dysfunctional family throughout devel-
   opmental stages
Related to dysfunctional communication patterns
Related to drug or alcohol abuse

OUTCOME CRITERIA

The person will:

1. Experience control of behavior with assistance from others
2. Have a decreased number of violent responses
3. Describe causation and possible preventive measures

GENERIC INTERVENTIONS

1. Acknowledge the individual's feelings; be genuine and empathetic.
2. Tell individual that you will help control behavior and not let him or her do anything destructive.
3. Set limits when individual presents a risk to others. Refer to *Anxiety* for further interventions on limit setting.

443

4. Offer the individual choices and options. At times, it is necessary to give in on some demands to avoid a power struggle.

5. Encourage individual to express anger and hostility verbally instead of "acting out."

6. Remain calm; if you are becoming upset, leave the situation in the hands of others, if possible.

7. Allow the acutely agitated individual space that is five times greater than that for an individual who is in control. Do not touch the person unless you have a trusting relationship. Avoid physical entrapment of individual or staff.

8. Do not approach a violent individual alone. Often the presence of three to four staff members will be enough to reassure the individual that you will not let him or her lose control.

9. When assault is imminent, quick, coordinated action is essential.

10. Approach individual in a calm, self-assured manner to avoid communicating your anxiety or fear.

11. Establish an environment that reduces agitation.
   a. Decrease noise level.
   b. Give short, concise explanations.
   c. Control the number of persons present at one time.
   d. Provide single or semiprivate room.

12. Establish the expectation that person can control behavior, and continue to reinforce the expectation.

13. Provide positive feedback when person is able to exercise restraint.

14. Allow appropriate verbal expressions of anger. Give positive feedback.

15. Set limits on verbal abuse. Do not take insults personally. Support others (clients, staff) who may be targets of abuse.

16. Plan for unpredictable violence.
   a. Assess person's potential for violence and history.
   b. Ensure availability of staff before potential violent behavior (never try to assist person alone when physical restraint is necessary).
   c. Determine who will be in charge of directing personnel to intervene in violent behavior if it occurs.
   d. Ensure protection for oneself (door nearby for withdrawal, pillow to protect face).

17. Use seclusion or restraint, according to policy.
   a. Remove individual from situation if environment is contributing to aggressive behavior, using the

least amount of control needed (*e.g.,* ask others to leave, and take individual to quiet room).

b. Reinforce that you are going to help person control self.

c. Repeatedly tell the person what is going to happen before external control is begun. When using seclusion, institutional policy will provide specific guidelines; the following are general.

- Observe individual at least every 15 minutes.
- Search the individual before secluding to remove harmful objects.
- Check seclusion room to see that safety is maintained.
- Offer fluids and food periodically (in nonbreakable containers).
- When approaching an individual to be secluded, have sufficient staff present.
- Explain concisely what is going to happen ("You will be placed in a room by yourself until you can better control your behavior."), and give person a chance to cooperate.
- Assist person in toileting and personal hygiene (assess ability to be out of seclusion; a urinal or commode may need to be used).
- If person is taken out of seclusion, someone must be present continually.
- Maintain verbal interaction during seclusion (provides information necessary to assess person's degree of control).
- When person is allowed out of seclusion, a staff member needs to be in constant attendance to determine whether person can handle additional stimulation.

18. Assist individual in developing alternative coping strategies when crisis has passed and learning can occur.

19. Teach negotiation skills with significant others and persons in authority.

20. Encourage an increase in recreational activities.

21. Use group therapy to decrease sense of aloneness and increase communication skills.

22. Consult with person's therapist or your supervisor if third parties need to be warned of danger from the client (*e.g.,* police, potential victim).

Section II

Diagnostic Clusters
(Medical Conditions With
Associated Nursing Diagnoses
and Collaborative Problems)

Medical Conditions

Cardiovascular/Hematological/ Peripheral Vascular Disorders

Cardiac Conditions

ANGINA PECTORIS

Nursing Diagnoses*

Anxiety related to chest pain secondary to effects of hypoxia

Fear related to present status and unknown future

Sleep Pattern Disturbance related to treatments and environment

Risk for Constipation related to bed rest, change in lifestyle, and medications

Activity Intolerance related to deconditioning secondary to fear of recurrent angina

Risk for Self-Concept Disturbance related to perceived and/or actual role changes

Risk for Impaired Home Maintenance Management related to angina or fear of angina

Risk for Altered Family Processes related to impaired ability of person to assume role responsibilities

Risk for Altered Sexuality Patterns related to fear of angina and altered self-concept

Grieving related to actual or perceived losses secondary to cardiac condition

Risk for Ineffective Management of Therapeutic Regimen related to insufficient knowledge of condition, home activities, diet, and medications

*List includes nursing diagnoses that may be associated with the medical diagnosis.

CONGESTIVE HEART FAILURE WITH PULMONARY EDEMA

Collaborative Problems

†△ *PC: Deep vein thrombosis*
▲ *PC: Severe hypoxia*
△ *PC: Cardiogenic shock*
  PC: Hepatic failure

Nursing Diagnoses

▲ Activity Intolerance related to insufficient oxygen for activities of daily living
△ Altered Nutrition: Less than body requirements related to nausea; anorexia secondary to venous congestion of gastrointestinal tract and fatigue
△ Altered Peripheral Tissue Perfusion related to venous congestion secondary to right-sided heart failure
▲ Anxiety related to breathlessness
* Fear related to progressive nature of condition
* Risk for Impaired Home Maintenance Management related to inability to perform activities of daily living secondary to breathlessness and fatigue
* (Specify) Self-Care Deficit related to dyspnea and fatigue
△ Sleep Pattern Disturbance related to nocturnal dyspnea and inability to assume usual sleep position
▲ Risk for Fluid Volume Excess: Edema related to decreased renal blood flow secondary to right-sided heart failure
△ Powerlessness related to progressive nature of condition
△ Risk for Ineffective Management of Therapeutic Regimen related to insufficient knowledge of low-salt diet, drug therapy (diuretic, digitalis), activity program, and signs and symptoms of complications

▲ This diagnosis was reported to be monitored for or managed frequently (75%–100%).
△ This diagnosis was reported to be monitored for or managed often (50%–74%).
* This diagnosis was not included in the validation study.
† PCs (potential complications) are collaborative problems, not nursing diagnoses.

449

ENDOCARDITIS, PERICARDITIS
(Rheumatic, Infectious)

See also *Corticosteroid Therapy*.
If child, see *Rheumatic Fever*.

Collaborative Problems

>PC: Congestive heart failure
>PC: Valvular stenosis
>PC: Cerebrovascular accident
>PC: Emboli (pulmonary, cerebral, renal, splenic, heart)
>PC: Cardiac tamponade

Nursing Diagnoses

>Activity Intolerance related to insufficient oxygen secondary to decreased cardiac output
>Risk for Altered Respiratory Function related to decreased respiratory depth secondary to pain
>Pain related to friction rub and inflammation process
>Risk for Ineffective Management of Therapeutic Regimen related to insufficient knowledge of etiology, prevention, antibiotic prophylaxis, and signs and symptoms of complications

MYOCARDIAL INFARCTION (Uncomplicated)

Collaborative Problems

>▲ PC: Dysrhythmias
>▲ PC: Cardiogenic shock
>▲ PC: Thromboembolism
>PC: Recurrent myocardial infarction

Nursing Diagnoses

>▲ Anxiety related to acute pain secondary to cardiac tissue ischemia
>* Fear related to pain, present status, and unknown future

▲ This diagnosis was reported to be monitored for or managed frequently (75%–100%).
* This diagnosis was not included in the validation study.

* Sleep Pattern Disturbances related to treatments and environment

  Risk for Constipation related to decreased peristalsis secondary to medication effects, decreased activity, and change in diet

▲ Activity Intolerance related to insufficient oxygen for activities of daily living secondary to cardiac tissue ischemia

* Risk for Self-Concept Disturbance related to perceived or actual role changes

  Risk for Impaired Home Maintenance Management related to angina or fear of angina

▲ Anxiety/Fear (individual, family) related to unfamiliar situation status, unpredictable nature of condition, negative effect on lifestyle, possible sexual dysfunction

* Risk for Altered Family Processes related to impaired ability of ill person to assume role responsibilities

* Risk for Altered Sexuality Patterns related to fear of angina and altered self-concept

△ Grieving related to actual or perceived losses secondary to cardiac condition

△ Risk for Ineffective Management of Therapeutic Regimen related to insufficient knowledge of hospital routines, treatments, conditions, medications, diet, activity progression, signs and symptoms of complications, reduction of risks, follow-up care, community resources

Hematological Conditions

ANEMIA

Collaborative Problems

PC: Bleeding
PC: Cardiac failure
PC: Iron overload (repeated transfusion)

▲ This diagnosis was reported to be monitored for or managed frequently (75%–100%).

△ This diagnosis was reported to be monitored for or managed often (50%–74%).

* This diagnosis was not included in the validation study.

Nursing Diagnoses

Activity Intolerance related to impaired oxygen transport secondary to diminished red blood cell count

Risk for Infection related to decreased resistance secondary to tissue hypoxia and/or abnormal white blood cells (neutropenia, leukopenia)

Risk for Injury: Bleeding tendencies related to thrombocytopenia and splenomegaly

Risk for Altered Oral Mucous Membrane related to gastrointestinal mucosal atrophy

Risk for Ineffective Management of Therapeutic Regimen related to insufficient knowledge of condition, nutritional requirements, and drug therapy

APLASTIC ANEMIA

Collaborative Problems

PC: Fatal aplasia
PC: Pancytopenia
PC: Hemorrhage
PC: Hypoxia
PC: Sepsis

Nursing Diagnoses

Activity Intolerance related to insufficient oxygen secondary to diminished red blood cell count

Risk for Infection related to increased susceptibility secondary to leukopenia

Risk for Altered Oral Mucous Membrane related to tissue hypoxia and vulnerability

Risk for Ineffective Management of Therapeutic Regimen related to insufficient knowledge of causes, prevention, and signs and symptoms of complications

PERNICIOUS ANEMIA

See also *Anemia.*

Nursing Diagnoses

Altered Oral Mucous Membrane related to sore red tongue secondary to papillary atrophy and inflammatory changes

Diarrhea/Constipation related to gastrointestinal
   mucosal atrophy
Risk for Altered Nutrition: Less than body requirements
   related to anorexia secondary to sore mouth
Risk for Ineffective Management of Therapeutic Regimen related to insufficient knowledge of chronicity of
   disease and vitamin B treatment

DISSEMINATED INTRAVASCULAR COAGULATION (DIC)

See also *Underlying Disorders* (*e.g.*, *Obstetric, Infections,
Burns*).
See also *Anticoagulant Therapy.*

Collaborative Problems

PC: Hemorrhage
PC: Renal failure
*PC: Microthrombi (renal, cardiac, pulmonary, cerebral,
   gastrointestinal)*

Nursing Diagnoses

Fear related to treatments, environment, and unpredictable outcome
Altered Family Processes related to critical nature of
   the situation and uncertain prognosis
Anxiety related to insufficient knowledge of causes and
   treatment

POLYCYTHEMIA VERA

Collaborative Problems

PC: Thrombus formation
PC: Hemorrhage
PC: Hypertension
PC: Congestive heart failure
PC: Peptic ulcer
PC: Gout

Nursing Diagnoses

Altered Nutrition: Less than body requirements related
   to anorexia, nausea, and vasocongestion

Activity Intolerance related to insufficient oxygen secondary to pulmonary congestion and tissue hypoxia

Risk for Infection related to hypoxia secondary to vasocongestion

Risk for Ineffective Management of Therapeutic Regimen related to insufficient knowledge of fluid requirements, exercise program, and signs and symptoms of complications

Peripheral Vascular Conditions

DEEP VEIN THROMBOSIS

See also *Anticoagulant Therapy,* if indicated.

Collaborative Problems

▲ *PC: Pulmonary embolism*
▲ *PC: Chronic leg edema*
△ *PC: Chronic stasis ulcers*

Nursing Diagnoses

Risk for Constipation related to decreased peristalsis secondary to immobility

△ Risk for Altered Respiratory Function related to immobility

△ Risk for Impaired Skin Integrity related to chronic ankle edema

▲ Acute pain related to impaired circulation for ambulation

△ Risk for Ineffective Management of Therapeutic Regimen related to insufficient knowledge of prevention of recurrence of deep vein thrombosis and signs and symptoms of complications

---

▲ This diagnosis was reported to be monitored for or managed frequently (75%–100%).
△ This diagnosis was reported to be monitored for or managed often (50%–74%).

HYPERTENSION

Collaborative Problems

PC: Retinal hemorrhage
PC: Cerebrovascular accident
PC: Cerebral hemorrhage
PC: Renal failure

Nursing Diagnoses

Risk for Noncompliance related to negative side effects of prescribed therapy versus the belief that no treatment is needed without the presence of symptoms

Risk for Altered Sexuality Patterns related to decreased libido or erectile dysfunction secondary to medication side effects

Risk for Ineffective Management of Therapeutic Regimen related to insufficient knowledge of condition, diet restrictions, medications, risk factors, and follow-up care

VARICOSE VEINS

Collaborative Problems

PC: Vascular rupture
PC: Hemorrhage

Nursing Diagnoses

Chronic Pain related to engorgement of veins
Risk for Ineffective Management of Therapeutic Regimen related to insufficient knowledge of condition, treatment options, and risk factors

PERIPHERAL ARTERIAL DISEASE

(Atherosclerosis, Arteriosclerosis)

Collaborative Problems

PC: Stroke (cerebrovascular accident)
PC: Ischemic ulcers
PC: Claudication
PC: Acute arterial thrombosis
PC: Hypertension

Nursing Diagnoses

Risk for Impaired Tissue Integrity related to compromised circulation

Chronic Pain related to muscle ischemia during prolonged activity

Risk for Injury related to decreased sensation secondary to chronic atherosclerosis

Risk for Infection related to compromised circulation

Risk for Injury related to effects of orthostatic hypotension

Activity Intolerance related to claudication

Risk for Ineffective Management of Therapeutic Regimen related to insufficient knowledge of condition, management of claudication, risk factors, foot care, and treatment plan

RAYNAUD'S DISEASE

Collaborative Problems

PC: Acute arterial occlusion
PC: Ischemic ulcers
PC: Gangrene

Nursing Diagnoses

Acute Pain related to ischemia secondary to acute vasospasm

Altered Peripheral Tissue Perfusion related to compromised blood flow and vasospasms secondary to cold environment

Risk for Impaired Tissue Integrity: Ischemic ulcers related to vasospasm

Fear related to potential loss of work secondary to work-related aggravating factors

Risk for Ineffective Management of Therapeutic Regimen related to insufficient knowledge of condition, risk factors, and self-care

VENOUS STASIS ULCERS (Postphlebitis Syndrome)

Collaborative Problem

▲ *PC: Cellulitis*

▲ This diagnosis was reported to be monitored for or managed frequently (75%–100%).

Nursing Diagnoses

* Altered Peripheral Tissue Perfusion related to dependent position of legs
* Risk for Infection related to compromised circulation
▲ Chronic Pain related to ulcers and débridement treatments
△ Risk for Body Image Disturbance related to chronic open wounds and response of others to appearance
△ Ineffective Management of Therapeutic Regimen related to lack of knowledge of condition, prevention of complications, risk factors, and treatment

Respiratory Disorders

ADULT RESPIRATORY DISTRESS SYNDROME

See also *Mechanical Ventilation* (under *Diagnostic and Therapeutic Procedures*).

Collaborative Problems

PC: Electrolyte imbalance
PC: Hypoxemia

Nursing Diagnoses

Anxiety related to implications of condition and critical care setting
Powerlessness related to condition and treatments (ventilator, monitoring)

CHRONIC OBSTRUCTIVE PULMONARY DISEASE (Emphysema, Bronchitis)

Collaborative Problems

▲ *PC: Hypoxemia*
△ *PC: Right-sided heart failure*

▲ This diagnosis was reported to be monitored for or managed frequently (75%–100%).
△ This diagnosis was reported to be monitored for or managed often (50%–74%).
* This diagnosis was not included in the validation study.

Nursing Diagnoses

▲ Ineffective Airway Clearance related to excessive and tenacious secretions

△ Risk for Altered Nutrition: Less than body requirements related to anorexia secondary to dyspnea, halitosis, and fatigue

▲ Activity Intolerance related to insufficient oxygen for activities and fatigue

Impaired Verbal Communication related to dyspnea

▲ Anxiety related to breathlessness and fear of suffocation

△ Powerlessness related to feeling of loss of control and lifestyle restrictions

△ Sleep Pattern Disturbance related to cough, inability to assume recumbent position, and environmental stimuli

△ Risk for Ineffective Management of Therapeutic Regimen related to insufficient knowledge of condition, treatments, prevention of infection, breathing exercises, risk factors, signs and symptoms of complications

PLEURAL EFFUSION

See also underlying disorders (*Congestive Heart Disease, Cirrhosis, Malignancy*).

Collaborative Problems

PC: Respiratory failure
PC: Pneumothorax (post-thoracentesis)
PC: Hypoxemia
PC: Hemothorax

Nursing Diagnoses

Activity Intolerance related to insufficient oxygen for activities of daily living

Risk for Altered Nutrition: Less than body requirements related to anorexia secondary to pressure on abdominal structures

---

▲ This diagnosis was reported to be monitored for or managed frequently (75%–100%).

△ This diagnosis was reported to be monitored for or managed often (50%–74%).

Altered Comfort related to accumulation of fluid in pleural space

(Specify) Self-Care Deficits related to fatigue and dyspnea

PNEUMONIA

Collaborative Problems

▲ *PC: Respiratory insufficiency*
PC: Septic shock
PC: Paralytic ileus

Nursing Diagnoses

Risk for Hyperthermia related to infectious process

▲ Activity Intolerance related to insufficient oxygen for activities of daily living

△ Risk for Altered Oral Mucous Membrane related to mouth breathing, frequent expectoration, and decreased fluid intake secondary to malaise

* Risk for Fluid Volume Deficit related to increased insensible fluid loss secondary to fever and hyperventilation

△ Risk for Altered Nutrition: Less than body requirements related to anorexia, dyspnea, and abdominal distention secondary to air swallowing

▲ Ineffective Airway Clearance related to pain, increased tracheobronchial secretions, and fatigue

* Risk for Infection Transmission related to communicable nature of the disease

* Altered Comfort related to hyperthermia and malaise

* Risk for Impaired Skin Integrity related to prescribed bed rest

△ Risk for Ineffective Management of Therapeutic Regimen related to lack of knowledge of condition, infection transmission, prevention of recurrence, diet, signs and symptoms of recurrence, and follow-up care

---

▲ This diagnosis was reported to be monitored for or managed frequently (75%–100%).
△ This diagnosis was reported to be monitored for or managed often (50%–74%).
* This diagnosis was not included in the validation study.

PULMONARY EMBOLISM

See also *Anticoagulant Therapy.*

Collaborative Problem

PC: Hypoxemia

Nursing Diagnoses

Risk for Impaired Skin Integrity related to immobility and prescribed bed rest

Risk for Ineffective Management of Therapeutic Regimen related to insufficient knowledge of anticoagulant therapy and signs and symptoms of complications

---

Metabolic/Endocrine Disorders

ADDISON'S DISEASE

Collaborative Problems

PC: Addisonian crisis (shock)
PC: Electrolyte imbalances (sodium, potassium)
PC: Hypoglycemia

Nursing Diagnoses

Risk for Altered Nutrition: Less than body requirements related to anorexia and nausea

Risk for Fluid Volume Deficit related to excessive loss of sodium and water secondary to polyuria

Diarrhea related to increased excretion of sodium and water

Risk for Self-Concept Disturbance related to appearance changes secondary to increased skin pigmentation and decreased axillary and pubic hair (female)

Risk for Injury related to postural hypotension secondary to fluid/electrolyte imbalances

Risk for Ineffective Management of Therapeutic Regimen related to insufficient knowledge of disease, signs and symptoms of complications, risks for crisis (infection, diarrhea, decreased sodium intake, diaphoresis), overexertion, dietary management, identification (card, medallion), emergency kit, and pharmacological management

ALDOSTERONISM, PRIMARY

Collaborative Problems

PC: Hypokalemia
PC: Alkalosis
PC: Hypertension
PC: Hypernatremia

Nursing Diagnoses

Altered Comfort related to excessive urine excretion and polydipsia

Risk for Fluid Volume Deficit related to excessive urinary excretion

Risk for Ineffective Management of Therapeutic Regimen related to insufficient knowledge of condition, surgical treatment, and effects of corticosteroid therapy

CIRRHOSIS (Laënnec's Disease)

See also *Substance Abuse,* if indicated.

Collaborative Problems

▲ PC: Hemorrhage
△ PC: Hypokalemia
△ PC: Portal systemic encephalopathy
* PC: Negative nitrogen balance
▲ PC: Drug toxicity (opiates, short-acting barbiturates, major tranquilizers)
△ PC: Renal failure
* PC: Anemia
* PC: Esophageal varices

▲ This diagnosis was reported to be monitored for or managed frequently (75%–100%).
△ This diagnosis was reported to be monitored for or managed often (50%–74%).
* This diagnosis was not included in the validation study.

Nursing Diagnoses

▲ Pain related to liver enlargement and ascites
△ Diarrhea related to excessive secretion of fats in stool secondary to liver dysfunction
* Risk for Injury related to decreased prothrombin production and synthesis of substances used in blood coagulation
▲ Altered Nutrition: Less than body requirements related to anorexia, impaired protein, fat, glucose metabolism, and impaired storage of vitamins (A, C, K, D, E)
* Risk for Altered Respiratory Function related to pressure on diaphragm secondary to ascites
* Risk for Self-Concept Disturbance related to appearance changes (jaundice, ascites)
△ Risk for Infection related to leukopenia secondary to enlarged, overactive spleen and hypoproteinemia
△ Altered Comfort: Pruritus related to accumulation of bilirubin pigment and bile salts on skin
▲ Fluid Volume Excess related to portal hypertension, lowered plasma colloidal osmotic pressure, and sodium retention
△ Risk for Ineffective Management of Therapeutic Regimen related to insufficient knowledge of pharmacological contraindications, nutritional requirements, signs and symptoms of complications, and risks of alcohol ingestion

CUSHING'S SYNDROME

Collaborative Problems

PC: Hypertension
PC: Congestive heart failure
PC: Psychosis
PC: Electrolyte imbalance (sodium, potassium)

Nursing Diagnoses

Self-Concept Disturbance related to physical changes secondary to disease process (moon face, thinning of hair, truncal obesity, virilism)

▲ This diagnosis was reported to be monitored for or managed frequently (75%–100%).
△ This diagnosis was reported to be monitored for or managed often (50%–74%).
* This diagnosis was not included in the validation study.

Risk for Infection related to excessive protein catabolism and depressed leukocytic phagocytosis secondary to hyperglycemia

Risk for Injury: Fractures related to osteoporosis

Risk for Impaired Skin Integrity related to loss of tissue, edema, and dryness

Altered Sexuality Patterns related to loss of libido and cessation of menses (female) secondary to excessive adrenocorticotropic hormone production

Risk for Ineffective Management of Therapeutic Regimen related to insufficient knowledge of disease and diet therapy (high protein, low cholesterol, low sodium)

DIABETES MELLITUS

Collaborative Problems

Acute complications:

▲ *PC: Ketoacidosis (DKA)*
△ *PC: Hyperosmolar hyperglycemic nonketotic coma (HHNR)*
▲ *PC: Hypoglycemia*
▲ *PC: Infections*

Chronic complications:

Macrovascular
▲ *PC: Cardiac artery disease*
▲ *PC: Peripheral vascular disease*
Microvascular
△ *PC: Retinopathy*
▲ *PC: Neuropathy*
△ *PC: Nephropathy*

Nursing Diagnoses

△ Risk for Injury related to decreased tactile sensation, diminished visual acuity, and hypoglycemia
△ Fear (client, family) related to diagnosis of diabetes, potential complications of diabetes, insulin injection, negative effect on lifestyle

▲ This diagnosis was reported to be monitored for or managed frequently (75%–100%).
△ This diagnosis was reported to be monitored for or managed often (50%–74%).

△ Risk for Ineffective Coping (client, family) related to chronic disease, complex self-care regimen, and uncertain future

▲ Altered Nutrition: More than body requirements related to intake in excess of activity expenditures, lack of knowledge, and ineffective coping

Risk for Altered Sexuality Patterns (male) related to erectile problems secondary to peripheral neuropathy or psychological conflicts

Risk for Altered Sexuality Patterns (female) related to frequent genitourinary problems and physical and psychological stressors of diabetes

△ Powerlessness related to the future development of complications of diabetes (blindness, amputations, kidney failure, painful neuropathy)

* Social Isolation related to visual impairment/blindness

△ Risk for Noncompliance related to the complexity and chronicity of the prescribed regimen

△ Risk for Ineffective Management of Therapeutic Regimen related to insufficient knowledge of condition, self-monitoring of blood glucose, medications, American Diabetes Association exchange diet, treatment of hypoglycemia, weight control, sick day care, exercise program, foot care, signs and symptoms of complications, and community resources

HEPATITIS (Viral)

Collaborative Problems

* PC: Hepatic failure
* PC: Coma
* PC: Subacute hepatic necrosis
* PC: Fulminant hepatitis
△ PC: Portal systemic encephalopathy
△ PC: Hypokalemia
△ PC: Hemorrhage
△ PC: Drug toxicity
△ PC: Renal failure
△ PC: Progressive liver degeneration

▲ This diagnosis was reported to be monitored for or managed frequently (75%–100%).
△ This diagnosis was reported to be monitored for or managed often (50%–74%).
* This diagnosis was not included in the validation study.

Nursing Diagnoses

* * Fatigue related to reduced metabolism by liver
* ▲ Risk for Infection Transmission related to contagious nature of virus type A and type B
* ▲ Altered Nutrition: Less than body requirements related to anorexia, epigastric distress, and nausea
* * Risk for Fluid Volume Deficit related to lack of desire to drink
* △ Altered Comfort related to accumulation of bilirubin pigment and bile salts
* * Risk for Injury related to reduced prothrombin synthesis and reduced vitamin K absorption
* △ Pain related to swelling of inflamed liver
* * Diversional Activity Deficit related to the monotony of confinement and isolation precautions
* △ Risk for Ineffective Management of Therapeutic Regimen related to insufficient knowledge of condition, rest requirements, precautions to prevent transmission, nutritional requirements, and contraindications

HYPERTHYROIDISM (Thyrotoxicosis, Graves' Disease)

Collaborative Problems

PC: Thyroid storm
PC: Cardiac dysrhythmias

Nursing Diagnoses

Altered Nutrition: Less than body requirements related to intake less than metabolic needs secondary to excessive metabolic rate

Activity Intolerance related to fatigue and exhaustion secondary to excessive metabolic rate

Diarrhea related to increased peristalsis secondary to excessive metabolic rate

Altered Comfort related to heat intolerance and profuse diaphoresis

---

▲ This diagnosis was reported to be monitored for or managed frequently (75%–100%).
△ This diagnosis was reported to be monitored for or managed often (50%–74%).
* This diagnosis was not included in the validation study.

Risk for Impaired Tissue Integrity: Corneal related to inability to close eyelids secondary to exophthalmos

Risk for Injury related to tremors

Risk for Hyperthermia related to lack of metabolic compensatory mechanism secondary to hyperthyroidism

Risk for Ineffective Management of Therapeutic Regimen related to insufficient knowledge of condition, treatment regimen, pharmacological therapy, eye care, dietary management, and signs and symptoms of complications

HYPOTHYROIDISM (Myxedema)

Collaborative Problems

PC: Atherosclerotic heart disease
PC: Normochromic, normocytic anemia
PC: Acute organic psychosis
PC: Myxedemic coma
PC: Metabolic
PC: Hematological

Nursing Diagnoses

Altered Nutrition: More than body requirements related to intake greater than metabolic needs secondary to slowed metabolic rate

Activity Intolerance related to insufficient oxygen secondary to slowed metabolic rate

Constipation related to decreased peristaltic action secondary to decreased metabolic rate and decreased physical activity

Impaired Skin Integrity related to edema and dryness secondary to decreased metabolic rate and infiltration of fluid into interstitial tissues

Altered Comfort related to cold intolerance secondary to decreased metabolic rate

Risk for Impaired Social Interactions related to listlessness and depression

Risk for Ineffective Management of Therapeutic Regimen related to insufficient knowledge of condition, treatment regimen, dietary management, signs and symptoms of complications, pharmacological therapy, and contraindications

OBESITY

Nursing Diagnoses

Altered Health Maintenance related to imbalance between caloric intake and energy expenditure

Ineffective Individual Coping related to increased food consumption secondary to response to external stressors

Chronic Low Self-Esteem related to feelings of self-degradation and the response of others to the condition

PANCREATITIS

Collaborative Problems

△ PC: Hypovolemia/shock
* PC: Hemorrhagic pancreatitis
* PC: Respiratory failure
* PC: Pleural effusion
△ PC: Hypocalcemia
▲ PC: Hyperglycemia
△ PC: Delirium tremens

Nursing Diagnoses

▲ Acute Pain related to nasogastric suction, distention of pancreatic capsule, and local peritonitis

Risk for Fluid Volume Deficit related to decreased intake secondary to nausea and vomiting

▲ Altered Nutrition: Less than body requirements related to vomiting, anorexia, and impaired digestion secondary to decreased pancreatic enzymes

△ Diarrhea related to excessive excretion of fats in stools secondary to insufficient pancreatic enzymes

△ Ineffective Denial related to acknowledgment of alcohol abuse or dependency

△ Risk for Ineffective Management of Therapeutic Regimen related to insufficient knowledge of disease process, treatments, contraindications, dietary management, and follow-up care

▲ This diagnosis was reported to be monitored for or managed frequently (75%–100%).
△ This diagnosis was reported to be monitored for or managed often (50%–74%).
* This diagnosis was not included in the validation study.

Gastrointestinal Disorders

ESOPHAGEAL DISORDERS (Esophagitis, Hiatal Hernia)

Collaborative Problems

PC: Hemorrhage
PC: Gastric ulcers

Nursing Diagnoses

Risk for Altered Nutrition: Less than body requirements related to anorexia, heartburn, and dysphagia

Altered Comfort: Heartburn related to regurgitation and eructation

Risk for Ineffective Management of Therapeutic Regimen related to insufficient knowledge of condition, dietary management, hazards of alcohol and tobacco, positioning after meals, pharmacological therapy, and weight reduction (if indicated)

GASTROENTERITIS

Collaborative Problem

PC: Fluid/electrolyte imbalance

Nursing Diagnoses

Risk for Fluid Volume Deficit related to vomiting and diarrhea

Altered Comfort related to abdominal cramping, diarrhea, and vomiting secondary to vascular dilatation and hyperperistalsis

Risk for Ineffective Management of Therapeutic Regimen related to insufficient knowledge of condition, dietary restrictions, and signs and symptoms of complications

HEMORRHOIDS/ANAL FISSURE (Nonsurgical)

Collaborative Problems

PC: Bleeding
PC: Bowel strangulation
PC: Thrombosis

Nursing Diagnoses

Altered Comfort related to pain on defecation

Risk for Constipation related to fear of pain on defecation

Risk for Ineffective Management of Therapeutic Regimen related to insufficient knowledge of condition, bowel routine, diet instructions, exercise program, and perianal care

INFLAMMATORY BOWEL DISEASE (Diverticulosis, Diverticulitis, Regional Enteritis, Ulcerative Colitis)

Collaborative Problems

▲ *PC: Gastrointestinal bleeding*
* *PC: Anal fissure*
* *PC: Perianal abscess, fissure, fistula*
▲ *PC: Fluid/electrolyte imbalances*
  PC: Toxic megacolon
▲ *PC: Anemia*
▲ *PC: Intestinal obstruction*
  PC: Urolithiasis
△ *PC: Fistula/fissure/abscess*

Nursing Diagnoses

▲ Chronic Pain related to intestinal inflammatory process
▲ Diarrhea related to intestinal inflammatory process
* Constipation related to inadequate dietary intake of fiber
* Risk for Impaired Skin Integrity (Perianal) related to diarrhea and chemical irritants
△ Risk for Ineffective Individual Coping related to chronicity of condition and lack of definitive treatment
▲ Altered Nutrition: Less than body requirements related to dietary restrictions, nausea, diarrhea, and abdominal cramping associated with eating or painful ulcers of the oral mucous membrane

▲ This diagnosis was reported to be monitored for or managed frequently (75%–100%).
△ This diagnosis was reported to be monitored for or managed often (50%–74%).
* This diagnosis was not included in the validation study.

△ Risk for Ineffective Management of Therapeutic Regimen related to insufficient knowledge of condition, diagnostic tests, prognosis, treatment, and signs and symptoms of complications

PEPTIC ULCER DISEASE
Collaborative Problems

▲ *PC: Hemorrhage*
▲ *PC: Perforation*
△ *PC: Pyloric obstruction*

Nursing Diagnoses

▲ Acute/Chronic Pain related to lesions secondary to increased gastric secretions
▲ Constipation/Diarrhea related to effects of medications on bowel function
△ Risk for Ineffective Management of Therapeutic Regimen related to insufficient knowledge of disease process, contraindications, signs and symptoms of complications, and treatment regimen

---

Renal/Urinary Tract Disorders

NEUROGENIC BLADDER
Collaborative Problems

PC: Renal calculi
PC: Autonomic dysreflexia

Nursing Diagnoses

Risk for Impaired Skin Integrity related to constant irritation from urine
Risk for Infection related to retention of urine or introduction of urinary catheter

---

▲ This diagnosis was reported to be monitored for or managed frequently (75%–100%).
△ This diagnosis was reported to be monitored for or managed often (50%–74%).

Risk for Social Isolation related to embarrassment from wetting self in front of others and fear of odor from urine

Urinary Retention related to chronically overfilled bladder with loss of sensation of bladder distention *or*

Reflex Incontinence related to absence of sensation to void and loss of ability to inhibit bladder contraction *or*

Urge Incontinence related to disruption of the inhibitory efferent impulses secondary to brain or spinal cord dysfunction

Risk for Dysreflexia related to reflex stimulation of sympathetic nervous system secondary to loss of autonomic control

Risk for Ineffective Management of Therapeutic Regimen related to insufficient knowledge of etiology of incontinence, management, bladder retraining programs, signs and symptoms of complications, and community resources

RENAL FAILURE (Acute)

Collaborative Problems

▲ *PC: Fluid overload*
▲ *PC: Metabolic acidosis*
▲ *PC: Electrolyte imbalances*

Nursing Diagnoses

△ Altered Nutrition: Less than body requirements related to anorexia, nausea, vomiting, loss of taste, loss of smell, stomatitis, and unpalatable diet

▲ Risk for Infection related to invasive procedures

* Anxiety related to present status and unknown prognosis

* Risk for Ineffective Management of Therapeutic Regimen related to insufficient knowledge of condition, dietary restriction, daily recording, pharmacological therapy, signs and symptoms of complications, follow-up visits, and community resources

---

▲ This diagnosis was reported to be monitored for or managed frequently (75%–100%).
△ This diagnosis was reported to be monitored for or managed often (50%–74%).
* This diagnosis was not included in the validation study.

RENAL FAILURE (Chronic, Uremia)

See also *Peritoneal Dialysis and Hemodialysis,* if indicated.

Collaborative Problems

▲ *PC: Fluid/electrolyte imbalance*
△ *PC: Gastrointestinal bleeding*
  PC: Hyperparathyroidism
  PC: Pathological fractures
* *PC: Malnutrition*
▲ *PC: Anemia*
▲ *PC: Fluid overload*
△ *PC: Hypoalbuminemia*
△ *PC: Polyneuropathy*
△ *PC: Congestive heart failure*
* *PC: Pulmonary edema*
△ *PC: Metabolic acidosis*
△ *PC: Pleural effusion*
  PC: Pericarditis, cardiac tamponade

Nursing Diagnoses

△ Altered Nutrition: Less than body requirements related to anorexia, nausea/vomiting, loss of taste/smell, stomatitis, and unpalatable diet
  Altered Sexuality Patterns related to decreased libido, impotence, amenorrhea, sterility, fatigue
* Self-Concept Disturbance related to effects of limitation on achievement of developmental tasks
* Risk for Caregiver Role Strain related to long-term care needs secondary to disability and treatment requirements
* Altered Comfort related to (examples) fatigue, headaches, fluid retention, anemia
* Fatigue related to insufficient oxygenation secondary to anemia
△ Altered Comfort related to calcium phosphate or urate crystals on skin

---

▲ This diagnosis was reported to be monitored for or managed frequently (75%–100%).
△ This diagnosis was reported to be monitored for or managed often (50%–74%).
* This diagnosis was not included in the validation study.

▲ Risk for Infection related to invasive procedures
△ Powerlessness related to progressively disabling nature of illness
▲ Risk for Ineffective Management of Therapeutic Regimen related to insufficient knowledge of condition, dietary restriction, daily recording, pharmacological therapy, signs and symptoms of complications, follow-up visits, and community resources

URINARY TRACT INFECTIONS (Cystitis, Pyelonephritis, Glomerulonephritis)

See also *Acute Renal Failure.*

Nursing Diagnoses

Chronic Pain related to inflammation and tissue trauma
Altered Comfort related to inflammation and infection
Risk for Altered Nutrition: Less than body requirements related to anorexia secondary to malaise
Risk for Ineffective Individual Coping related to the chronicity of the condition
Risk for Ineffective Management of Therapeutic Regimen related to insufficient knowledge of prevention of recurrence (adequate fluid intake, frequent voiding, hygiene measures [personal post-toileting], and voiding after sexual activity), signs and symptoms of recurrence, and pharmacological therapy

UROLITHIASIS (Renal Calculi)

Collaborative Problems

△ *PC: Pyelonephritis*
▲ *PC: Renal insufficiency*

Nursing Diagnoses

▲ Acute Pain related to inflammation secondary to irritation of calculi and smooth muscle spasms
* Diarrhea related to renointestinal reflexes

▲ This diagnosis was reported to be monitored for or managed frequently (75%–100%).
△ This diagnosis was reported to be monitored for or managed often (50%–74%).
* This diagnosis was not included in the validation study.

* Activity Intolerance related to deconditioning secondary to fatigue and weakness

* Disuse Syndrome

△ Total Incontinence related to loss of bladder tone, loss of sphincter control, or inability to perceive bladder cues

▲ Self-Care Deficit related to impaired physical mobility or confusion

▲ Impaired Swallowing related to muscle paralysis or paresis secondary to damage to upper motor neurons

△ Grieving (Family, Individual) related to loss of function and inability to meet role responsibilities

△ Risk for Impaired Social Interactions related to difficulty communicating and embarrassment regarding disabilities

△ Risk for Fluid Volume Deficit related to dysphagia, difficulty in obtaining fluids secondary to weakness or motor deficits

△ Risk for Impaired Home Maintenance Management related to altered ability to maintain self at home secondary to sensory/-motor/cognitive deficits and lack of knowledge of caregivers of home care, reality orientation, bowel/bladder program, skin care and signs and symptoms of complications, and community resources

▲ *Functional Incontinence related to inability or difficulty in reaching toilet secondary to decreased mobility or motivation*

△ *Unilateral Neglect related to (specify site) secondary to right hemispheric brain damage*

* *Risk for Caregiver Role Strain related to complex care requirements secondary to (specify sensory or motor deficits)*

△ *Risk for Self-Concept Disturbance related to effects of prolonged debilitating condition on achieving developmental tasks and lifestyle*

* *Risk for Ineffective Management of Therapeutic Regimen related to insufficient knowledge of condition,*

▲ This diagnosis was reported to be monitored for or managed frequently (75%–100%).

△ This diagnosis was reported to be monitored for or managed often (50%–74%).

* This diagnosis was not included in the validation study.

pharmacological therapy, self-care activities of daily living, home care, speech therapy, exercise program, community resources, self-help groups, and signs and symptoms of complications

NERVOUS SYSTEM DISORDERS (Degenerative, Demyelinating, Inflammatory, Myasthenia Gravis, Multiple Sclerosis, Muscular Dystrophy, Parkinson's Disease, Guillain-Barré Syndrome, Amyotrophic Lateral Sclerosis)

Because the responses associated with these disorders can range from minimal to profound, the following possible diagnoses reflect individuals with varying degrees of involvement.

Collaborative Problems

PC: Renal failure
PC: Pneumonia
PC: Atelectasis

Nursing Diagnoses

Risk for Self-Concept Disturbance related to the effects of prolonged debilitating condition on lifestyle and on achieving developmental tasks

Risk for Injury related to visual disturbances, unsteady gait, sensory losses, weakness, or uncontrolled movements

Impaired Verbal Communication related to dysarthrias secondary to ataxia of muscles of speech

Risk for Altered Nutrition: Less than body requirements related to dysphagia/chewing difficulties secondary to cranial nerve impairment

Activity Intolerance related to fatigue and difficulty in performing activities of daily living

Disuse Syndrome

Impaired Physical Mobility related to effects of muscle rigidity, tremors, and slowness of movement on activities of daily living

Impaired Swallowing related to cerebellar lesions

Fatigue related to extremity weakness, spasticity, fear of injury, and stressors

477

Urinary Retention related to sensory/motor deficits

Chronic Sorrow (Client, Family) related to nature of disease and uncertain prognosis

Altered Sexuality Patterns (female) related to loss of libido, fatigue, and decreased perineal sensation

Altered Family Processes related to nature of disorder, role disturbances, and uncertain future

Risk for Diversional Activity Deficit related to inability to perform usual job-related/recreational activities

Risk for Social Isolation related to mobility difficulties and associated embarrassment

Impaired Home Maintenance Management related to inability to care for/difficulty in caring for self/home secondary to disability or unavailable or inadequate caregiver

Parental Role Conflict related to disruptions secondary to disability

Caregiver Role Strain related to continuous, multiple care needs

(Specify) Self-Care Deficits related to (examples) headaches, muscular spasms, joint pain, fatigue, paresis/paralysis

Powerlessness related to the unpredictable nature of the condition (*i.e.,* remissions/exacerbations)

Incontinence: (specify) related to poor sphincter control and spastic bladder

Ineffective Airway Clearance related to impaired ability to cough

Risk for Ineffective Management of Therapeutic Regimen related to insufficient knowledge of condition, treatments, prevention of infection, stress management, aggravating factors, signs and symptoms of complications, and community resources

PRESENILE DEMENTIA (Alzheimer's Disease, Huntington's Disease)

See also *Nervous System Diseases.**

Because these disorders can cause alterations similar to those in the nervous system disorder category, the reader is referred to the latter section to review additional possible diagnoses.

Nursing Diagnoses

Risk for Injury related to lack of awareness of environmental hazards

Chronic Confusion related to an inability to evaluate reality secondary to cerebral neuron degeneration

Impaired Physical Mobility related to gait instability

Risk for Altered Family Processes related to effects of condition on relationships, role responsibilities, and finances

Impaired Home Maintenance Management related to inability to care for/difficulty in caring for self/home or inadequate or unavailable caregiver

Unilateral Neglect related to (specify site) secondary to neurological pathology

(Specify) Self-Care Deficit related to (specify)

Decisional Conflict related to placement of person in a care facility

Caregiver Role Strain related to multiple care needs and insufficient resources

SEIZURE DISORDERS (Epilepsy)

If the client is a child, see also *Developmental Problems/Needs*.

Nursing Diagnoses

* Risk for Injury related to uncontrolled tonic-clonic movements during seizure episode

▲ Risk for Ineffective Airway Clearance related to relaxation of tongue and gag reflexes secondary to disruption in muscle innervation

Risk for Social Isolation related to fear of embarrassment secondary to having a seizure in public

* Risk for Altered Growth and Development related to interruption in achieving/failure to achieve developmental tasks (adolescence, young adulthood, middle age)

▲ This diagnosis was reported to be monitored for or managed frequently (75%–100%).

* This diagnosis was not included in the validation study.

* Risk for Altered Oral Mucous Membrane related to effects of drug therapy on oral tissue
* Fear related to unpredictable nature of seizures and embarrassment
△ Risk for Ineffective Management of Therapeutic Regimen related to insufficient knowledge of condition, medication, activity, care during seizures, environmental hazards, and community resources

SPINAL CORD INJURY†

Collaborative Problems

△ *PC: Electrolyte imbalance*
* *PC: Spinal shock*
△ *PC: Hemorrhage*
* *PC: Respiratory complications*
△ *PC: Paralytic ileus*
* *PC: Sepsis*
* *PC: Hydronephrosis*
△ *PC: Gastrointestinal bleeding*
▲ *PC: Thrombophlebitis*
* *PC: Postural hypotension*
△ *PC: Fracture dislocation*
△ *PC: Cardiovascular*
▲ *PC: Hypoxemia*
▲ *PC: Urinary retention*
△ *PC: Renal insufficiency*

Nursing Diagnoses

▲ Self-Care Deficit related to sensory/motor deficits secondary to level of spinal cord injury
* Impaired Verbal Communication related to impaired ability to speak words secondary to tracheostomy

---

▲ This diagnosis was reported to be monitored for or managed frequently (75%–100%).
△ This diagnosis was reported to be monitored for or managed often (50%–74%).
* This diagnosis was not included in the validation study.
† Because disabilities associated with spinal cord injuries can be varied (hemiparesis quadriparesis, diplegia, monoplegia, triplegia, paraplegia), the nurse will have to specify clearly the individual's limitations in the diagnostic statment.

* Fear related to possible abandonment by others, changes in role responsibilities, effects of injury on lifestyle, multiple tests, and procedures, or separation from support systems

△ Altered Family Processes related to adjustment requirements, role disturbances, and uncertain future

* Risk for Aspiration related to inability to cough secondary to level of injury

△ Risk for Impaired Home Maintenance Management related to insufficient knowledge of the effects of altered skin, bowel, bladder, respiratory, thermoregulation, and sexual function and their management; signs and symptoms of complications; follow-up care; and community resources

▲ Anxiety related to perceived effects of injury on lifestyle and unknown future

▲ Chronic Grieving related to loss of body function and its effects on lifestyle

* Risk for Social Isolation (individual/family) related to disability or requirements for the caregiver(s)

* Risk for Caregiver Role Strain related to continuous, multiple care needs; inadequate resources; and coping mechanisms

△ Risk for Self-Concept Disturbance related to effects of disability on achieving developmental tasks and lifestyle

* Risk for Fluid Volume Deficit related to difficulty obtaining liquids

* Risk for Altered Nutrition: More than body requirements related to imbalance of intake versus activity expenditures

* Risk for Altered Nutrition: Less than body requirements related to anorexia and increased metabolic requirements

* Risk for Diversional Activity Deficit related to effects of limitations on ability to participate in recreational activities

---

▲ This diagnosis was reported to be monitored for or managed frequently (75%–100%).

△ This diagnosis was reported to be monitored for or managed often (50%–74%).

* This diagnosis was not included in the validation study.

* Reflex Incontinence or Urinary Retention related to bladder atony secondary to sensory–motor deficits
* Disuse Syndrome
* Risk for Injury related to impaired ability to control movements and sensory–motor deficits
* Risk for Infection related to urinary stasis, repeated catheterizations, and invasive procedures (skeletal tongs, tracheostomy, venous lines, surgical sites)
△ Risk for Altered Sexuality Patterns related to physiological, sensory, and psychological effects of disability on sexuality or function
△ Bowel Incontinence: Reflexic related to lack of voluntary sphincter control secondary to spinal cord injury of the 11th thoracic vertebra (T_{11})
△ Bowel Incontinence: Areflexia related to lack of voluntary sphincter secondary to spinal cord injury involving sacral reflex arc (S_2–S_4)
△ Risk for Dysreflexia related to reflex stimulation of sympathetic nervous system secondary to loss of autonomic control
* Risk for Ineffective Management of Therapeutic Regimen related to insufficient knowledge of condition, treatment regimen, rehabilitation, and assistance devices

UNCONSCIOUS INDIVIDUAL

See also *Mechanical Ventilation,* if indicated.

Collaborative Problems

* *PC: Respiratory insufficiency*
▲ *PC: Pneumonia*
▲ *PC: Atelectasis*
▲ *PC: Fluid/electrolyte imbalance*
   PC: Negative nitrogen balance
* *PC: Bladder distention*
* *PC: Seizures*
* *PC: Stress ulcers*

▲ This diagnosis was reported to be monitored for or managed frequently (75%–100%).
△ This diagnosis was reported to be monitored for or managed often (50%–74%).
* This diagnosis was not included in the validation study.

* *PC: Increased intracranial pressure*
△ *PC: Sepsis*
▲ *PC: Thrombophlebitis*
  PC: Renal calculi
△ *PC: Urinary tract infection*

Nursing Diagnoses

* Risk for Infection related to immobility and invasive devices (tracheostomy, Foley catheter, venous lines)
* Risk for Impaired Tissue Integrity: Corneal related to corneal drying secondary to open eyes and lower tear production
* Family Anxiety/Fear related to present state of individual and uncertain prognosis
* Risk for Altered Oral Mucous Membrane related to inability to perform own mouth care and pooling of secretions
▲ Total Incontinence related to unconscious state
△ Disuse Syndrome
△ Powerlessness (family) related to feelings of loss of control and the restrictions that are placed on lifestyle
▲ Risk for Ineffective Airway Clearance related to stasis of secretions secondary to inadequate cough and decreased mobility

Sensory Disorders

OPHTHALMIC DISORDERS (Cataracts, Detached Retina, Glaucoma, Inflammations)

See also *Cataract Extractions.*
See also *Scleral Buckle/Vitrectomy.*

Collaborative Problem

PC: Increased intraocular pressure

▲ This diagnosis was reported to be monitored for or managed frequently (75%–100%).
△ This diagnosis was reported to be monitored for or managed often (50%–74%).
* This diagnosis was not included in the validation study.

Nursing Diagnoses

Risk for Injury related to visual limitations

Acute Pain related to (examples) inflammation (lid, lacrimal structures, conjunctiva, uveal tract, retina, cornea, sclera), infection, increased intraocular pressure, ocular tumors

Risk for Noncompliance related to negative side effects of prescribed therapy versus the belief that no treatment is needed without the presence of symptoms

Risk for Social Isolation related to fear of injury or embarrassment outside home environment

Risk for Impaired Home Maintenance Management related to impaired ability to perform activities of daily living secondary to impaired vision

(Specify) Self-Care Deficit related to impaired vision

Anxiety related to actual or possible vision loss and perceived impact of chronic illness on lifestyle

Risk for Self-Concept Disturbance related to effects of visual limitations

Risk for Ineffective Management of Therapeutic Regimen related to insufficient knowledge of condition, eye care, medications, safety measures, activity restrictions, and follow-up care

OTIC DISORDERS (Infections, Mastoiditis, Trauma)

Nursing Diagnoses

Risk for Injury related to disturbances of balance and impaired ability to detect environmental hazards

Impaired Verbal Communication related to difficulty understanding others secondary to impaired hearing

Risk for Impaired Social Interactions related to difficulty in participating in conversations

Social Isolation related to the lack of contact with others secondary to fear and embarrassment of hearing losses

Acute Pain related to inflammation, infection, tinnitus, or vertigo

Fear related to actual or possible loss of hearing

Risk for Ineffective Management of Therapeutic Regimen related to insufficient knowledge of condition, medications, prevention of recurrence, hazards (swimming, air travel, showers), signs and symptoms of complications, and hearing aids

Integumentary Disorders

DERMATOLOGICAL DISORDERS (Dermatitis, Psoriasis, Eczema)

Nursing Diagnoses

Impaired Skin Integrity related to lesions and inflammatory response

Pruritus related to dermal eruptions

Risk for Impaired Social Interaction related to fear of embarrassment and negative reactions of others

Risk for Self-Concept Disturbance related to appearance and response of others

Risk for Ineffective Management of Therapeutic Regimen related to insufficient knowledge of condition, topical agents, and contraindications

PRESSURE ULCERS†

Collaborative Problem

△ PC: Sepsis

Nursing Diagnoses

▲ Risk for Infection related to exposure of ulcer base to fecal/urinary drainage

▲ Impaired Tissue Integrity related to mechanical destruction of tissue secondary to pressure, shear, and friction

* Impaired Home Maintenance Management related to complexity of care or unavailable caregiver

---

▲ This diagnosis was reported to be monitored for or managed frequently (75%–100%).

△ This diagnosis was reported to be monitored for or managed often (50%–74%).

* This diagnosis was not included in the validation study.

† The factors that can contribute to the development of pressure sores are varied and complex; therefore, the nurse must assess for and identify the specific related factors for the individual.

▲ Altered Nutrition: Less than body requirements related to anorexia secondary to (specify)
▲ Impaired Physical Mobility related to imposed restrictions, deconditioned status, loss of motor control, or altered mental status
* Fluid Volume Excess: Edema related to (specify)
* Total Incontinence related to (specify)
△ Risk for Ineffective Management of Therapeutic Regimen related to insufficient knowledge of etiology, prevention, treatment, and home care

SKIN INFECTIONS (Impetigo, Herpes Zoster, Fungal Infections)

Collaborative Problems (Herpes Zoster)

PC: Postherpetic neuralgia
PC: Keratitis
PC: Uveitis
PC: Corneal ulceration
PC: Blindness

Nursing Diagnoses

Impaired Skin Integrity related to lesions and pruritus
Altered Comfort related to dermal eruptions and pruritus
Risk for Infection Transmission related to contagious nature of the organism
Risk for Ineffective Management of Therapeutic Regimen related to insufficient knowledge of condition (causes, course), prevention, treatment, and skin care

THERMAL INJURIES (Burns, Severe Hypothermia)

Acute Period

Collaborative Problems

▲ *PC: Hypovolemic shock*

▲ This diagnosis was reported to be monitored for or managed frequently (75%–100%).
△ This diagnosis was reported to be monitored for or managed often (50%–74%).
* This diagnosis was not included in the validation study.

△ *PC: Hypervolemia*
* *PC: Fluid overload*
* *PC: Anemia*
△ *PC: Negative nitrogen balance*
▲ *PC: Electrolyte imbalance*
△ *PC: Metabolic acidosis*
▲ *PC: Respiratory*
△ *PC: Thromboembolism*
▲ *PC: Sepsis*
* *PC: Emboli*
▲ *PC: Graft rejection/infection*
* *PC: Hypothermia*
* *PC: Hypokalemia/hyperkalemia*
△ *PC: Curling's ulcer*
△ *PC: Paralytic ileus*
* *PC: Convulsive disorders*
* *PC: Stress diabetes*
  PC: Adrenocortical insufficiency
* *PC: Pneumonia*
△ *PC: Renal insufficiency*
* *PC: Compartmental syndrome*
* *PC: Adrenal insufficiency*

Nursing Diagnoses

▲ Risk for Infection related to loss of protective layer
   secondary to thermal injury
▲ Altered Nutrition: Less than body requirements related
   to increased caloric requirement secondary to thermal injury and inability to ingest sufficient quantities
   to meet increased requirements
* Impaired Physical Mobility related to acute pain
   secondary to thermal injury and treatments
△ (Specify) Self-Care Deficit related to impaired range-of-
   motion ability secondary to pain
* Fear related to painful procedures and possibility of
   death

▲ This diagnosis was reported to be monitored for or managed
   frequently (75%–100%).
△ This diagnosis was reported to be monitored for or managed
   often (50%–74%).
* This diagnosis was not included in the validation study.

* Risk for Social Isolation related to infection control measures and separation from family and support systems
△ Disuse Syndrome
* Sleep Pattern Disturbances related to position restrictions, pain, and treatment interruptions
* Risk for Sensory/Perceptual Alterations related to (examples) excessive environmental stimuli, stress, imposed immobility, sleep deprivation, protective isolation
▲ Grieving (family, individual) related to actual or perceived impact of injury on life, appearance, relationships, lifestyle
▲ Anxiety related to sudden injury, treatments, uncertainty of outcome, and pain
* Anxiety related to pain secondary to thermal injury treatments and immobility
▲ Altered Comfort related to thermal injury treatments and immobility

Postacute Period

If individual is a child, see also *Developmental Problems/Needs.*

Collaborative Problem

PC: Same as in acute period

Nursing Diagnoses

△ Diversional Activity Deficit related to monotony of confinement
* Risk for Social Isolation related to embarrassment and the response of others to injury
* Powerlessness related to inability to control present situation
△ Risk for Self-Concept Disturbance related to effects of thermal injury on achieving developmental tasks (child, adolescent, adult)

▲ This diagnosis was reported to be monitored for or managed frequently (75%–100%).
△ This diagnosis was reported to be monitored for or managed often (50%–74%).
* This diagnosis was not included in the validation study.

* Fear related to uncertain future and effects of injury on lifestyle, relationships, occupation
* Impaired Home Maintenance Management related to long-term requirements of treatments
△ Risk for Ineffective Management of Therapeutic Regimen related to insufficient knowledge of exercise program, wound care, nutritional requirements, pain management, signs and symptoms of complications, and burn prevention and follow-up care

Musculoskeletal/Connective Tissue Disorders

FRACTURED JAW

Nursing Diagnoses

Risk for Aspiration related to inadequate cough secondary to pain and fixative devices

Altered Oral Mucous Membrane related to difficulty in performing oral hygiene secondary to fixation devices

Impaired Verbal Communication related to fixation devices

Altered Comfort related to tissue trauma and fixation device

Risk for Altered Nutrition: Less than body requirements related to inability to ingest solid food secondary to fixation devices

Risk for Ineffective Management of Therapeutic Regimen related to insufficient knowledge of mouth care, nutritional requirements, signs and symptoms of infection, and procedure for emergency wire cutting (*e.g.*, vomiting)

FRACTURES

See also *Casts*.

___

△ This diagnosis was reported to be monitored for or managed often (50%–74%).
* This diagnosis was not included in the validation study.

Collaborative Problems

▲ *PC: Neurovascular compromise*
▲ *PC: Fat embolism*
▲ *PC: Hemorrhage/hematoma formation*
* *PC: Osteomyelitis*
* *PC: Compartmental syndrome*
* *PC: Contracture*
▲ *PC: Thromboemboli*

Nursing Diagnoses

* Altered Comfort related to tissue trauma and immobility
▲ Impaired Physical Mobility related to tissue trauma secondary to fracture
* Disuse Syndrome
* Risk for Infection related to invasive fixation devices
▲ Self-Care Deficit (specify) related to limitation of movement secondary to fracture
ᴬ Diversional Activity Deficit related to boredom of confinement secondary to immobilization devices
* Risk for Impaired Home Maintenance Management related to (examples) fixation device, impaired physical mobility, unavailable support system
* Altered Family Processes related to difficulty of ill person in assuming role responsibilities secondary to limited motion
△ Risk for Ineffective Management of Therapeutic Regimen related to insufficient knowledge of condition, signs and symptoms of complications, activity restrictions

LOW BACK PAIN

Collaborative Problems

PC: Pulposus
PC: Herniated nucleus pulposus

▲ This diagnosis was reported to be monitored for or managed frequently (75%–100%).
△ This diagnosis was reported to be monitored for or managed often (50%–74%).
* This diagnosis was not included in the validation study.

Nursing Diagnoses

Pain related to (examples) acute lumbosacral strain, weak muscles, osteoarthritis of spine, unstable lumbosacral ligaments, spinal stenosis, intervertebral disk problem

Impaired Physical Mobility related to decreased mobility and flexibility secondary to muscle spasm

Risk for Ineffective Individual Coping related to effects of chronic pain on lifestyle

Risk for Altered Family Processes related to impaired ability to meet role responsibilities (financial, home, social)

Risk for Ineffective Management of Therapeutic Regimen related to insufficient knowledge of condition, exercise program, noninvasive pain relief methods (relaxation, imagery), proper posture and body mechanics, and risk factors (smoking, inactivity, overweight)

OSTEOPOROSIS

Collaborative Problems

PC: Fractures
PC: Kyphosis
PC: Paralytic ileus

Nursing Diagnoses

Pain related to muscle spasm and fractures

Altered Health Maintenance related to insufficient daily physical activity

Altered Nutrition: Less than body requirements related to inadequate dietary intake of calcium, protein, and vitamin D

Impaired Physical Mobility related to limited range of motion secondary to skeletal changes

Fear related to unpredictable nature of condition

Risk for Ineffective Management of Therapeutic Regimen related to insufficient knowledge of condition, risk factors, nutritional therapy, and prevention

INFLAMMATORY JOINT DISEASE

Collaborative Problems

PC: Septic arthritis
PC: Sjögren's syndrome
PC: Neuropathy
PC: Anemia, leukopenia

Nursing Diagnoses

Chronic Pain related to local and systemic inflammatory lesions

(Specify) Self-Care Deficits related to loss of motion, muscle weakness, pain, stiffness, or fatigue

Powerlessness related to physical and psychological changes imposed by the disease

Ineffective Individual Coping related to the stress imposed by unpredictable exacerbations

(Specify) Self-Care Deficit related to limitations secondary to disease process

Fatigue related to effects of chronic inflammatory process

Risk for Altered Oral Mucous Membrane related to effects of medications or Sjögren's syndrome

Impaired Home Maintenance Management related to impaired ability to perform household responsibilities secondary to limited mobility and pain

Sleep Pattern Disturbance related to pain or secondary to fibrositis

Impaired Physical Mobility related to pain and limited joint motion

Altered Sexuality Patterns related to pain, fatigue, difficulty in assuming positions, and lack of adequate lubrication (female) secondary to disease process

Risk for Social Isolation related to ambulation difficulties and fatigue

Altered Family Processes related to difficulty/inability of ill person to assume role responsibilities secondary to fatigue and limited motion

Risk for Ineffective Management of Therapeutic Regimen related to insufficient knowledge of condition, pharmacological therapy, home care, stress management, and quackery

Infectious/Immunodeficient Disorders

LUPUS ERYTHEMATOSUS (Systemic)

See also *Rheumatic Diseases.*
See also *Corticosteroid Therapy.*

Collaborative Problems

PC: Polymyositis
PC: Vasculitis
PC: Hematological problem
PC: Raynaud's disease
PC: Renal failure secondary to corticosteroid therapy
PC: Pericarditis
PC: Pleuritis

Nursing Diagnoses

Powerlessness related to unpredictable course of disease

Ineffective Individual Coping related to unpredictable course and altered appearance

Risk for Social Isolation related to embarrassment and the response of others to appearance

Risk for Self-Concept Disturbance related to inability to achieve developmental tasks secondary to disabling condition and changes in appearance

Risk for Injury related to increased dermal vulnerability secondary to disease process

Fatigue related to decreased mobility and effects of chronic inflammation

Risk for Ineffective Management of Therapeutic Regimen related to insufficient knowledge of condition, rest versus activity requirements, pharmacological therapy, signs and symptoms of complications, risk factors, and community resources

MENINGITIS / ENCEPHALITIS

Collaborative Problems

PC: Fluid/electrolyte imbalance

493

PC: Cerebral edema
PC: Adrenal damage
PC: Circulatory collapse
PC: Hemorrhage
PC: Seizures
PC: Sepsis
PC: Alkalosis
PC: Increased intracranial pressure

Nursing Diagnoses

Risk for Infection Transmission related to contagious nature of organism

Altered Comfort related to headache, fever, neck pain secondary to meningeal irritation

Activity Intolerance related to fatigue and malaise secondary to infection

Risk for Impaired Skin Integrity related to immobility, dehydration, and diaphoresis

Risk for Altered Oral Mucous Membrane related to dehydration and impaired ability to perform mouth care

Risk for Altered Nutrition: Less than body requirements related to anorexia, fatigue, nausea, and vomiting

Risk for Altered Respiratory Function related to immobility and pain

Risk for Injury related to restlessness and disorientation secondary to meningeal irritation

Altered Family Processes related to critical nature of situation and uncertain prognosis

Anxiety related to treatments, environment, and risk of death

Risk for Ineffective Management of Therapeutic Regimen related to insufficient knowledge of condition, treatments, pharmacological therapy, rest/activity balance, signs and symptoms of complications, follow-up care, and prevention of recurrence

SEXUALLY TRANSMITTED DISEASES

Nursing Diagnoses

Risk for Infection Transmission related to lack of knowledge of the contagious nature of the disease and reports of high risk behaviors

Fear related to nature of the condition and its implications for lifestyle

Altered Comfort related to inflammatory process

Social Isolation related to fear of transmitting disease to others

Risk for Ineffective Management of Therapeutic Regimen related to insufficient knowledge of condition, modes of transmission, consequences of repeated infections, and prevention of recurrences

ACQUIRED IMMUNODEFICIENCY SYNDROME (AIDS) (Adult)

See also *End-Stage Cancer.*

Collaborative Problems

* *PC: Encephalopathy*
▲ *PC: Sepsis*
* *PC: Gastrointestinal bleeding*
* *PC: Pneumocystis carinii pneumonia*
* *PC: Meningitis*
* *PC: Esophagitis*
* *PC: Electrolyte imbalances*
▲ *PC: Opportunistic infections*
△ *PC: Myelosuppression*

Nursing Diagnoses

* Altered Comfort related to headache, fever secondary to inflammation of cerebral tissue
▲ Fatigue related to effects of disease, stress, chronic infections, and nutritional deficiency
* Risk for Impaired Skin Integrity related to perineal and anal tissue excoriation secondary to diarrhea and chronic genital candidal or herpes lesions
* Altered Nutrition: Less than body requirements related to chronic diarrhea, gastrointestinal malabsorption, fatigue, anorexia, or oral/esophageal lesions

▲ This diagnosis was reported to be monitored for or managed frequently (75%–100%).
△ This diagnosis was reported to be monitored for or managed often (50%–74%).
* This diagnosis was not included in the validation study.

▲ Risk for Infection Transmission related to contagious nature of blood and body secretions

△ Social Isolation related to fear of rejection or actual rejection of others secondary to fear

* Hopelessness related to nature of the condition and poor prognosis

△ Powerlessness related to unpredictable nature of condition

▲ Altered Family Processes related to the nature of the AIDS condition, role disturbance, and uncertain future

△ Anxiety related to perceived effects of illness on lifestyle and unknown future

△ Chronic Sorrow related to loss of body function and its effects on lifestyle

▲ Risk for Infection related to increased susceptibility secondary to compromised immune system

▲ Risk for Altered Oral Mucous Membrane related to compromised immune system

* Risk for Caregiver Role Strain related to multiple needs of ill person and chronicity

△ Risk for Ineffective Management of Therapeutic Regimen related to insufficient knowledge of condition, medications, home care, infection control, and community resources

---

Neoplastic Disorders

CANCER (Initial Diagnosis)

See also specific types.

Nursing Diagnoses

▲ Anxiety related to unfamiliar hospital environment, uncertainty about outcomes, feelings of helplessness and hopelessness, and insufficient knowledge about cancer and treatment

---

▲ This diagnosis was reported to be monitored for or managed frequently (75%–100%).

△ This diagnosis was reported to be monitored for or managed often (50%–74%).

* This diagnosis was not included in the validation study.

▲ Grieving related to potential loss of body function and the perceived losses associated with cancer on lifestyle

* Powerlessness related to uncertainty about prognosis and outcome of cancer treatment

▲ Altered Family Processes related to fears associated with recent cancer diagnosis, disruptions associated with treatments, financial problems, and uncertain future

△ Decisional Conflict related to treatment modality choices

△ Risk for Self-Concept Disturbance related to changes in lifestyle, role responsibilities, and appearance

△ Risk for Social Isolation related to fear of rejection or actual rejection secondary to fear

△ Risk for Spiritual Distress related to conflicts centering on the meaning of life, cancer, spiritual beliefs, and death

* Risk for Ineffective Management of Therapeutic Regimen related to insufficient knowledge of cancer, cancer treatment options, diagnostic tests, effects of treatment, treatment plan, and support services

CANCER (General; Applies to Malignancies in Varied Sites and Stages)

Nursing Diagnoses

Altered Oral Mucous Membranes related to (examples) disease process, therapy, radiation, chemotherapy, inadequate oral hygiene, and altered nutritional/hydration status

Risk for Altered Sexuality Patterns related to (examples) fear, grieving, changes in body image, anatomical changes, pain, fatigue (treatments, disease), or change in role responsibilities

---

▲ This diagnosis was reported to be monitored for or managed frequently (75%–100%).

△ This diagnosis was reported to be monitored for or managed often (50%–74%).

* This diagnosis was not included in the validation study.

Altered Comfort related to disease process and treatments

Diarrhea related to (examples) disease process, chemotherapy, radiation, and medications

Constipation related to (examples) disease process, chemotherapy, radiation therapy, immobility, dietary intake, and medications

Self-Concept Disturbance related to (examples) anatomical changes, role disturbances, uncertain future, disruption of lifestyle

(Specify) Self-Care Deficits related to fatigue, pain, or depression

Risk for Infection related to altered immune system

Altered Nutrition: Less than body requirements related to anorexia, fatigue, nausea, and vomiting secondary to disease process and treatments

Risk for Injury related to disorientation, weakness, sensory/perceptual deterioration, or skeletal/muscle deterioration

Disuse Syndrome

Risk for Fluid Volume Deficit related to (examples) altered ability/desire to obtain fluids, weakness, vomiting, diarrhea, depression, and fatigue

Risk for Impaired Home Maintenance Management related to (examples) lack of knowledge, lack of resources (support system, equipment, finances), motor deficits, sensory deficits, cognitive deficits, and emotional deficits

Risk for Impaired Social Interactions related to fear of rejection or actual rejection of others after diagnosis

Powerlessness related to inability to control situation

Altered Family Process related to (examples) stress of diagnosis/treatments, role disturbances, and uncertain future

Grieving (Family, Individual) related to actual, perceived, or anticipated losses associated with diagnosis

Risk for Ineffective Management of Therapeutic Regimen related to insufficient knowledge of disease, misconceptions, treatments, home care, and support agencies

CANCER (End-Stage)

See also specific types.

Collaborative Problems

PC: Hypercalcemia
PC: Intracerebral metastasis
PC: Malignant effusions
PC: Narcotic toxicity
PC: Pathological fractures
PC: Spinal cord compression
PC: Superior vena cava syndrome
PC: Negative nitrogen imbalance
PC: Myelosuppression

Nursing Diagnoses

See also *Cancer (General)*.

Altered Nutrition: Less than body requirements related to decreased oral intake, increased metabolic demands of tumor, and altered lipid metabolism

Altered Comfort related to pruritus secondary to dry skin and biliary obstruction

Ineffective Airway Clearance related to inability to cough up secretions secondary to weakness, increased viscosity, and pain

Impaired Physical Mobility related to pain, sedation, weakness, fatigue, and edema

(Specify) Self-Care Deficit related to fatigue, weakness, sedation, pain, or decreased sensory/perceptual capacity

Activity Intolerance related to hypoxia, fatigue, malnutrition, and decreased mobility

Grieving related to terminal illness, impending death, functional losses, and withdrawal of or from others

Hopelessness related to overwhelming functional losses or impending death

Self-Concept Disturbance related to dependence on others to meet basic needs and decrease in functional ability

Powerlessness related to change from curative status to palliative status

Caregiver Role Strain related to multiple care needs and concern about ability to manage home care

Risk for Spiritual Distress related to fear of death, overwhelming grief, belief system conflicts, and unresolved conflicts

Death Anxiety related to effects of disease process and inadequate relief from pain-relief measures

Risk for Impaired Home Maintenance Management related to insufficient knowledge of home care, pain management, signs and symptoms of complications, and community resources available

COLORECTAL CANCER (Additional Nursing Diagnoses)

See also *Cancer (General)*.

Nursing Diagnoses

Risk for Altered Sexuality Patterns (Male) related to inability to have or sustain an erection secondary to surgical procedure on perineal structures

Risk for Ineffective Management of Therapeutic Regimen related to insufficient knowledge of ostomy care, supplies, dietary management, signs and symptoms of complications, and community services

---

Surgical Procedures

GENERAL SURGERY

Preoperative Period

Nursing Diagnoses

Fear related to surgical experience, loss of control, and the unpredictable outcome

Anxiety related to preoperative procedures (surgical permit, diagnostic studies, Foley catheter, diet and fluid restrictions, medications, skin preparation, wait-

ing area for family) and postoperative procedure
(disposition [recovery room, intensive care unit],
medications for pain, coughing/turning/leg exercises, tube/drain placement, nothing by mouth
[NPO]/diet restrictions, bed rest)

Postoperative Period

Collaborative Problems

PC: Urinary retention
PC: Hemorrhage
PC: Hypovolemia/shock
PC: Renal failure
PC: Pneumonia (stasis)
PC: Peritonitis
PC: Thrombophlebitis
PC: Paralytic ileus
PC: Evisceration
PC: Dehiscence

Nursing Diagnoses

Risk for Infection related to site for bacterial invasion
Risk for Altered Respiratory Function related to
postanesthesia state, postoperative immobility, and
pain
Acute Pain related to incision, flatus, and immobility
Risk for Constipation related to decreased peristalsis
secondary to the effects of anesthesia, immobility,
and pain medication
Risk for Altered Nutrition: Less than body requirements
related to increased protein/vitamin requirements for
wound healing and decreased intake secondary to
pain, nausea, vomiting, and diet restrictions
Risk for Ineffective Management of Therapeutic Regimen related to insufficient knowledge of home care,
incisional care, signs and symptoms of complications, activity restriction, and follow-up care

AMPUTATION (Lower Extremity)

Preoperative Period

See also *Surgery (General).*

Nursing Diagnoses

▲ Anxiety related to insufficient knowledge of postoperative routines, postoperative sensations, and crutch-walking techniques

Postoperative Period

Collaborative Problems

▲ *PC: Edema of stump*
▲ *PC: Hemorrhage*
▲ *PC: Hematoma site*

Nursing Diagnoses

* Disuse Syndrome
▲ Grieving related to loss of limb and its effects on lifestyle
▲ Altered Comfort related to phantom limb sensations secondary to peripheral nerve stimulation or abnormal impulses to central nervous system
▲ Risk for Injury related to altered gait and hazards of assistive devices
△ Risk for Impaired Home Maintenance Management related to architectural barriers
△ Risk for Body Image Disturbance related to perceived negative effects of amputation and response of others to appearance
▲ Risk for Contractures related to impaired movement secondary to pain
△ Risk for Ineffective Management of Therapeutic Regimen related to insufficient knowledge of activities of daily living adaptations, stump care, prosthesis care, gait training, and follow-up care

ANEURYSM RESECTION (Abdominal Aortic)

See also *Surgery (General)*.

▲ This diagnosis was reported to be monitored for or managed frequently (75%–100%).
△ This diagnosis was reported to be monitored for or managed often (50%–74%).
* This diagnosis was not included in the validation study.

Preoperative Period

Collaborative Problems

▲ *PC: Rupture of aneurysm*

Postoperative Period

Collaborative Problems

▲ *PC: Distal vessel thrombosis or emboli*
▲ *PC: Renal failure*
△ *PC: Mesenteric ischemia/thrombosis*
△ *PC: Spinal cord ischemia*

Nursing Diagnoses

▲ Risk for Infection related to location of surgical incision
   Risk for Altered Sexuality Patterns (male) related to possible loss of ejaculate and erections secondary to surgery
△ Risk for Ineffective Management of Therapeutic Regimen related to insufficient knowledge of home care, activity restrictions, signs and symptoms of complications, and follow-up care

ANORECTAL SURGERY

See also *Surgery (General)*.

Preoperative Period

See also *Hemorrhoids* or *Anal Fissure*.

Postoperative Period

Collaborative Problems

PC: Hemorrhage
PC: Urinary retention

▲ This diagnosis was reported to be monitored for or managed frequently (75%–100%).
△ This diagnosis was reported to be monitored for or managed often (50%–74%).

Nursing Diagnoses

Risk for Constipation related to fear of pain

Risk for Infection related to surgical incision and fecal contamination

Risk for Ineffective Management of Therapeutic Regimen related to insufficient knowledge of wound care, prevention of recurrence, nutritional requirements (diet, fluid), exercise program, and signs and symptoms of complications

ARTERIAL BYPASS GRAFT OF LOWER EXTREMITY (Aortic, Iliac, Femoral, Popliteal)

See also *Surgery (General)*.
See also *Anticoagulant Therapy*.

Postoperative Period

Collaborative Problems

▲ *PC: Thrombosis of graft*
△ *PC: Compartmental syndrome*
   PC: Lymphocele
▲ *PC: Disruption of anastomosis*

Nursing Diagnoses

▲ Risk for Infection related to location of surgical incision
▲ Altered Comfort related to increased tissue perfusion to previous ischemic tissue
△ Risk for Impaired Tissue Integrity related to immobility and vulnerability of heels
△ Risk for Ineffective Management of Therapeutic Regimen related to insufficient knowledge of wound care, signs and symptoms of complications, activity restrictions, and follow-up care

---

▲ This diagnosis was reported to be monitored for or managed frequently (75%–100%).
△ This diagnosis was reported to be monitored for or managed often (50%–74%).

▲ *PC: Hypoglossal*
▲ *PC: Glossopharyngeal*
△ *PC: Vagus*
△ *PC: Local nerve impairment (peri-incisional numbness
    of skin)*
▲ *PC: Respiratory obstruction*

Nursing Diagnoses

△ Risk for Injury related to syncope secondary to vascular insufficiency
△ Risk for Ineffective Management of Therapeutic
   Regimen related to insufficient knowledge of home
   care, signs and symptoms of complications, risk factors, activity restrictions, and follow-up care

CATARACT EXTRACTION

Postoperative Period

Collaborative Problem

▲ *PC: Hemorrhage*

Nursing Diagnoses

△ Acute Pain related to surgical procedure
▲ Risk for Infection related to increased susceptibility
   secondary to surgical interruption of eye surface
▲ Risk for Injury related to visual limitations, presence in
   unfamiliar environment, limited mobility, and postoperative presence of eye patch
   Risk for Social Isolation related to altered visual acuity
   and fear of falling
△ Risk for Impaired Home Maintenance Management
   related to inability to perform activities of daily living
   secondary to activity restrictions and visual limitations
▲ Risk for Ineffective Management of Therapeutic Regimen related to insufficient knowledge of activities

---

▲ This diagnosis was reported to be monitored for or managed
  frequently (75%–100%).
△ This diagnosis was reported to be monitored for or managed
  often (50%–74%).

permitted and restricted, medications, complications, and follow-up care

CESAREAN SECTION

See also *Surgery (General)*.
See also *Postpartum Period*.

CHOLECYSTECTOMY

See also *Surgery (General)*.

Postoperative Period

Collaborative Problem

PC: Peritonitis

Nursing Diagnoses

Risk for Altered Respiratory Function related to high abdominal incision and splinting secondary to pain

Risk for Altered Oral Mucous Membrane related to NPO state and mouth breathing secondary to nasogastric intubation

COLOSTOMY

See also *Surgery (General)*.

Postoperative Period

Collaborative Problems

▲ *PC: Peristomal ulceration/herniation*
▲ *PC: Stomal necrosis, retraction prolapse, stenosis, obstruction*

Nursing Diagnoses

△ Grieving related to implications of cancer diagnosis
▲ Risk for Self-Concept Disturbance related to effects of ostomy on body image and lifestyle

---

▲ This diagnosis was reported to be monitored for or managed frequently (75%–100%).
△ This diagnosis was reported to be monitored for or managed often (50%–74%).

△ Risk for Altered Sexuality Patterns related to perceived negative impact of ostomy on sexual functioning and attractiveness

Risk for Sexual Dysfunction related to physiological impotence secondary to damaged sympathetic nerves (male) or inadequate vaginal lubrication (female)

△ Risk for Social Isolation related to anxiety about possible odor and leakage from appliance

▲ Risk for Ineffective Management of Therapeutic Regimen related to insufficient knowledge of stoma pouching procedure, colostomy irrigation, peristomal skin care, perineal wound care, and incorporation of ostomy care into activities of daily living

CORNEAL TRANSPLANT (Penetrating Keratoplasty)

See also *Surgery (General)*.

Postoperative Period

Collaborative Problems

PC: Endophthalmitis
▲ *PC: Increased intraocular pressure*
PC: Epithelial defects
PC: Graft failure

Nursing Diagnoses

△ Risk for Infection related to nonintact ocular tissue
▲ Altered Comfort related to surgical procedure
▲ Risk for Ineffective Management of Therapeutic Regimen related to insufficient knowledge of eye care, resumption of activities, medications/medication administration, signs and symptoms of complications, and long-term follow-up care

---

▲ This diagnosis was reported to be monitored for or managed frequently (75%–100%).
△ This diagnosis was reported to be monitored for or managed often (50%–74%).

CORONARY ARTERY BYPASS GRAFT (CABG)

See also *Surgery (General).*

Postoperative Period
Collaborative Problems

▲ *PC: Cardiovascular insufficiency*
▲ *PC: Respiratory insufficiency*
▲ *PC: Renal insufficiency*

Nursing Diagnoses

▲ Acute Pain related to surgical incisions, chest tubes, and immobility secondary to lengthy surgery
Impaired Physical Mobility related to surgical incisions, chest tubes, and fatigue
△ Fear related to transfer from intensive environment of the critical care unit and potential for complications
Impaired Verbal Communication related to endotracheal tube (temporary)
△ Altered Family Process related to disruption of family life, fear of outcome (death, disability), and stressful environment (intensive care unit)
△ Risk for Self-Concept Disturbance related to the symbolic meaning of the heart and changes in lifestyle
△ Risk for Ineffective Management of Therapeutic Regimen related to insufficient knowledge of incisional care, pain management (angina, incisions), signs and symptoms of complications, condition, pharmacological care, risk factors, restrictions, stress management techniques, and follow-up care

CRANIAL SURGERY

See also *Surgery (General).*
See also *Brain Tumor* for preoperative and postoperative care.

▲ This diagnosis was reported to be monitored for or managed frequently (75%–100%).
△ This diagnosis was reported to be monitored for or managed often (50%–74%).

Postoperative Period

Collaborative Problems

▲ *PC: Increased intracranial pressure*
▲ *PC: Cerebral/cerebellar dysfunction*
* *PC: Hypoxemia*
▲ *PC: Seizures*
▲ *PC: Brain hemorrhage, hematomas*
▲ *PC: Cranial nerve dysfunctions*
* *PC: Cardiac dysrhythmias*
▲ *PC: Fluid/electrolyte imbalances*
△ *PC: Meningitis/encephalitis*
▲ *PC: Sensory–motor losses*
▲ *PC: Hypothermia/hyperthermia*
△ *PC: Antidiuretic hormone secretion disorders*
▲ *PC: Cerebrospinal fluid leaks*
▲ *PC: Hygromas*
* *PC: Brain shifts/herniations*
* *PC: Hydrocephalus*
* *PC: Gastrointestinal bleeding*

Nursing Diagnoses

▲ Altered Comfort related to compression/displacement of brain tissue and increased intracranial pressure
△ Risk for Impaired Corneal Tissue Integrity related to inadequate lubrication secondary to tissue edema
△ Risk for Ineffective Management of Therapeutic Regimen related to insufficient knowledge of wound care, signs and symptoms of complications, restrictions, and follow-up care

DILATATION AND CURETTAGE

See also *Surgery (General)—Preoperative and Postoperative.*

▲ This diagnosis was reported to be monitored for or managed frequently (75%–100%).
△ This diagnosis was reported to be monitored for or managed often (50%–74%).
* This diagnosis was not included in the validation study.

Postoperative Period

Collaborative Problem

PC: Hemorrhage

Nursing Diagnoses

Risk for Ineffective Management of Therapeutic Regimen related to insufficient knowledge of condition, home care, signs and symptoms of complications, and activity restrictions.

ENUCLEATION

Postoperative Period

Collaborative Problems

▲ *PC: Hemorrhage*
PC: Abscess

Nursing Diagnoses

△ Risk for Injury related to visual limitations and presence in unfamiliar environment
△ Grieving related to loss of eye and its effects on lifestyle
△ Risk for Self-Concept Disturbance related to effects of change in appearance on lifestyle
△ Risk for Social Isolation related to changes in body image and altered vision
△ Risk for Impaired Home Maintenance Management related to inability to perform activities of daily living secondary to change in visual abilities
△ Risk for Ineffective Management of Therapeutic Regimen related to insufficient knowledge of activities permitted, self-care activities, medications, complications, and plans for follow-up care

▲ This diagnosis was reported to be monitored for or managed frequently (75%–100%).
△ This diagnosis was reported to be monitored for or managed often (50%–74%).

FRACTURED HIP AND FEMUR

See also *Surgery (General)*.

Postoperative Period

Collaborative Problems

- ▲ *PC: Hemorrhage/shock*
- ▲ *PC: Pulmonary embolism*
- ▲ *PC: Sepsis*
- ▲ *PC: Fat emboli*
- ▲ *PC: Compartmental syndrome*
- △ *PC: Peroneal nerve palsy*
- ▲ *PC: Displacement of hip joint*
- ▲ *PC: Venous stasis/thrombosis*
- *PC: Avascular necrosis of femoral head*

Nursing Diagnoses

- ▲ (Specify) Self-Care Deficit related to prescribed activity restriction
- ▲ Disuse syndrome
- △ Fear related to anticipated postoperative dependence
- △ Risk for Sensory/Perceptual Alterations related to increased age, pain, and immobility
- △ Risk for Ineffective Management of Therapeutic Regimen related to insufficient knowledge of activity restrictions, assistive devices, home care, follow-up care, and supportive services

HYSTERECTOMY (Vaginal, Abdominal)

See also *Surgery (General)*.

Postoperative Period

Collaborative Problems

- ▲ *PC: Vaginal bleeding*
- * *PC: Urinary retention (postcatheter removal)*

▲ This diagnosis was reported to be monitored for or managed frequently (75%–100%).
△ This diagnosis was reported to be monitored for or managed often (50%–74%).
* This diagnosis was not included in the validation study.

PC: Fistula formation
▲ PC: Deep vein thrombosis
▲ PC: Trauma (ureter, bladder, rectum)

Nursing Diagnoses

* Risk for Infection related to surgical intervention and presence of urinary catheter
△ Risk for Self-Concept Disturbance related to significance of loss
* Grieving related to loss of body part and childbearing ability
△ Risk for Ineffective Management of Therapeutic Regimen related to insufficient knowledge of perineal/incisional care, signs of complications, activity restrictions, loss of menses, hormone therapy, and follow-up care

ILEOSTOMY

Postoperative Period

Collaborative Problems

▲ PC: Peristomal ulceration/herniation
▲ PC: Stomal necrosis, retraction prolapse, stenosis, obstruction
▲ PC: Fluid and electrolyte imbalances
PC: Pouchitis

Nursing Diagnoses

▲ Risk for Self-Concept Disturbance related to effects of ostomy on body image
△ Risk for Altered Sexuality Patterns related to perceived negative impact of ostomy on sexual functioning and attractiveness
△ Risk for Social Isolation related to anxiety about possible odor and leakage from appliance

---

▲ This diagnosis was reported to be monitored for or managed frequently (75%–100%).
△ This diagnosis was reported to be monitored for or managed often (50%–74%).
* This diagnosis was not included in the validation study.

△ Risk for Ineffective Management of Therapeutic Regimen related to insufficient knowledge of stoma pouching procedure, peristomal skin care, perineal wound care, and incorporation of ostomy care into activities of daily living
△ Risk for Ineffective Management of Therapeutic Regimen related to insufficient knowledge of care of ileoanal reservoir
Risk for Ineffective Management of Therapeutic Regimen related to insufficient knowledge of intermittent intubation of Kock continent ileostomy

LAMINECTOMY

See also *Surgery (General)*.

Postoperative Period

Collaborative Problems

- ▲ *PC: Neurosensory impairments*
- * *PC: Bowel/bladder dysfunction*
- ▲ *PC: Paralytic ileus*
- * *PC: Cord edema*
- * *PC: Skeletal misalignment*
- △ *PC: Cerebrospinal fistula*
- * *PC: Hematoma*
- ▲ *PC: Urinary retention*

Nursing Diagnoses

- * Risk for Injury related to vertigo secondary to postural hypotension
- ▲ Acute Pain related to muscle spasms (back, thigh) secondary to surgical trauma
- * (Specify) Self-Care Deficit related to activity restrictions
- ▲ Risk for Ineffective Management of Therapeutic Regimen related to insufficient knowledge of home care, brace care, activity restrictions, and exercise program

---

▲ This diagnosis was reported to be monitored for or managed frequently (75%–100%).
△ This diagnosis was reported to be monitored for or managed often (50%–74%).
* This diagnosis was not included in the validation study.

MASTECTOMY

See also *Cancer (General)*.
See also *Surgery (General)*.

Postoperative Period
Collaborative Problem

▲ *PC: Neurovascular compromise*

Nursing Diagnoses

▲ Risk for Impaired Physical Mobility (shoulder, arm)
    related to lymphedema, nerve/muscle damage, and
    pain
▲ Risk for Injury related to compromised lymph, motor,
    and sensory function in affected arm
▲ Grieving related to loss of breast and change in
    appearance
▲ Risk for Ineffective Management of Therapeutic Regi-
    men related to insufficient knowledge of wound care,
    exercises, breast prosthesis, signs and symptoms of
    complications, hand/arm precautions, community
    resources, and follow-up care

OPHTHALMIC SURGERY

See also *Surgery (General)*.

Postoperative Period
Collaborative Problems

△ *PC: Wound dehiscence/evisceration*
△ *PC: Increased intraocular pressure*
△ *PC: Retinal detachment*
   PC: Dislocation of lens implant
   PC: Choroidal hemorrhage
   PC: Endophthalmitis
   PC: Hyphema
   PC: Hypopyon
△ *PC: Blindness*

▲ This diagnosis was reported to be monitored for or managed
   frequently (75%–100%).
△ This diagnosis was reported to be monitored for or managed
   often (50%–74%).

Nursing Diagnoses

△ Risk for Infection related to increased susceptibility
    secondary to surgical trauma

▲ Risk for Injury related to visual limitations, presence in
    unfamiliar environment, and presence of postopera-
    tive eye patches

▲ Feeding, Bathing/Hygiene Self-Care Deficit related to
    activity restrictions, visual impairment, or presence of
    eye patch(es)

▲ Risk for Sensory/Perceptual Alterations related to insuf-
    ficient input secondary to impaired vision or pres-
    ence of unilateral/bilateral eye patches

△ Risk for Ineffective Management of Therapeutic Regi-
    men related to insufficient knowledge of activities
    permitted and restricted, medications, complica-
    tions, and follow-up care

OTIC SURGERY (Stapedectomy, Tympanoplasty, Myringotomy, Tympanic Mastoidectomy)

See also *Surgery (General)*.

Postoperative Period

Collaborative Problems

    PC: Hemorrhage
    PC: Facial paralysis
    PC: Infection
    PC: Impaired hearing/deafness

Nursing Diagnoses

    Impaired Communication related to decreased hearing
    Risk for Social Isolation related to embarrassment of
        not being able to hear in a social setting
    Risk for Injury related to vertigo
    Risk for Ineffective Management of Therapeutic Regi-
        men related to insufficient knowledge of signs and

▲ This diagnosis was reported to be monitored for or managed
   frequently (75%–100%).

△ This diagnosis was reported to be monitored for or managed
   often (50%–74%).

symptoms of complications (facial nerve injury, vertigo, tinnitus, gait disturbances, and ear discharge), ear care, contraindications, and follow-up care

RADICAL NECK DISSECTION (Laryngectomy)

See also *Surgery (General)*.
See also *Cancer (General)*.
See also *Tracheostomy*.

Postoperative Period

Collaborative Problems

* * PC: Hypoxemia
* ▲ PC: Flap rejection
* ▲ PC: Hemorrhage
* ▲ PC: Carotid artery rupture
* * PC: Cranial nerve injury
* * PC: Infection

Nursing Diagnoses

* ▲ Risk for Impaired Physical Mobility: Shoulder, head related to removal of muscles, nerves, flap graft reconstruction and surgical trauma
* ▲ Risk for Self-Concept Disturbance related to change in appearance
* ▲ Risk for Ineffective Management of Therapeutic Regimen related to insufficient knowledge of wound care, signs and symptoms of complications, exercises, and follow-up care

RADICAL VULVECTOMY

See also *Surgery (General)*.
See also *Anticoagulant Therapy*.

---

* ▲ This diagnosis was reported to be monitored for or managed frequently (75%–100%).
* * This diagnosis was not included in the validation study.

Postoperative Period

Collaborative Problems

▲ *PC: Hemorrhage/shock*
▲ *PC: Urinary retention*
▲ *PC: Sepsis*
△ *PC: Pulmonary embolism*
▲ *PC: Thrombophlebitis*

Nursing Diagnoses

▲ Altered Comfort related to effects of surgery and immobility
▲ Grieving related to loss of body function and its effects on lifestyle
△ Risk for Altered Sexuality Patterns related to negative impact of surgery on sexual functioning and attractiveness
△ Risk for Ineffective Management of Therapeutic Regimen related to insufficient knowledge of home care, wound care, self-catheterization, and follow-up care

RENAL SURGERY (General, Percutaneous Nephrostomy/Extracorporeal Renal Surgery, Nephrectomy)

See also *Surgery (General)*.

Collaborative Problems

▲ *PC: Hemorrhage*
▲ *PC: Shock*
▲ *PC: Paralytic ileus*
* *PC: Pneumothorax*
* *PC: Fistulae*
▲ *PC: Renal insufficiency*
△ *PC: Pyelonephritis*
△ *PC: Ureteral stent dislodgement*
△ *PC: Pneumothorax secondary to thoracic approach*

▲ This diagnosis was reported to be monitored for or managed frequently (75%–100%).
△ This diagnosis was reported to be monitored for or managed often (50%–74%).
* This diagnosis was not included in the validation study.

Nursing Diagnoses

△ Impaired Physical Mobility related to distention of renal capsule and incision

▲ Risk for Altered Respiratory Function related to pain on breathing and coughing secondary to location of incision

▲ Risk for Ineffective Management of Therapeutic Regimen related to insufficient knowledge of hydration requirements, nephrostomy care, and signs and symptoms of complications

RENAL TRANSPLANT

See also *Corticosteroid Therapy*.
See also *Surgery (General)*.

Collaborative Problems

▲ *PC: Hemodynamic instability*
▲ *PC: Hypervolemia/hypovolemia*
▲ *PC: Hypertension/hypotension*
▲ *PC: Renal insufficiency (donor kidney)*
    Examples:
        Ischemic damage before implantation
        Hematoma
        Rupture of anastomosis
        Bleeding at anastomosis
        Renal vein thrombosis
        Renal artery stenosis
        Blockage of ureter (kinks, clots)
        Kinking of ureter, renal artery
▲ *PC: Rejection of donor tissue*
▲ *PC: Excessive immunosuppression*
▲ *PC: Electrolyte imbalances (potassium, phosphate)*
▲ *PC: Deep vein thrombosis*
▲ *PC: Sepsis*

▲ This diagnosis was reported to be monitored for or managed frequently (75%–100%).
△ This diagnosis was reported to be monitored for or managed often (50%–74%).

Nursing Diagnoses

▲ Risk for Infection related to altered immune system secondary to medications
▲ Risk for Altered Oral Mucous Membrane related to increased susceptibility to infection secondary to immunosuppression
△ Risk for Self-Concept Disturbance related to transplant experience and potential for rejection
▲ Fear related to possibility of rejection and dying
▲ Risk for Noncompliance related to complexity of treatment regimen (diet, medications, record-keeping, weight, blood pressure, urine testing) and euphoria (post-transplant)
▲ Risk for Ineffective Management of Therapeutic Regimen related to insufficient knowledge of prevention of infection, activity progression, dietary management, daily recording (intake, output, weights, urine testing, blood pressure, temperature), pharmacological therapy, daily urine testing (protein), signs and symptoms of rejection/infection, avoidance of pregnancy, follow-up care, and community resources

THORACIC SURGERY

See also *Surgery (General)*.
See also *Mechanical Ventilation*.

Postoperative Period

Collaborative Problems

* *PC: Atelectasis*
* *PC: Pneumonia*
▲ *PC: Respiratory insufficiency*
▲ *PC: Pneumothorax, hemothorax*
* *PC: Hemorrhage*
▲ *PC: Pulmonary embolism*
▲ *PC: Subcutaneous emphysema*

▲ This diagnosis was reported to be monitored for or managed frequently (75%–100%).
△ This diagnosis was reported to be monitored for or managed often (50%–74%).
* This diagnosis was not included in the validation study.

△ *PC: Mediastinal shift*
▲ *PC: Acute pulmonary edema*
△ *PC: Thrombophlebitis*

Nursing Diagnoses

▲ Altered Comfort related to surgical incision, chest tube sites, and immobility secondary to lengthy surgery
▲ Ineffective Airway Clearance related to increased secretions and diminished cough secondary to pain and fatigue
　Activity Intolerance related to reduction in exercise capacity secondary to loss of alveolar ventilation
▲ Impaired Physical Mobility related to restricted arm and shoulder movement secondary to pain and muscle dissection and imposed position restrictions
　Grieving related to loss of body part and its perceived effects on lifestyle
* Risk for Ineffective Management of Therapeutic Regimen related to insufficient knowledge of condition, pain management, shoulder/arm exercises, incisional care, breathing exercises, splinting, prevention of infection, nutritional needs, rest versus activity, respiratory toilet, and follow-up care

TONSILLECTOMY

See also *Surgery (General)*.

Collaborative Problems

　PC: Airway obstruction
　PC: Aspiration
　PC: Bleeding

▲ This diagnosis was reported to be monitored for or managed frequently (75%–100%).
△ This diagnosis was reported to be monitored for or managed often (50%–74%).
* This diagnosis was not included in the validation study.

Nursing Diagnoses

Risk for Fluid Volume Deficit related to decreased fluid intake secondary to pain on swallowing

Risk for Altered Nutrition: Less than body requirements related to decreased intake secondary to pain on swallowing

Risk for Ineffective Management of Therapeutic Regimen related to insufficient knowledge of rest requirements, nutritional needs, signs and symptoms of complications, pain management, positioning, and activity restrictions

TRANSURETHRAL RESECTION (Prostate [Benign Hypertrophy or Cancer], Bladder Tumor)

See also *Surgery (General)*.

Postoperative Period

Collaborative Problems

PC: Oliguria/anuria
PC: Hemorrhage
PC: Perforated bladder (intraoperative)
PC: Hyponatremia
PC: Sepsis
PC: Occlusion of drainage devices
PC: Prostatectomy
PC: Clot formation

Nursing Diagnoses

Altered Comfort related to bladder spasms, clot retention, or back and leg pain

Risk for Ineffective Management of Therapeutic Regimen related to insufficient knowledge of fluid requirements, activity restrictions, catheter care, urinary control, and follow-up and signs and symptoms of complications

UROSTOMY

See also *Surgery (General)*.

Postoperative Period

Collaborative Problems

△ *PC: Internal urine leakage*
▲ *PC: Urinary tract infection*
▲ *PC: Peristomal ulceration/herniation*
▲ *PC: Stomal necrosis, retraction, prolapse, stenosis, obstruction*

Nursing Diagnoses

△ Risk for Self-Concept Disturbance related to effects of ostomy on body image
  Risk for Altered Sexuality Patterns related to perceived negative impact of ostomy on sexual functioning and attractiveness
  Risk for Altered Sexuality Patterns related to erectile dysfunction (male) or inadequate vaginal lubrication (female)
△ Risk for Social Isolation related to anxiety about possible odor and leakage from appliance
▲ Risk for Ineffective Management of Therapeutic Regimen related to insufficient knowledge of stoma pouching procedure, colostomy irrigation, peristomal skin care, perineal wound care, incorporation of ostomy care into activities of daily living
△ Risk for Ineffective Management of Therapeutic Regimen related to insufficient knowledge of intermittent self-catheterization of Kock continent urostomy

▲ This diagnosis was reported to be monitored for or managed frequently (75%–100%).
△ This diagnosis was reported to be monitored for or managed often (50%–74%).

Obstetrical/Gynecological Conditions

Obstetrical Conditions

PRENATAL PERIOD (General)

Nursing Diagnoses

Nausea related to elevated estrogen levels, decreased blood sugar, or decreased gastric motility and pressure on cardiac sphincter from enlarged uterus

Constipation related to decreased gastric motility and pressure of uterus on lower colon

Activity Intolerance related to fatigue and dyspnea secondary to pressure of enlarging uterus on diaphragm and increased blood volume

Risk for Altered Oral Mucous Membranes related to hyperemic gums secondary to estrogen and progesterone levels

Risk for Injury related to syncope/hypotension secondary to peripheral venous pooling

Risk for Altered Health Maintenance related to insufficient knowledge of (examples) effects of pregnancy on body systems (cardiovascular, integumentary, gastrointestinal, urinary, pulmonary, musculoskeletal), psychosocial domain, sexuality/sexual function, family unit (spouse, children), fetal growth and development, nutritional requirements, hazards of smoking, excessive alcohol intake, drug abuse, excessive caffeine intake, excessive weight gain, signs and symptoms of complications (vaginal bleeding, cramping, gestational diabetes, excessive edema, preeclampsia), preparation for childbirth (classes, printed references)

ABORTION, INDUCED

Preprocedure Period

Nursing Diagnoses

Anxiety related to significance of decision, procedure and postprocedure care

Postprocedure Period

Collaborative Problems

PC: Hemorrhage
PC: Infection

Nursing Diagnoses

Risk for Ineffective Individual Coping related to unresolved emotional responses (guilt) to societal, moral, religious, and familial opposition

Risk for Altered Family Processes related to effects of procedure on relationships (disagreement about decisions, previous conflicts [personal, marital], or adolescent identity problems)

Risk for Altered Health Maintenance related to insufficient knowledge of self-care (hygiene, breast care), nutritional needs, expected bleeding, cramping, signs and symptoms of complications, resumption of sexual activity, contraception, sex education as indicated, comfort measures, expected emotional responses, follow-up appointment, and community resources

ABORTION, SPONTANEOUS

Nursing Diagnoses

Fear related to possibility of subsequent abortions
Grieving related to loss of pregnancy

EXTRAUTERINE PREGNANCY (Ectopic Pregnancy)

Collaborative Problems

PC: Hemorrhage
PC: Shock
PC: Sepsis
PC: Acute pain

Nursing Diagnoses

Grieving related to loss of fetus
Fear related to possibility of not being able to carry subsequent pregnancies

526

HYPEREMESIS GRAVIDARUM

Collaborative Problems

PC: Negative nitrogen balance

Nursing Diagnoses

Risk for Altered Nutrition: Less than body requirements related to loss of nutrients and fluid secondary to vomiting

PREGNANCY-INDUCED HYPERTENSION

See also *Prenatal Period.*
See also *Postpartum Period.*

Collaborative Problems

PC: Malignant hypertension
PC: Seizures
PC: Proteinuria
PC: Visual disturbances
PC: Coma
PC: Renal failure
PC: Cerebral edema
PC: Fetal compromise

Nursing Diagnoses

Fear related to the effects of condition on self, pregnancy, and infant

Risk for Injury related to vertigo, visual disturbances, or seizures

Risk for Ineffective Management of Therapeutic Regimen related to insufficient knowledge of dietary restrictions, signs and symptoms of complications, conservation of energy, pharmacological therapy, and comfort measures for headaches and backaches

PREGNANT ADOLESCENT

See also *General Prenatal, Intrapartum Period,* and *Postpartum Period.*

Prenatal

Collaborative Problems

PC: Pregnancy-induced hypertension

Nursing Diagnoses

Altered Family Process related to stressors associated with adolescent pregnancy and future implications for family

Risk for Altered Nutrition: Less than body requirements related to maternal growth needs and lower nutritional stores secondary to adolescence

Self-Concept Disturbance related to pregnancy-associated body changes and conflict with adolescent and parenting roles

Risk for Social Isolation related to negative response of peer group to pregnancy

Risk for Urinary Tract Infection related to insufficient knowledge of prevention of infection and increased vulnerability secondary to effects of pregnancy on renal and ureter anatomy

Postpartum

Nursing Diagnoses

Risk for Altered Parenting related to conflicting developmental task of adolescence and parenthood

Decisional Conflict related to caregiver of infant, adoption options, or living arrangements

UTERINE BLEEDING DURING PREGNANCY

(Placenta Previa, Abruptio Placentae, Uterine Rupture, Nonmalignant Lesions, Hydatidiform Mole)

See also *Postpartum Period*.

Collaborative Problems

PC: Hemorrhage
PC: Shock
PC: Disseminated intravascular coagulation
PC: Renal failure
PC: Fetal death

PC: *Anemia*
PC: *Sepsis*

Nursing Diagnoses

Fear related to effects of bleeding on pregnancy and infant

Impaired Physical Mobility related to increased bleeding in response to activity

Grieving related to anticipated possible loss of pregnancy and loss of expected child

Fear related to possibility of subsequent future complications of pregnancy

INTRAPARTUM PERIOD (General)

Collaborative Problems

PC: *Hemorrhage (placenta previa, abruptio placentae)*
PC: *Fetal distress*
PC: *Hypertension*
PC: *Uterine rupture*
PC: *Dystocia*

Nursing Diagnoses

Acute Pain related to uterine contractions during labor

Fear related to unpredictability of uterine contractions and possibility of having an impaired baby

Anxiety related to insufficient knowledge of relaxation/breathing exercises, positioning and procedures (preparations [bowel, skin], frequent assessments, anesthesia [regional, inhalation])

POSTPARTUM PERIOD

General Postpartum Period

Collaborative Problems

PC: *Hemorrhage*
PC: *Uterine atony*
PC: *Retained placental fragments*
PC: *Lacerations*
PC: *Hematomas*
PC: *Urinary retention*

Nursing Diagnoses

Risk for Infection related to bacterial invasion secondary to trauma during labor, delivery, and episiotomy

Risk for Ineffective Breastfeeding related to inexperience or engorged breasts

Altered Comfort related to trauma to perineum during labor and delivery, hemorrhoids, engorged breasts, and involution of uterus

Risk for Constipation related to decreased intestinal peristalsis (postdelivery) and decreased activity

Risk for Altered Parenting related to (examples) inexperience, feelings of incompetence, powerlessness, unwanted child, disappointment with child, or lack of role models

Stress Incontinence related to tissue trauma during delivery

Risk for Situational Low Self-Esteem related to changes that persist after delivery (skin, weight, lifestyle)

Risk for Altered Health Maintenance related to insufficient knowledge of postpartum routines, hygiene (breast, perineum), exercises, sexual counseling (contraception), nutritional requirements (infant, maternal), infant care, stresses of parenthood, adaptation of father, sibling, parent–infant bonding, postpartum emotional responses, sleep/rest requirements, household management, community resources, management of discomforts (breast, perineum), and signs and symptoms of complications

Mastitis (Lactational)

Collaborative Problem

PC: Abscess

Nursing Diagnoses

Altered Comfort related to inflammation of breast tissue

Risk for Ineffective Breastfeeding related to interruption secondary to inflammation

Risk for Altered Health Maintenance related to insufficient knowledge of need for breast support, breast

hygiene, breastfeeding restrictions, and signs and
symptoms of abscess formation

Fetal/Newborn Death

Nursing Diagnoses

Altered Family Processes related to emotional trauma
of loss on each family member
Grieving related to loss of infant
Fear related to the possibility of future fetal deaths

CONCOMITANT MEDICAL CONDITIONS (Cardiac
Disease [Prenatal, Postpartum], Diabetes [Prenatal,
Postpartum])

Cardiac Disease

See also *Cardiac Disorders.*
See also *Prenatal Period.*
See also *Postpartum Period.*

Collaborative Problems

PC: Congestive heart failure
*PC: Pregnancy-induced hypertension (preeclampsia,
eclampsia)*
PC: Valvular damage

Nursing Diagnoses

Fear related to effects of condition on self, pregnancy,
and infant
Activity Intolerance related to increased metabolic
requirements (pregnancy) in presence of compromised cardiac function
Impaired Home Maintenance Management related to
impaired ability to perform role responsibilities
during and after pregnancy
Risk for Altered Family Processes related to disruption
of activity restrictions and fears of effects on lifestyle
Risk for Ineffective Management of Therapeutic Regimen related to insufficient knowledge of dietary
requirements, prevention of infection, conservation of
energy, signs and symptoms of complications, and
community resources

Diabetes (Prenatal)

See also *Prenatal Period*.
See also *Diabetes Mellitus*.
See also *Postpartum Period*.

Collaborative Problems

PC: Hypoglycemia/hyperglycemia
PC: Hydramnios
PC: Acidosis
PC: Pregnancy-induced hypertension

Nursing Diagnoses

Risk for Impaired Skin Integrity related to excessive skin stretching secondary to hydramnios

Risk for Vaginal Infection related to susceptibility to monilial infection

Altered Comfort: Headaches related to cerebral edema or hyperirritability

Risk for Ineffective Management of Therapeutic Regimen related to insufficient knowledge of effects of pregnancy on diabetes, effects of diabetes on pregnancy, nutritional requirements, insulin requirements, signs and symptoms of complications, and need for frequent blood/urine samples

Diabetes (Postpartum)

See also *Postpartum Period (General)*.

Collaborative Problems

PC: Hypoglycemia
PC: Hyperglycemia
PC: Hemorrhage (secondary to uterine atony from excessive amniotic fluid)
PC: Pregnancy-induced hypertension

Nursing Diagnoses

Anxiety related to separation from infant secondary to the special care needs of infant

Risk for Infection of Perineal area related to depleted host defenses and depressed leukocytic phagocytosis secondary to hyperglycemia

Risk for Ineffective Management of Therapeutic Regimen related to insufficient knowledge of risks of future pregnancies, birth control methods, types contraindicated, and special care requirements for infant

Gynecological Conditions

ENDOMETRIOSIS

Collaborative Problems

PC: Hypermenorrhea
PC: Polymenorrhea

Nursing Diagnoses

Chronic Pain related to response of displaced endometrial tissue (abdominal, peritoneal) to cyclic ovarian hormonal stimulation

Altered Sexuality Patterns related to painful intercourse or infertility

Anxiety related to unpredictable nature of disease

Risk for Ineffective Management of Therapeutic Regimen related to insufficient knowledge of condition, myths, pharmacological therapy, and potential for pregnancy

PELVIC INFLAMMATORY DISEASE

Collaborative Problems

PC: Septicemia
PC: Abscess formation
PC: Pneumonia
PC: Pulmonary embolism

Nursing Diagnoses

Altered Comfort related to malaise, increased temperature secondary to infectious process

Risk for Fluid Volume Deficit related to inadequate intake, fatigue, pain, and fluid losses secondary to elevated temperature

Chronic pain related to inflammatory process

Risk for Ineffective Individual Coping: Depression related to chronicity of condition and lack of definitive diagnosis/treatment

Risk for Ineffective Management of Therapeutic Regimen related to insufficient knowledge of condition, nutritional requirements, signs and symptoms of complications, prevention of sexually transmitted diseases, and sleep/rest requirements

Neonatal Conditions

NEONATE, NORMAL

Collaborative Problems

PC: Hypothermia
PC: Hypoglycemia
PC: Hyperbilirubinemia
PC: Bradycardia

Nursing Diagnoses

Risk for Infection related to vulnerability of infant, lack of normal flora, environmental hazards, and open wound (umbilical cord, circumcision)

Risk for Ineffective Airway Clearance related to oropharynx secretions

Risk for Impaired Skin Integrity related to susceptibility to nosocomial infection and lack of normal skin flora

Ineffective Thermoregulation related to newborn extrauterine transition

Risk for Ineffective Management of Therapeutic Regimen related to insufficient knowledge of (specify) (see Postpartum Period)

NEONATE, PREMATURE

See also *Family of High-Risk Neonate.*

Collaborative Problems

PC: Cold stress
PC: Apnea
PC: Bradycardia
PC: Hypoglycemia
PC: Acidosis
PC: Hypocalcemia
PC: Sepsis
PC: Seizures
PC: Pneumonia
PC: Hyperbilirubinemia

Nursing Diagnoses

Risk for Constipation related to decreased intestinal motility and immobility

Risk for Aspiration related to immobility and increased secretions

Risk for Infection related to vulnerability of infant, lack of normal flora, environmental hazards, and open wounds (umbilical cord, circumcision)

Risk for Impaired Skin Integrity related to susceptibility to nosocomial infection (lack of normal skin flora)

Ineffective Thermoregulation related to newborn transition to extrauterine environment

Ineffective Infant Feeding Pattern related to lethargy secondary to prematurity

NEONATE, POSTMATURE (Small for Gestational Age [SGA], Large for Gestational Age [LGA])

Collaborative Problems

PC: Asphyxia at birth
PC: Meconium aspiration
PC: Hypoglycemia
PC: Polycythemia (SGA)
PC: Edema (generalized, cerebral)
PC: Central nervous system depression
PC: Renal tubular necrosis
PC: Impaired intestinal absorption
PC: Birth injuries (LGA)

Nursing Diagnoses

Risk for Impaired Skin Integrity related to absence of protective vernix and prolonged exposure to amniotic fluid (LGA)

Ineffective Infant Feeding Pattern related to lethargy

NEONATE WITH SPECIAL PROBLEM (Congenital Infections—Cytomegalovirus, Rubella, Toxoplasmosis, Syphilis, Herpes)

See also *High-Risk Neonate.*
See also *Family of High-Risk Neonate.*
See also *Developmental Problems/Needs* under *Pediatric Disorders.*

Collaborative Problems

PC: Hyperbilirubinemia
PC: Hepatosplenomegaly
PC: Anemia
PC: Hydrocephalus
PC: Microcephaly
PC: Mental retardation
PC: Congenital heart disease (rubella)
PC: Cataracts (rubella)
PC: Retinitis
PC: Thrombocytopenic purpura (rubella)
PC: Sensory–motor deafness (cytomegalovirus)
PC: Periostitis (syphilis)
PC: Seizures

Nursing Diagnoses

Risk for Infection Transmission related to contagious nature of organism

Risk for Injury related to uncontrolled tonic-clonic movements

NEONATE WITH MENINGOMYELOCELE

See also *Normal Neonate.*
See also *Family of High-Risk Neonate.*

Collaborative Problems

PC: Hydrocephalus
PC: Neurovascular insufficiency (below lesion)

Nursing Diagnoses

Risk for Trauma related to vulnerability of meningomyelocele

Altered Bowel Elimination related to effects of spinal cord disorder on anal sphincter

Urinary Retention related to effects of spinal cord injury on bladder function

Risk for Impaired Skin Integrity related to inability to move lower extremities

NEONATE WITH CONGENITAL HEART DISEASE
(Preoperative)

See also *Normal Neonate.*
See also *Family of High-Risk Neonate.*

Collaborative Problems

PC: Congestive heart failure
PC: Dysrhythmias
PC: Decreased cardiac output

Nursing Diagnoses

Risk for Ineffective Infant Feeding Pattern related to difficulty breathing and fatigue

NEONATE OF A DIABETIC MOTHER

See also *Neonate, Normal.*
See also *Family of High-Risk Neonate.*

Collaborative Problems

PC: Hypoglycemia
PC: Hypocalcemia
PC: Polycythemia
PC: Hyperbilirubinemia
PC: Sepsis
PC: Acidosis
PC: Birth injury (macrosomia)

PC: Hyaline membrane disease
PC: Respiratory distress syndrome
PC: Venous thrombosis

Nursing Diagnoses

Risk for Fluid Volume Deficit related to increased urinary excretion and osmotic diuresis

HIGH-RISK NEONATE

See also *Family of High-Risk Neonate*.

Collaborative Problems

PC: Hypoxemia
PC: Shock
PC: Respiratory distress
PC: Seizures
PC: Hypotension
PC: Septicemia

Nursing Diagnoses

Disorganized Infant Behavior related to immature central nervous system and excess stimulation

Risk for Infection related to vulnerability of infant, lack of normal flora, environmental hazards, open wounds (umbilical cord, circumcision), and invasive lines

Ineffective Infant Feeding Pattern related to (specify)

Risk for Altered Respiratory Function related to increased oropharyngeal secretions

Risk for Impaired Skin Integrity related to susceptibility to nosocomial infection secondary to lack of normal skin flora

Ineffective Thermoregulation related to newborn transition to extrauterine environment

FAMILY OF HIGH-RISK NEONATE

Nursing Diagnoses

Chronic Sorrow related to realization of possible present or future loss for family or child

Altered Family Processes related to effect of extended hospitalization on family (role responsibilities, finances)

Anxiety related to unpredictable prognosis

Risk for Altered Parenting related to inadequate bonding secondary to parent–child separation or failure to accept impaired child

HYPERBILIRUBINEMIA (Rh Incompatibility, ABO Incompatibility)

See also *Family of High-Risk Neonate.*
See also *Neonate, Normal.*

Collaborative Problems

PC: Anemia
PC: Jaundice
PC: Kernicterus
PC: Hepatosplenomegaly
PC: Hydrops fetalis (cardiac failure, hypoxia, anasarca, and pericardial, pleural, and peritoneal effusions)
PC: Renal failure (phototherapy complications, hyperthermia/hypothermia, dehydration, priapism, "bronze baby" syndrome)

Nursing Diagnoses

Risk for Impaired Corneal Tissue Integrity related to exposure to phototherapy light and continuous wearing of eye pads

Risk for Impaired Skin Integrity related to diarrhea, urinary excretions of bilirubin, and exposure to phototherapy light

NEONATE OF NARCOTIC-ADDICTED MOTHER

See also *Family of High-Risk Neonate.*
See also *Neonate, Normal.*
See also *Substance Abuse for Mother.*

Collaborative Problems

PC: Hyperirritability/seizures
PC: Withdrawal
PC: Hypocalcemia
PC: Hypoglycemia
PC: Sepsis

PC: Dehydration
PC: Electrolyte imbalances

Nursing Diagnoses

Risk for Impaired Skin Integrity related to generalized diaphoresis and marked rigidity

Diarrhea related to increased peristalsis secondary to hyperirritability

Sleep Pattern Disturbance related to hyperirritability

Risk for Injury related to frantic sucking of fists

Risk for Injury related to uncontrolled tremors or tonic-clonic movements

Sensory/Perceptual Alterations related to hypersensitivity to environmental stimuli

Ineffective Infant Feeding Pattern related to lethargy

RESPIRATORY DISTRESS SYNDROME

See also *High-Risk Neonate*.
See also *Mechanical Ventilation*.

Collaborative Problems

PC: Hypoxemia
PC: Atelectasis
PC: Acidosis
PC: Sepsis
PC: Hyperthermia

Nursing Diagnoses

Activity Intolerance related to insufficient oxygenation of tissues secondary to impaired respirations

Risk for Infection related to vulnerability of infant, lack of normal flora, environmental hazards (personnel, other newborns, parents), and open wounds (umbilical cord, circumcision)

Risk for Impaired Skin Integrity related to susceptibility to nosocomial infection and lack of normal skin flora

SEPSIS (Septicemia)

See also *Neonate, Normal*.
See also *Family of High-Risk Neonate*.
See also *High-Risk Neonate*.

Collaborative Problems

PC: *Anemia*
PC: *Respiratory distress*
PC: *Hypothermia/hyperthermia*
PC: *Hypotension*
PC: *Edema*
PC: *Seizures*
PC: *Hepatosplenomegaly*
PC: *Hemorrhage*
PC: *Jaundice*
PC: *Meningitis*
PC: *Pyarthrosis*

Nursing Diagnoses

Risk for Impaired Skin Integrity related to edema and immobility

Diarrhea related to intestinal irritation secondary to infecting organism

Risk for Injury related to uncontrolled tonic-clonic movements and hematopoietic insufficiency

Pediatric/Adolescent Disorders*

DEVELOPMENTAL PROBLEMS/NEEDS RELATED TO CHRONIC ILLNESS (*e.g.,* Permanent Disability, Multiple Handicaps, Developmental Disability [Mental/Physical], Life-Threatening Illness)

*For additional pediatric medical diagnoses, see the adult diagnoses and Developmental Problems/Needs. For example:

Diabetes mellitus	Neoplastic disorders
Anorexia nervosa (psychiatric disorders)	Fractures
	Congestive heart failure
Spinal cord injury	Pneumonia
Head trauma	

Nursing Diagnoses

Chronic Sorrow (parental) related to anticipated losses secondary to condition

Altered Family Processes related to adjustment requirements for situation: (examples) time, energy (emotional, physical), financial, and physical care

Risk for Impaired Home Maintenance Management related to inadequate resources, housing, or impaired caregiver(s)

Risk for Parental Role Conflict related to separations secondary to frequent hospitalizations

Risk for Social Isolation (child/family) related to the disability and the requirements of the caregiver(s)

Risk for Altered Parenting related to abuse, rejection, overprotection secondary to inadequate resources or coping mechanisms

Decisional Conflict related to illness, health care interventions, and parent–child separation

(Specify) Self-Care Deficit related to illness limitations or hospitalization

Risk for Altered Growth and Development related to impaired ability to achieve developmental tasks

Caregiver Role Strain related to multiple ongoing care needs secondary to restrictions imposed by disease, disability, or treatments

ANXIETY/SCHOOL PHOBIA

Nursing Diagnoses

Anxiety related to altered self-esteem, change in environment, fear of separation, and negative responses (peers, family)

Ineffective Individual Coping related to inadequate problem-solving skills and denial of problem

Self-Esteem Disturbance related to negative peer responses, perceived mental deficits, and unrealistic expectations in performance

ACQUIRED IMMUNODEFICIENCY SYNDROME
(Child)

See also *Acquired Immunodeficiency Syndrome (Adult)*.
See also *Developmental Problems/Needs Related to Chronic Illness*.

Nursing Diagnoses

Risk for Infection Transmission related to exposure to stool and other secretions during diaper changes or failure of child to follow handwashing procedure after toileting

Altered Nutrition: Less than body requirements related to lactose intolerance, need for double the usual recommended daily allowance, anorexia secondary to oral lesions, and malaise

Altered Growth and Development related to decreased muscle tone secondary to encephalopathy

Impaired Physical Mobility related to hypotonia or hypertonia secondary to cortical atrophy

Altered Family Processes related to the impact of the child's condition on role responsibilities, siblings, and finances and negative responses of relatives, friends, and community

Risk for Ineffective Management of Therapeutic Regimen related to insufficient knowledge of modes of transmission, risks of live virus vaccines, avoidance of infections, school attendance, and community resources

ASTHMA

See also *Developmental Problems/Needs*.

Collaborative Problems

PC: Hypoxemia
PC: Corticosteroid therapy
PC: Respiratory acidosis

Nursing Diagnoses

Ineffective Airway Clearance related to bronchospasm and increased pulmonary secretions

Fear related to breathlessness and recurrences

Risk for Ineffective Management of Therapeutic Regimen related to insufficient knowledge of condition, environmental hazards (smoking, allergens, weather), prevention of infection, breathing/relaxation exercises, signs and symptoms of complications, pharmacological therapy, fluid requirements, behavioral modification, and daily diary recording of peak flaws

ATTENTION DEFICIT DISORDER (Hootman, 1993)

Collaborative Problems

PC: Adverse effects of central nervous system stimulants

Nursing Diagnoses

Activity Intolerance related to delayed physical, emotional, or mental capacity and fatigue

Ineffective Individual Coping related to fatigue and delayed development

Altered Growth and Development related to delayed maturation secondary to genetic, physical, and mental disability

Risk for Injury related to motor deficits and hyperactivity

Self-Esteem Disturbance related to lack of success in school and negative peer interactions

Impaired Social Interaction related to delayed social development and poor peer acceptance

CELIAC DISEASE

See also *Developmental Problems/Needs*.

Collaborative Problems

PC: Severe malnutrition/dehydration
PC: Anemia
PC: Altered blood coagulation
PC: Osteoporosis
PC: Electrolyte imbalances
PC: Metabolic acidosis
PC: Shock
PC: Delayed growth

Nursing Diagnoses

Risk for Altered Nutrition: Less than body requirements related to malabsorption, dietary restrictions, and anorexia

544

Diarrhea related to decreased absorption in small
intestines secondary to damaged villi resulting from
toxins from undigested gliadin

Risk for Fluid Volume Deficit related to fluid loss in diarrhea

Risk for Ineffective Management of Therapeutic Regimen related to insufficient knowledge of dietary management, restrictions, and requirements

CEREBRAL PALSY*

See also *Developmental Problems/Needs.*

Collaborative Problems

PC: Contractures
PC: Seizures
PC: Respiratory infections

Nursing Diagnoses

Risk for Injury related to inability to control movements

Risk for Altered Nutrition: Less than body requirements
related to sucking difficulties (infant) and dysphagia

(Specify) Self-Care Deficit related to sensory–motor
impairments

Impaired Verbal Communication related to impaired
ability to speak words related to facial muscle
involvement

Risk for Fluid Volume Deficit related to difficulty obtaining or swallowing liquids

Risk for Diversional Activity Deficit related to effects of
limitations on ability to participate in recreational
activities

Risk for Ineffective Management of Therapeutic Regimen related to insufficient knowledge of disease,
pharmacological regimen, activity program, education, community services, and orthopedic appliances

*Because disabilities associated with cerebral palsy can be var-
ied (hemparesis, quadriparesis, diplegia, monoplegia, triplegia,
paraplegia), the nurse will have to specify the child's limitations
clearly in the diagnostic statements.

CHILD ABUSE (Battered Child Syndrome, Child Neglect)

See also *Fractures, Burns*.
See also *Failure to Thrive*.

Collaborative Problems

PC: Failure to thrive
PC: Malnutrition

Nursing Diagnoses

Ineffective Family Coping: Disabling related to presence of factors that contribute to child abuse: (examples) lack of or unavailability of extended family, economic problems (inflation, unemployment); lack of role model as a child, high-risk children (unwanted, of undesired gender or appearance, physically or mentally handicapped, hyperactive, terminally ill); and high-risk parents (single, adolescent, emotionally disturbed, alcoholic, drug-addicted, or physically ill)

Ineffective Individual Coping (child abuser) related to (examples) history of abuse by own parents and lack of warmth and affection from them, social isolation (few friends or outlets for tensions), marked lack of self-esteem with low tolerance for criticism, emotional immaturity and dependency, distrust of others, inability to admit need for help, high expectations for/of child (perceiving child as a source of emotional gratification), and unrealistic desire for child to give pleasure

Ineffective Individual Coping (nonabusing parent) related to passive and compliant response to abuse

Fear related to possibility of placement in a shelter or foster home

Parental Fear related to responses of others, possible loss of child, and criminal prosecution

Risk for Altered Nutrition: Less than body requirements related to inadequate intake secondary to lack of knowledge or neglect

Risk for Ineffective Management of Therapeutic Regimen related to insufficient knowledge of parenting skills (discipline, expectations), constructive stress management, signs and symptoms of abuse, high-risk groups, child protection laws, and community services

CLEFT LIP AND PALATE

See also *Developmental Problems/Needs.*
See also *Surgery (General).*

Preoperative Period

Nursing Diagnosis

Risk for Altered Nutrition: Less than body requirements related to impaired sucking secondary to cleft lip

Postoperative Period

Collaborative Problems

PC: Respiratory distress
PC: Failure to thrive (organic)

Nursing Diagnoses

Impaired Physical Mobility related to restricted activity secondary to use of restraints
Risk for Impaired Verbal Communication related to impaired muscle development, insufficient palate function, faulty dentition, or hearing loss
Risk for Aspiration related to impaired sucking
Risk for Ineffective Management of Therapeutic Regimen related to insufficient knowledge of condition, feeding and suctioning techniques, surgical site care, risks for otitis media (dental/oral problems), and referral to speech therapist

COMMUNICABLE DISEASES

See also *Developmental Problems/Needs.*

Nursing Diagnoses

Altered Comfort related to pruritus, fatigue, malaise, sore throat, and elevated temperature
Risk for Infection Transmission related to contagious agents

Risk for Fluid Volume Deficit related to increased fluid loss secondary to elevated temperature or insufficient oral intake secondary to malaise

Risk for Altered Nutrition: Less than body requirements related to anorexia and sore throat or pain on chewing (mumps)

Risk for Ineffective Airway Clearance related to increased mucus production (whooping cough)

Risk for Ineffective Management of Therapeutic Regimen related to insufficient knowledge of condition, transmission, prevention, immunizations, and skin care

CONGENITAL HEART DISEASE

See also *Developmental Problems/Needs Related to Chronic Illness.*

Collaborative Problems

PC: Congestive heart failure
PC: Pneumonia
PC: Hypoxemia
PC: Cerebral thrombosis
PC: Digoxin toxicity

Nursing Diagnoses

Activity Intolerance related to insufficient oxygenation secondary to heart defects

Risk for Altered Nutrition: Less than body requirements related to inadequate sucking, fatigue, and dyspnea

Risk for Ineffective Management of Therapeutic Regimen related to insufficient knowledge of condition, prevention of infection, signs and symptoms of complications, digoxin therapy, nutrition requirements, and community services

CONVULSIVE DISORDERS

See also *Developmental Problems/Needs.*
See also *Mental Disabilities,* if indicated.

Collaborative Problem

PC: Respiratory arrest

Nursing Diagnoses

Risk for Injury related to uncontrolled movements of seizure activity

Anxiety related to embarrassment and fear of seizure episodes

Risk for Ineffective Individual Coping related to restrictions, parental overprotection, and parental indulgence

Risk for Ineffective Management of Therapeutic Regimen related to insufficient knowledge of condition/cause, pharmacological therapy, treatment during seizures, and environmental hazards (water, driving, heights)

CRANIOCEREBRAL TRAUMA

Collaborative Problems

PC: Increased intracranial pressure
PC: Hemorrhage
PC: Tentorial herniation
PC: Cranial nerve dysfunction

Nursing Diagnoses

Acute Pain related to compression/displacement of cerebral tissue

Risk for Injury related to uncontrolled tonic-clonic movements during seizure episode or somnolence

Risk for Ineffective Management of Therapeutic Regimen related to insufficient knowledge of condition, signs and symptoms of complications, post-traumatic syndrome, activity restrictions, and follow-up care

CYSTIC FIBROSIS

See also *Developmental Problems/Needs*.

Collaborative Problems

PC: Bronchopneumonia, atelectasis
PC: Paralytic ileus

Nursing Diagnoses

Ineffective Airway Clearance related to mucopurulent secretions

Risk for Altered Nutrition: Less than body requirements related to need for increased calories and protein secondary to impaired intestinal absorption, loss of fat, and fat-soluble vitamins in stools

Constipation/Diarrhea related to excessive or insufficient pancreatic enzyme replacement

Activity Intolerance related to impaired oxygen transport secondary to mucopurulent secretions

Risk for Ineffective Management of Therapeutic Regimen related to insufficient knowledge of condition (genetic transmission), risk of infection, pharmacological therapy (side effects, ototoxicity, renal toxicity), equipment, nutritional therapy, salt replacement requirements, breathing exercises, postural drainage, exercise program, and community resources (Cystic Fibrosis Foundation)

DOWN SYNDROME

See also *Developmental Problems/Needs.*
See also *Mental Disabilities,* if indicated.

Nursing Diagnoses

Risk for Altered Respiratory Function related to decreased respiratory expansion secondary to decreased muscle tone, inadequate mucus drainage, and mouth breathing

Risk for Impaired Skin Integrity related to rough, dry skin surface, and flaccid extremities

Risk for Constipation related to decreased gastric motility

Risk for Altered Nutrition: More than body requirements related to increased caloric consumption secondary to boredom in the presence of limited physical activity and decreased metabolic rate

(Specify) Self-Care Deficits related to physical limitations

Ineffective Infant Feeding Pattern related to neurological impairment

Risk for Ineffective Management of Therapeutic Regimen related to insufficient knowledge of condition, home care, education, and community services

DYSMENORRHEA

Nursing Diagnoses

Acute Pain related to insufficient knowledge of comfort measures, menstrual physiology, and nutritional management

FAILURE TO THRIVE (Nonorganic)

See also *Developmental Problems/Needs*.

Collaborative Problems

PC: Metabolic dysfunction
PC: Dehydration

Nursing Diagnoses

Altered Nutrition: Less than body requirements related to inadequate intake secondary to lack of emotional and sensory stimulation or lack of knowledge of caregiver

Sensory/Perceptual Alterations related to history of insufficient sensory input from primary caregiver

Sleep Pattern Disturbance related to anxiety and apprehension secondary to parental deprivation

Altered Parenting related to (examples) insufficient knowledge of parenting skills, impaired caregiver, impaired child, lack of support system, lack of role model, relationship problems, unrealistic expectations for child, unmet psychological needs

Impaired Home Maintenance Management related to difficulty of caregiver with maintaining a safe home environment

Risk for Ineffective Management of Therapeutic Regimen related to insufficient knowledge of growth and development requirements, feeding guidelines, risk for child abuse, parenting skills, and community agencies

GLOMERULAR DISORDERS (Glomerulonephritis: Acute, Chronic; Nephrotic Syndrome: Congenital, Secondary, Idiopathic)

See also *Developmental Problems/Needs.*
See also *Corticosteroid Therapy.*

Collaborative Problems

PC: Anasarca (generalized edema)
PC: Hypertension
PC: Azotemia
PC: Sepsis
PC: Malnutrition
PC: Ascites
PC: Pleural effusion
PC: Hypoalbuminemia

Nursing Diagnoses

Risk for Infection related to increased susceptibility during edematous phase and lowered resistance secondary to corticosteroid therapy

Risk for Impaired Skin Integrity related to (examples) immobility, lowered resistance, edema, or frequent application of collection bags

Altered Nutrition: Less than body requirements related to dietary restrictions, anorexia secondary to fatigue, malaise, and pressure on abdominal structures (edema)

Fatigue related to circulatory toxins, fluid, and electrolytic imbalance

Diversional Activity Deficit related to hospitalization and impaired ability to perform usual activities

Risk for Ineffective Management of Therapeutic Regimen related to insufficient knowledge of condition, etiology, course, treatments, signs and symptoms of complications, pharmacological therapy, nutritional/fluid requirements, prevention of infection, home care, follow-up care, and community services

HEMOPHILIA

See also *Developmental Problems/Needs.*

Collaborative Problem

PC: Hemorrhage

Nursing Diagnoses

Pain related to joint swelling and limitations secondary to hemarthrosis

Risk for Impaired Physical Mobility related to joint swelling and limitations secondary to hemarthrosis

Risk for Altered Oral Mucous Membranes related to trauma from coarse food and insufficient dental hygiene

Risk for Ineffective Management of Therapeutic Regimen related to insufficient knowledge of condition, contraindications (*e.g.*, aspirin), genetic transmission, environmental hazards, and emergency treatment to control bleeding

HYDROCEPHALUS

See also *Developmental Problems/Needs Related to Chronic Illness*.

Collaborative Problems

PC: Increased intracranial pressure
PC: Sepsis (postshunt procedure)

Nursing Diagnoses

Risk for Impaired Skin Integrity related to impaired ability to move head secondary to size

Risk for Injury related to inability to support large head and strain on neck

Risk for Altered Nutrition: Less than body requirements related to vomiting secondary to cerebral compression and irritability

Risk for Ineffective Management of Therapeutic Regimen related to insufficient knowledge of condition, home care, signs and symptoms of infection, increased intracranial pressure, and emergency treatment of shunt

INFECTIOUS MONONUCLEOSIS (Adolescent)

Collaborative Problems

PC: Enlarged spleen
PC: Hepatic dysfunction

Nursing Diagnoses

Activity Intolerance related to fatigue secondary to infectious process

Altered Comfort related to sore throat, malaise, and headaches

Risk for Altered Nutrition: Less than body requirements related to sore throat and malaise

Risk for Infection Transmission related to contagious condition

Risk for Ineffective Management of Therapeutic Regimen related to insufficient knowledge of condition, communicable nature, diet therapy, risks of alcohol ingestion (with hepatic dysfunction), signs and symptoms of complications (hepatic, splenic, neurological, hematological), and activity restrictions

LEGG-CALVÉ-PERTHES DISEASE

See also *Developmental Problems/Needs.*

Collaborative Problem

PC: Permanently deformed femoral head

Nursing Diagnoses

Pain related to joint dysfunction

Risk for Impaired Skin Integrity related to immobilization devices (casts, braces)

(Specify) Self-Care Deficits related to pain and immobilization devices

Risk for Ineffective Management of Therapeutic Regimen related to insufficient knowledge of disease, weight-bearing restrictions, application/maintenance of devices, and pain management at home

LEUKEMIA

See also *Chemotherapy.*
See also *Radiation Therapy.*

See also *Cancer (General)*.
See also *Developmental Problems/Needs*.

Collaborative Problems

PC: Hepatosplenomegaly
PC: Increased intracranial edema
PC: Metastasis (brain, lungs, kidneys, gastrointestinal tract, spleen, liver)
PC: Hypermetabolism
PC: Hemorrhage
PC: Dehydration
PC: Myelosuppression
PC: Lymphadenopathy
PC: Central nervous system involvement
PC: Electrolyte imbalance

Nursing Diagnoses

Risk for Infection related to increased susceptibility secondary to leukemic process and side effects of chemotherapy

Risk for Social Isolation related to effects of disease and treatments on appearance and embarrassment

Risk for Injury related to bleeding tendencies secondary to leukemic process and side effects of chemotherapy

Powerlessness related to inability to control situation

Risk for Altered Growth and Development related to impaired ability to achieve developmental tasks secondary to limitations of disease and treatments

Risk for Ineffective Management of Therapeutic Regimen related to insufficient knowledge of disease process, treatment, signs and symptoms of complications, reduction of risk factors, and community resources

MENINGITIS (Bacterial)

See also *Developmental Problems/Needs*.

Collaborative Problems

PC: Peripheral circulatory collapse
PC: Disseminated intravascular coagulation

PC: *Increased intracranial pressure/hydrocephalus*
PC: *Visual/auditory nerve palsies*
PC: *Paresis (hemiparesis, quadriparesis)*
PC: *Subdural effusions*
PC: *Respiratory distress*
PC: *Seizures*
PC: *Fluid/electrolyte imbalances*

Nursing Diagnoses

Risk for Injury related to seizure activity secondary to infectious process

Altered Comfort related to nuchal rigidity, muscle aches, immobility, and increased sensitivity to external stimuli secondary to infectious process

Impaired Physical Mobility related to intravenous infusion, nuchal rigidity, and restraining devices

Risk for Impaired Skin Integrity related to immobility

Risk for Ineffective Management of Therapeutic Regimen related to insufficient knowledge of condition, antibiotic therapy, and diagnostic procedures

MENINGOMYELOCELE

See also *Developmental Problems/Needs.*

Collaborative Problems

PC: *Hydrocephalus/shunt infections*
PC: *Increased intracranial pressure*
PC: *Urinary tract infections*

Nursing Diagnoses

Reflex Incontinence related to sensory–motor dysfunction

Risk for Infection related to vulnerability of meningomyelocele sac

Risk for Impaired Skin Integrity related to sensory–motor impairments and orthopedic appliances

(Specify) Self-Care Deficit related to sensory–motor impairments

Impaired Physical Mobility related to lower limb impairments

Parental Grieving related to birth of infant with defects
Risk for Ineffective Management of Therapeutic Regimen related to insufficient knowledge of condition, home care, orthopedic appliances, self-catheterization, activity program, and community services

MENTAL DISABILITIES

See also *Developmental Problems/Needs*.

Nursing Diagnoses

(Specify) Self-Care Deficit related to sensory–motor deficits
Impaired Communication related to impaired receptive skills or impaired expressive skills
Risk for Social Isolation (family, child) related to fear and embarrassment of child's behavior/appearance
Risk for Ineffective Management of Therapeutic Regimen related to insufficient knowledge of condition, child's potential, home care, and community services

MUSCULAR DYSTROPHY

See also *Developmental Problems/Needs*.

Collaborative Problems

PC: Seizures
PC: Respiratory infections
PC: Metabolic failure

Nursing Diagnoses

Risk for Injury related to inability to control movements
Risk for Altered Nutrition: Less than body requirements related to sucking difficulties (infant) and dysphagia
Ineffective Infant Feeding Pattern related to muscle weakness and impaired coordination
(Specify) Self-Care Deficits related to sensory–motor impairments
Impaired Verbal Communication related to impaired ability to speak words secondary to facial muscle involvement

Risk for Impaired Physical Mobility related to muscle weakness

Risk for Altered Nutrition: More than body requirements related to increased caloric consumption in presence of decreased metabolic needs secondary to limited physical activity

Chronic Sorrow (parental) related to progressive, terminal nature of disease

Impaired Swallowing related to sensory–motor deficits

Risk for Hopelessness related to progressive nature of disease

Risk for Diversional Activity Deficit related to effects of limitations on ability to participate in recreational activities

Risk for Ineffective Management of Therapeutic Regimen related to insufficient knowledge of disease, pharmacological regimen, activity program, education, and community services

OBESITY

See also *Developmental Problems/Needs*.

Nursing Diagnoses

Ineffective Individual Coping related to increased food consumption in response to stressors

Altered Health Maintenance related to the need for exercise program, nutrition counseling, and behavioral modification

Self-Concept Disturbance related to feelings of self-degradation and response of others (peers, family, others) to obesity

Altered Family Processes related to responses to and effects of weight loss therapy on parent–child relationship

Risk for Impaired Social Interaction related to inability to initiate and maintain relationships secondary to feelings of embarrassment and negative responses of others

Risk for Ineffective Management of Therapeutic Regimen related to insufficient knowledge of condition, etiology, course, risks, therapies available, destructive versus constructive eating patterns, and self-help groups

OSTEOMYELITIS

See also *Developmental Problems/Needs.*

Collaborative Problems

PC: Infective emboli
PC: Side effects of antibiotic therapy (hematological, renal, hepatic)

Nursing Diagnoses

Altered Comfort related to swelling, hyperthermia, and infectious process of bone

Diversional Activity Deficit related to impaired mobility and long-term hospitalization

Risk for Altered Nutrition: Less than body requirements related to anorexia secondary to infectious process

Risk for Constipation related to immobility

Risk for Impaired Skin Integrity related to mechanical irritation of cast/splint

Risk for Injury: Pathological fractures related to disease process

Risk for Ineffective Management of Therapeutic Regimen related to insufficient knowledge of condition, wound care, activity restrictions, signs and symptoms of complications, pharmacological therapy, and follow-up care

PARASITIC DISORDERS

See also *Developmental Problems/Needs.*

Nursing Diagnoses

Risk for Altered Nutrition: Less than body requirements related to anorexia, nausea, vomiting, and deprivation of host nutrients by parasites

Impaired Skin Integrity related to pruritus secondary to emergence of parasites (pinworms) onto perianal skin, lytic necrosis, and tissue digestion

Diarrhea related to parasitic irritation to intestinal mucosa

Acute Pain related to parasitic invasion of small intestines

Risk for Infection Transmission related to contagious nature of parasites

559

Risk for Ineffective Management of Therapeutic Regimen related to insufficient knowledge of condition, mode of transmission, and prevention of reinfection

PEDICULOSIS (Hootman, 1993)

Nursing Diagnoses

Risk for Infection related to lesions

Altered Comfort related to pruritus

Risk for Infection Transmission related to insufficient knowledge of modes of transmission, treatment, and prevention

Risk for Ineffective Management of Therapeutic Regimen related to insufficient resources, low prioritization of problem, or repeated infections

POISONING

See also *Dialysis,* if indicated.

See also *Unconscious Individual.*

Collaborative Problems

PC: Respiratory alkalosis

PC: Metabolic acidosis

PC: Hemorrhage

PC: Fluid/electrolyte imbalance

PC: Burns (acid/alkaline)

PC: Aspiration

PC: Blindness

Nursing Diagnoses

Altered Comfort related to heat production secondary to poisoning (*e.g.*, salicylate)

Fear related to invasive nature of treatments (gastric lavage, dialysis)

Anxiety (parental) related to uncertainty of situation and feelings of guilt

Risk for Ineffective Management of Therapeutic Regimen related to insufficient knowledge of condition, treatments, home treatment of accidental poisoning, and poison prevention (storage, teaching, poisonous plants, locks)

RESPIRATORY TRACT INFECTION (Lower)

See also *Developmental Problems/Needs*.
See also *Adult Pneumonia*.

Collaborative Problems

PC: Hyperthermia
PC: Respiratory insufficiency
PC: Septic shock
PC: Paralytic ileus

Nursing Diagnoses

Altered Comfort related to hyperthermia, malaise, and respiratory distress
Risk for Altered Nutrition: Less than body requirements related to anorexia secondary to dyspnea and malaise
Anxiety related to breathlessness and apprehension
Risk for Fluid Volume Deficit related to insufficient intake secondary to dyspnea and malaise
Altered Comfort related to malaise and fever secondary to infectious process
Risk for Ineffective Management of Therapeutic Regimen related to insufficient knowledge of condition, prevention of recurrence, and treatment

RHEUMATIC FEVER

See also *Developmental Problems/Needs*.

Collaborative Problem

PC: Endocarditis

Nursing Diagnoses

Diversional Activity Deficit related to prescribed bed rest
Altered Nutrition: Less than body requirements related to anorexia and malaise
Altered Comfort related to arthralgia
Risk for Injury related to choreic movements
Risk for Noncompliance related to difficulty maintaining preventive drug therapy when illness is resolved

Risk for Ineffective Management of Therapeutic Regimen related to insufficient knowledge of condition, signs and symptoms of complications, long-term antibiotic therapy, prevention of recurrence, and risk factors (surgery, *e.g., dental)*

RHEUMATOID ARTHRITIS (Juvenile)

See also *Developmental Problems/Needs.*
See also *Corticosteroid Therapy.*

Collaborative Problems

PC: Pericarditis
PC: Iridocyclitis

Nursing Diagnoses

Impaired Physical Mobility related to pain and restricted joint movement
Pain related to swollen, inflamed joints and restricted movement
Fatigue related to chronic inflammatory process
Risk for Ineffective Management of Therapeutic Regimen related to insufficient knowledge of condition, pharmacological therapy, exercise program, rest versus activity, myths, and community resources

REYE'S SYNDROME

See also *Unconscious Individual,* if indicated.

Collaborative Problems

PC: Renal failure
PC: Increased intracranial pressure
PC: Fluid/electrolyte imbalance
PC: Hepatic failure
PC: Shock
PC: Seizures
PC: Coma
PC: Respiratory distress
PC: Diabetes insipidus

Nursing Diagnoses

Parental Anxiety related to diagnosis and uncertain prognosis

Risk for Injury related to uncontrolled tonic-clonic movements

Risk for Infection related to invasive monitoring procedures

Altered Comfort related to hyperpyrexia and malaise secondary to disease process

Fear related to separation from family, sensory bombardment (intensive care, treatments), and unfamiliar experiences

Altered Family Process related to critical nature of syndrome, hospitalization of child, and separation of family members

Grieving related to actual, anticipated, or possible death of child

Risk for Impaired Skin Integrity related to immobility

Risk for Ineffective Management of Therapeutic Regimen related to insufficient knowledge of condition, treatment, and complications

SCOLIOSIS

See also *Developmental Problems/Needs*.

Nursing Diagnoses

Impaired Physical Mobility related to restricted movement secondary to braces

Risk for Impaired Skin Integrity related to mechanical irritation of brace

Risk for Noncompliance related to chronicity and complexity of treatment regimen

Risk for Falls related to restricted range of motion

Risk for Ineffective Management of Therapeutic Regimen related to insufficient knowledge of condition, treatment, exercises, environmental hazards, care of appliances, follow-up care, and community services

SICKLE CELL ANEMIA

See also *Developmental Problems/Needs* if the individual is a child.

Collaborative Problems

PC: Sickling crisis of transfusion therapy
PC: Thrombosis and infarction
PC: Cholelithiasis

Nursing Diagnoses

Altered Peripheral Tissue Perfusion related to viscous blood and occlusion of microcirculation
Pain related to viscous blood and tissue hypoxia
(Specify) Self-Care Deficit related to pain and immobility of exacerbations
Risk for Ineffective Management of Therapeutic Regimen related to insufficient knowledge of hazards, signs and symptoms of complications, fluid requirements, and hereditary factors

TONSILLITIS

See also *Tonsillectomy,* if indicated.

Collaborative Problems

PC: Otitis media
PC: Rheumatic fever (β-hemolytic streptococci)

Nursing Diagnoses

Risk for Fluid Volume Deficit related to inadequate fluid intake secondary to pain
Risk for Ineffective Management of Therapeutic Regimen related to insufficient knowledge of condition, treatments, nutritional/fluid requirements, and signs and symptoms of complications

WILMS' TUMOR

See also *Developmental Problems/Needs.*
See also *Nephrectomy.*
See also *Cancer (General).*

Collaborative Problems

PC: Metastases to liver, lung, bone, brain
PC: Sepsis
PC: Tumor rupture

Nursing Diagnoses

Anxiety related to (examples) age-related concerns (separation, strangers, pain), response of others to visible signs (alopecia), and uncertain future

Parental Anxiety related to (examples) unknown prognosis, painful procedures, treatments (chemotherapy), and feelings of inadequacy

Grieving related to actual, anticipated, or possible death of child

Spiritual Distress related to nature of disease and its possible disturbances on belief systems

Risk for Ineffective Management of Therapeutic Regimen related to insufficient knowledge of condition, prognosis, treatments (side effects), home care, nutritional requirements, follow-up care, and community services

Mental Health Disorders

AFFECTIVE DISORDERS (Depression)

Nursing Diagnoses

Dressing/Grooming Self-Care Deficit related to decreased interest in body, inability to make decisions, and feelings of worthlessness

Ineffective Individual Coping related to internal conflicts (guilt, low self-esteem) or feelings of rejection

Social Isolation related to inability to initiate activities to reduce isolation secondary to low energy levels

Dysfunctional Grieving related to unresolved grief, prolonged denial, and repression

Chronic Low Self-Esteem related to feelings of worthlessness and failure secondary to (specify)

Ineffective Family Coping related to marital discord and role conflicts secondary to effects of chronic depression

Powerlessness related to unrealistic negative beliefs about self-worth or abilities

Altered Thought Processes related to negative cognitive set (overgeneralizing, polarized thinking, selected abstraction, arbitrary inference)

Altered Sexuality Patterns related to decreased sex drive, loss of interest and pleasure

Diversional Activity Deficit related to a loss of interest or pleasure in usual activities and low energy levels

Impaired Home Maintenance Management related to inability to make decisions or concentrate

Risk for Self-Harm related to feelings of hopelessness and loneliness

Sleep Pattern Disturbance related to difficulty falling asleep or early morning awakening secondary to emotional stress

Constipation related to sedentary lifestyle, insufficient exercise, or inadequate diet

Risk for Altered Nutrition: More than body requirements related to increased intake versus decreased activity expenditures secondary to boredom and frustrations

Risk for Altered Nutrition: Less than body requirements related to anorexia secondary to emotional stress

Risk for Ineffective Management of Therapeutic Regimen related to insufficient knowledge of condition, behavior modification, therapy options (pharmacological, electroshock), and community resources

ANOREXIA NERVOSA

Collaborative Problems

PC: Anemia
PC: Hypotension
PC: Dysrhythmias
PC: Amenorrhea

Nursing Diagnoses

Altered Nutrition: Less than body requirements related to exercise in excess of caloric intake, refusal to eat, self-induced vomiting following eating, or laxative abuse

Self-Concept Disturbance related to inaccurate perception of self as obese

Risk for Fluid Volume Deficit related to vomiting and excessive weight loss

Sleep Pattern Disturbance related to fears and anxiety concerning weight status

Activity Intolerance related to fatigue secondary to malnutrition

Ineffective Individual Coping related to self-induced vomiting, denial of hunger, and insufficient food intake secondary to feelings of loss of control and inaccurate perceptions of body states

Ineffective Family Coping related to marital discord and its effect on family members

Constipation related to insufficient food and fluid intake

Impaired Social Interactions related to inability to form relationships with others or fear of trusting relationships with others

Fear related to implications of a maturing body and dissatisfaction with relationships with others

ANXIETY AND ADJUSTMENT DISORDERS

(Phobias, Anxiety States, Traumatic Stress Disorders, Adjustment Reactions)

See also *Substance Abuse Disorders,* if indicated.

Nursing Diagnoses

Impaired Social Interactions related to effects of behavior and actions on forming and maintaining relationships

Anxiety related to irrational thoughts or guilt

Ineffective Individual Coping related to inadequate psychological resources to adapt to a traumatic event

Sleep Pattern Disturbance related to recurrent nightmares

Ineffective Individual Coping related to altered ability to manage stressors constructively secondary to (examples) physical illness, marital discord, business crisis, natural disasters, or developmental crisis

Risk for Ineffective Management of Therapeutic Regimen related to insufficient knowledge of condition, pharmacological therapy, and legal system regarding violence

BIPOLAR DISORDER (Mania)

Nursing Diagnoses

Defensive Coping related to exaggerated sense of self-importance and abilities secondary to feelings of inadequacy and inferiority

Impaired Social Interaction related to overt hostility, overconfidence, or manipulation of others

Risk for Violence: Directed at others related to impaired reality testing, impaired judgment, or inability to control behavior

Sleep Pattern Disturbance related to hyperactivity

Altered Thought Processes related to flight of ideas, delusions, or hallucinations

Impaired Verbal Communication related to pressured speech and hyperactivity

Risk for Fluid Volume Deficit related to altered sodium excretion secondary to lithium therapy

Noncompliance related to feelings of no longer requiring medication

Risk for Ineffective Management of Therapeutic Regimen related to insufficient knowledge of condition, pharmacological therapy, and follow-up care

CHILDHOOD BEHAVIORAL DISORDERS
(Attention Deficit Disorders, Learning Disabilities)

Nursing Diagnoses

Impaired Social Interactions related to inattention, impulsivity, or hyperactivity

Chronic Sorrow (parental) related to anticipated losses secondary to condition

Altered Family Process related to adjustment requirements for situation: (examples) time, energy, money, physical care, and prognosis

Risk for Violence related to history of aggressive acts and (specify)

Risk for Impaired Home Maintenance Management related to inadequate resources, inadequate housing, or impaired caregivers

Risk for Social Isolation (child, family) related to disability and requirements for caregivers

Risk for Altered Parenting related to inadequate resources or inadequate coping mechanisms

Self-Concept Disturbance related to effects of limitations on achievement of developmental tasks

OBSESSIVE-COMPULSIVE DISORDER

Nursing Diagnoses

(Specify) Self-Care Deficit related to ritualistic obsessions interfering with performance of activities of daily living

Noncompliance related to poor concentration and poor impulse control secondary to obsessive thought patterns

Social Isolation related to fear of vulnerability associated with need for closeness and embarrassment about ritualistic behavior

Anxiety related to the perceived threat of actual or anticipated events

PARANOID DISORDERS

Nursing Diagnoses

Impaired Social Interactions related to feelings of mistrust and suspicions of others

Ineffective Denial related to inability to accept own feelings and responsibility for actions secondary to low self-esteem

Risk for Altered Nutrition: Less than body requirements related to reluctance to eat secondary to fear of poisoning

Altered Thought Processes related to inability to evaluate reality secondary to feelings of mistrust

Social Isolation related to fear and mistrust of situations and others

PERSONALITY DISORDERS

Examples:

Schizoid
Antisocial
Borderline
Narcissistic
Avoidant
Compulsive

Histrionic
Passive-aggressive
Paranoid
Schizotypal
Dependent

Nursing Diagnoses

Ineffective Individual Coping: related to subordinating one's needs to decisions of others

Ineffective Individual Coping:
    Inappropriate intense anger
    Poor impulse control
    Marked mood shifts
    Habitual disregard for social norms related to altered ability to meet responsibilities (role, social) secondary to (specify)

Impaired Social Interaction related to inability to maintain enduring attachments secondary to (specify)

Ineffective Individual Coping related to resistance (procrastination, stubbornness, intentional inefficiency) in responses to responsibilities (role, social)

SCHIZOPHRENIC DISORDERS

Nursing Diagnoses

Risk for Violence: Self-directed or directed at others related to responding to delusional thoughts or hallucinations

Impaired Verbal Communication related to incoherent/illogical speech pattern and side effects of medications

Impaired Social Interactions related to preoccupation with egocentric and illogical ideas and extreme suspiciousness

Impaired Home Maintenance Management related to impaired judgment, inability to self-initiate activity, and loss of skills over long course of illness

SOMATOFORM DISORDERS (Somatization, Hypochondriasis, Conversion Reactions)

See also *Affective Disorders,* if indicated.

Nursing Diagnoses

Impaired Social Interaction related to effects of multiple somatic complaints and complaining on relationships

Ineffective Individual Coping related to unrealistic fear of having a disease despite reassurance to contrary

Ineffective Individual Coping: Depression related to belief of not getting proper care or sufficient response from others for complaints

Ineffective Family Coping related to chronicity of illness

Noncompliance related to impaired judgments and thought disturbances

Dressing/Grooming Self-Care Deficit related to loss of skills and lack of interest in body and appearance

Diversional Activity Deficit related to apathy, inability to initiate goal-directed activities, and loss of skills

Self-Concept Disturbance related to feelings of worthlessness and lack of ego boundaries

Risk for Ineffective Management of Therapeutic Regimen related to insufficient knowledge of condition, pharmacological therapy, tardive dyskinesia, occupational skills, and follow-up care

SUBSTANCE ABUSE DISORDERS

Collaborative Problems

PC: Delirium tremens
PC: Autonomic hyperactivity
PC: Seizures
PC: Alcohol hallucinosis
PC: Hypertension (alcohol, opiates, heroin)
PC: Sepsis (intravenous drug use)

Nursing Diagnoses

Altered Nutrition: Less than body requirements related to anorexia

Risk for Fluid Volume Deficit related to abnormal fluid loss secondary to vomiting and diarrhea

Risk for Injury related to disorientation, tremors, or impaired judgment

Risk for Self-Harm related to disorientation, tremors, or impaired judgment

Risk for Violence related to (examples) impulsive behavior, disorientation, tremors, or impaired judgment

Sleep Pattern Disturbances related to irritability, tremors, and nightmares

Anxiety related to loss of control, memory losses, and fear of withdrawal

Ineffective Individual Coping: Anger, dependence, or denial related to inability to manage stressors constructively without drugs/alcohol

Self-Concept Disturbance related to guilt, mistrust, or ambivalence

Impaired Social Interaction related to (examples) emotional immaturity, irritability, high anxiety, impulsive behavior, or aggressive responses

Social Isolation related to loss of work or withdrawal from others

Altered Sexuality Patterns related to impotence/loss of libido secondary to altered self-concept and substance abuse

Ineffective Family Coping related to disruption in marital dyad and inconsistent limit setting

Risk for Ineffective Management of Therapeutic Regimen related to insufficient knowledge of condition, treatments available, high-risk situations, and community resources

Diagnostic and Therapeutic Procedures

ANGIOPLASTY (Percutaneous, Transluminal, Coronary, Peripheral)

Preprocedure Period

Nursing Diagnoses

▲ Anxiety/Fear (individual, family) related to health status, angioplasty procedure, routines, outcome, and possible need for cardiac surgery

▲ This diagnosis was reported to be monitored for or managed frequently (75%–100%).

Postprocedure Period

Collaborative Problems

▲ PC: Dysrhythmias
▲ PC: Acute coronary occlusion *(clot, spasm, collapse)*
▲ PC: Myocardial infarction
▲ PC: Arterial dissection or rupture
▲ PC: Hemorrhage/hematoma at angioplasty site
* PC: Paresthesia distal to site
* PC: Arterial thrombosis
* PC: Embolization *(peripheral)*

Nursing Diagnoses

▲ Impaired Physical Mobility related to prescribed bed rest and restricted movement of involved extremity
▲ Risk for Ineffective Management of Therapeutic Regimen related to insufficient knowledge of care of insertion site, discharge activities, diet, medications, signs and symptoms of complications, exercises, and follow-up care

ANTICOAGULANT THERAPY

Collaborative Problem

▲ PC: Hemorrhage

Nursing Diagnoses

△ Risk for Ineffective Management of Therapeutic Regimen related to insufficient knowledge of administration schedule, identification card/band, contraindications, and signs and symptoms of bleeding

---

▲ This diagnosis was reported to be monitored for or managed frequently (75%–100%).
△ This diagnosis was reported to be monitored for or managed often (50%–74%).
* This diagnosis was not included in the validation study.

ARTERIOGRAM

Preprocedure Period

Nursing Diagnoses

△ Fear related to potential negative findings of arteriogram and insufficient knowledge of routines and expected sensations

Postprocedure Period

Collaborative Problems

▲ *PC: Hematoma*
▲ *PC: Hemorrhage*
* *PC: Stroke*
▲ *PC: Thrombosis (arterial site)*
△ *PC: Urinary retention*
△ *PC: Renal failure*
▲ *PC: Paresthesia*
▲ *PC: Embolism*
▲ *PC: Allergic reaction*

Nursing Diagnoses

▲ Risk for Ineffective Management of Therapeutic Regimen related to insufficient knowledge of activity restrictions and signs and symptoms of complications

CARDIAC CATHETERIZATION

Postprocedure Period

Collaborative Problems

▲ *PC: Systemic (allergic reaction)*
▲ *PC: Cardiac (dysrhythmias, myocardial infarction, pulmonary edema)*
* *PC: CVA*

▲ This diagnosis was reported to be monitored for or managed frequently (75%–100%).
△ This diagnosis was reported to be monitored for or managed often (50%–74%).
* This diagnosis was not included in the validation study.

▲ *PC: Circulatory (hematoma formation or hemorrhage at entry site, hypovolemia, thromboembolic phenomenon)*

Nursing Diagnoses

* Altered Comfort related to tissue trauma and pre-scribed postprocedure immobilization

△ Risk for Ineffective Management of Therapeutic Regimen related to insufficient knowledge of site care, signs and symptoms of complications, and follow-up care

CASTS

Collaborative Problems

* *PC: Pressure (edema, mechanical)*

▲ *PC: Compartmental syndrome*

* *PC: Ulcer formation*

▲ *PC: Infection*

Nursing Diagnoses

* Risk for Injury related to hazards of crutch-walking and impaired mobility secondary to cast

▲ Risk for Impaired Skin Integrity related to pressure of cast on skin surface

△ Risk for Impaired Home Maintenance Management related to the restrictions imposed by cast on performing activities of daily living and role responsibilities

▲ (Specify) Self-Care Deficits related to limitation of movement secondary to cast

* Risk for Altered Respiratory Function related to imposed immobility or restricted respiratory movement secondary to cast (body)

* Diversional Activity Deficit related to boredom and inability to perform usual recreational activities

---

▲ This diagnosis was reported to be monitored for or managed frequently (75%–100%).

△ This diagnosis was reported to be monitored for or managed often (50%–74%).

* This diagnosis was not included in the validation study.

▲ Risk for Ineffective Management of Therapeutic Regimen related to insufficient knowledge of cast care, signs and symptoms of complications, use of assistive devices, and hazards

CESIUM IMPLANT

Postprocedure Period

Collaborative Problems

▲ *PC: Bleeding*
▲ *PC: Infection*
△ *PC: Pulmonary complications*
  PC: Vaginal stenosis
▲ *PC: Radiation cystitis*
▲ *PC: Displacement of radioactive source*
△ *PC: Thrombophlebitis*
▲ *PC: Bowel dysfunction*

Nursing Diagnoses

▲ Anxiety related to fear of radiation and its effects, uncertainty of outcome, feelings of isolation, and pain or discomfort
▲ Bathing/Hygiene, Toileting Self-Care Deficit related to activity restrictions and isolation
▲ Risk for Impaired Skin Integrity related to immobility secondary to prescribed activity restrictions
▲ Social Isolation related to restrictions necessitated by cesium implant safety precautions
△ Risk for Ineffective Management of Therapeutic Regimen related to insufficient knowledge of home care, reportable signs and symptoms, activity restrictions, and follow-up care

CHEMOTHERAPY

See also *Cancer (General)*.

▲ This diagnosis was reported to be monitored for or managed frequently (75%–100%).
△ This diagnosis was reported to be monitored for or managed often (50%–74%).

Collaborative Problems

* PC: *Necrosis/phlebitis at intravenous site*
* PC: *Thrombocytopenia*
* PC: *Anemia*
* PC: *Leukopenia*
△ PC: *Peripheral nerve toxicosis*
▲ PC: *Anaphylactic reaction*
△ PC: *Central nervous system toxicity*
△ PC: *Congestive heart failure*
▲ PC: *Electrolyte imbalance*
▲ PC: *Extravasation of vesicant drugs*
△ PC: *Hemorrhagic cystitis*
▲ PC: *Myelosuppression*
▲ PC: *Renal insufficiency*

Nursing Diagnoses

* Risk for Fluid Volume Deficit related to gastrointestinal fluid losses secondary to vomiting
* Risk for Infection related to altered immune system secondary to effects of cytotoxic agents or disease process
* Risk for Altered Family Processes related to interruptions imposed by treatment and schedule on patterns of living
* Risk for Altered Sexuality Patterns related to amenorrhea and sterility (temporary/permanent) secondary to effects of chemotherapy on testes/ovaries
* Risk for Injury related to bleeding tendencies
▲ Anxiety related to prescribed chemotherapy, insufficient knowledge of chemotherapy, and self-care measures
▲ Fatigue related to effects of anemia, malnutrition, persistent vomiting, and sleep pattern disturbance
△ Risk for Constipation related to autonomic nerve dysfunction secondary to vinca alkaloid administration and inactivity
▲ Diarrhea related to intestinal cell damage, inflammation, and increased intestinal mobility

▲ This diagnosis was reported to be monitored for or managed frequently (75%–100%).
△ This diagnosis was reported to be monitored for or managed often (50%–74%).
* This diagnosis was not included in the validation study.

▲ Altered Comfort related to gastrointestinal cell damage, stimulation of vomiting center, fear, and anxiety
▲ Risk for Impaired Skin Integrity related to persistent diarrhea, malnutrition, prolonged sedation, and fatigue
▲ Altered Nutrition: Less than body requirements related to anorexia, taste changes, persistent nausea/vomiting, and increased metabolic rate
▲ Altered Oral Mucous Membrane related to dryness and epithelial cell damage secondary to chemotherapy
△ Self-Concept Disturbance related to change in lifestyle, role, alopecia, and weight loss or gain

CORTICOSTEROID THERAPY

Collaborative Problems

△ *PC: Peptic ulcer*
* *PC: Pseudotumor cerebri*
▲ *PC: Steroid-induced diabetes*
△ *PC: Osteoporosis*
△ *PC: Hypertension*
△ *PC: Hypokalemia*

Nursing Diagnoses

▲ Risk for Fluid Volume Excess related to sodium and water retention
▲ Risk for Infection related to immunosuppression
△ Risk for Altered Nutrition: More than body requirements related to increased appetite
△ Risk for Situational Low Self-Esteem related to appearance changes (*e.g.*, abnormal fat distribution, increased production of androgens)
△ Risk for Ineffective Management of Therapeutic Regimen related to insufficient knowledge of administration schedule, adverse reactions, signs and symptoms of complications, hazards of adrenal insufficiency, and potential causes of adrenal insufficiency

---

▲ This diagnosis was reported to be monitored for or managed frequently (75%–100%).
△ This diagnosis was reported to be monitored for or managed often (50%–74%).
* This diagnosis was not included in the validation study.

ELECTROCONVULSIVE THERAPY (ECT)

Postprocedure Period

Collaborative Problems

PC: Hypertension
PC: Dysrhythmias

Nursing Diagnoses

Risk for Injury related to uncontrolled tonic-clonic movements and disorientation, confusion post-treatment

Altered Comfort: Headaches, muscle aches, nausea related to seizure activity and tissue trauma secondary to electrical current

Risk for Aspiration related to post-ECT somnolence

Anxiety related to memory losses and disorientation secondary to effects of ECT on cerebral function

ELECTRONIC FETAL MONITORING (Internal)

See also *Intrapartum Period (General)*.

Postinsertion

Collaborative Problems

PC: Fetal scalp laceration
PC: Perforated uterus

Nursing Diagnosis

Impaired Physical Mobility related to restrictions secondary to monitor cords

ENTERAL NUTRITION

Collaborative Problems

▲ *PC: Hypoglycemia/hyperglycemia*
▲ *PC: Hypervolemia*

▲ This diagnosis was reported to be monitored for or managed frequently (75%–100%).

△ PC: *Hypertonic dehydration*
▲ PC: *Electrolyte and trace mineral imbalances*
△ PC: *Mucosal erosion*

Nursing Diagnoses

▲ Risk for Infection related to gastrostomy incision and enzymatic action of gastric juices on skin
▲ Altered Comfort: Cramping, distention, nausea, vomiting related to type of formula, administration rate, temperature, or route
▲ Diarrhea related to adverse response to formula, rate, or temperature
▲ Risk for Aspiration related to position of tube and of individual
△ Risk for Ineffective Management of Therapeutic Regimen related to insufficient knowledge of nutritional indications/requirements, home care, and signs and symptoms of complications

EXTERNAL ARTERIOVENOUS SHUNTING

Collaborative Problems

▲ PC: *Thrombosis*
▲ PC: *Bleeding*

Nursing Diagnoses

▲ Risk for Ineffective Management of Therapeutic Regimen related to insufficient knowledge of catheter care, precautions, emergency measures, prevention of infection, and activity limitations

HEMODIALYSIS

See also *Chronic Renal Failure.*

▲ This diagnosis was reported to be monitored for or managed frequently (75%–100%).
△ This diagnosis was reported to be monitored for or managed often (50%–74%).

Collaborative Problems

▲ *PC: Fluid imbalances*
▲ *PC: Electrolyte imbalance (potassium, sodium)*
▲ *PC: Nausea/vomiting*
△ *PC: Transfusion reaction*
* *PC: Aneurysm*
▲ *PC: Hemorrhage*
* *PC: Disruption of vascular access*
△ *PC: Dialysate leakage*
▲ *PC: Clotting*
* *PC: Infection*
* *PC: Hepatitis B*
* *PC: Fever/chills*
* *PC: Hemolysis*
△ *PC: Seizures*
▲ *PC: Hypertension/hypotension*
△ *PC: Dialysis disequilibrium syndrome*
▲ *PC: Air embolism*
▲ *PC: Sepsis*
△ *PC: Hyperthermia*

Nursing Diagnoses

* Risk for Injury to (vascular) access site related to vulnerability
* Risk for Infection related to direct access to bloodstream secondary to vascular access
△ Powerlessness related to need for treatments to live despite effects on lifestyle
△ Altered Family Processes related to the interruptions of role responsibilities caused by the treatment schedule
▲ Risk for Infection Transmission related to frequent contacts with blood and high risk for hepatitis B
* Risk for Ineffective Management of Therapeutic Regimen related to insufficient knowledge of rationale of treatment, care of site, precautions, emergency

▲ This diagnosis was reported to be monitored for or managed frequently (75%–100%).
△ This diagnosis was reported to be monitored for or managed often (50%–74%).
* This diagnosis was not included in the validation study.

treatments (disconnected, bleeding, clotting), pre-treatment instructions, and daily assessments (bruit, blood pressure, weights)

HEMODYNAMIC MONITORING

See also *Medical Conditions* for the specific medical diagnosis.

Collaborative Problems

* * *PC: Sepsis*
* ▲ *PC: Hemorrhage*
* * *PC: Bleeding back*
* * *PC: Vasospasm*
* * *PC: Tissue ischemia/hypoxia*
* ▲ *PC: Thrombosis/thrombophlebitis*
* ▲ *PC: Pulmonary embolism, air embolism*
* △ *PC: Arterial spasm*

Nursing Diagnoses

* ▲ Risk for Infection related to invasive lines
* △ Impaired Physical Mobility related to position restrictions secondary to hemodynamic monitoring
* △ Anxiety related to impending procedure, loss of control, and unpredictable outcome
* * Risk for Ineffective Management of Therapeutic Regimen related to insufficient knowledge of purpose, procedure, and associated care

HICKMAN CATHETER

Collaborative Problems

PC: Air embolism
PC: Bleeding
PC: Thrombosis

▲ This diagnosis was reported to be monitored for or managed frequently (75%–100%).
△ This diagnosis was reported to be monitored for or managed often (50%–74%).
* This diagnosis was not included in the validation study.

Nursing Diagnoses

> Risk for Infection related to direct access to bloodstream
> Risk for Impaired Home Maintenance Management related to lack of knowledge of catheter management

LONG-TERM VENOUS CATHETER

Collaborative Problems

△ PC: Pneumothorax
▲ PC: Hemorrhage
△ PC: Embolism/thrombosis
▲ PC: Sepsis

Nursing Diagnoses

▲ Anxiety related to upcoming insertion of catheter and insufficient knowledge of procedure
▲ Risk for Infection related to catheter's direct access to bloodstream
△ Risk for Ineffective Management of Therapeutic Regimen related to insufficient knowledge of home care, signs and symptoms of complications, and community resources

INTRA-AORTIC BALLOON PUMPING

Intraprocedure/Postprocedure Period

Collaborative Problems

> PC: Arterial insufficiency/thrombosis
> PC: Sepsis/infection
> PC: Peripheral neuropathy/claudication
> PC: Thrombocytopenia
> PC: Bleeding
> PC: Emboli
> PC: Gastrointestinal bleeding
> PC: Disseminated intravascular coagulation
> PC: Dysrhythmias

▲ This diagnosis was reported to be monitored for or managed frequently (75%–100%).
△ This diagnosis was reported to be monitored for or managed often (50%–74%).

Nursing Diagnoses

Impaired Physical Mobility related to prescribed immobility and restricted movement of involved extremity

Risk for Infection related to direct access to bloodstream

Risk for Constipation related to immobility and restricted movement of involved limb

Fear related to treatments, environment, and risk of death

Altered Family Processes related to the critical nature of situation and uncertain prognosis

MECHANICAL VENTILATION

See also *Tracheostomy.*

Collaborative Problems

* * *PC: Acidosis/alkalosis*
* * *PC: Airway obstruction/atelectasis*
* * *PC: Tracheal necrosis*
* * *PC: Infection*
* △ *PC: Gastrointestinal bleeding*
* * *PC: Tension pneumothorax*
* △ *PC: Oxygen toxicity*
* ▲ *PC: Respiratory insufficiency*
* ▲ *PC: Atelectasis*
* △ *PC: Decreased cardiac output*

Nursing Diagnoses

* ▲ Impaired Verbal Communication related to effects of intubation on ability to speak
* △ Disuse Syndrome
* ▲ Risk for Infection related to disruption of skin layer secondary to tracheostomy

  Altered Family Processes related to critical nature of situation and uncertain prognosis

---

▲ This diagnosis was reported to be monitored for or managed frequently (75%–100%).

△ This diagnosis was reported to be monitored for or managed often (50%–74%).

* This diagnosis was not included in the validation study.

△ Fear related to the nature of the situation, uncertain prognosis of ventilator dependence, or weaning

* Risk for Sensory/Perceptual Alterations related to excessive environmental stimuli and decreased input of meaningful stimuli secondary to treatment and critical care unit

▲ Risk for Ineffective Airway Clearance related to increased secretions secondary to tracheostomy, obstruction of inner cannula, or displacement of tracheostomy tube

△ Powerlessness related to dependency on respirator, inability to talk, and loss of mobility

△ Risk for Dysfunctional Ventilatory Weaning Response related to unsatisfactory weaning attempts, respiratory muscle fatigue secondary to mechanical ventilation, increased work of breathing, supine position, protein-calorie malnutrition, inactivity, and/or fatigue

* Risk for Self-Concept Disturbance related to mechanical ventilation, dependence on achieving developmental tasks, and lifestyle changes

PACEMAKER INSERTION

Postprocedure Period

Collaborative Problems

▲ *PC: Cardiac*
▲ *PC: Pacemaker malfunction*
△ *PC: Rejection of unit*
△ *PC: Necrosis over pulse generator*
* *PC: Site (hemorrhage)*

Nursing Diagnoses

* Altered Comfort related to pain at insertion site and prescribed postprocedure immobilization

△ Self-Concept Disturbance related to perceived loss of health and dependence on pacemaker

▲ This diagnosis was reported to be monitored for or managed frequently (75%–100%).
△ This diagnosis was reported to be monitored for or managed often (50%–74%).
* This diagnosis was not included in the validation study.

△ Impaired Physical Mobility related to incisional site pain, activity restrictions, and fear of lead displacements

* Risk for Infection related to operative site

△ Risk for Ineffective Management of Therapeutic Regimen related to insufficient knowledge of activity restrictions, precautions, signs and symptoms of complications, electromagnetic interference (microwave ovens, arc welding equipment, gasoline engines, electric motors, antitheft devices, power transmitters), pacemaker function (daily pulse taking, signs of impending battery failure), activity restrictions, and follow-up care

PERITONEAL DIALYSIS

Collaborative Problems

* PC: Fluid imbalances
▲ PC: Electrolyte imbalances
△ PC: Hemorrhage
* PC: Negative nitrogen balance
△ PC: Bowel/bladder perforation
△ PC: Hyperglycemia
* PC: Peritonitis
▲ PC: Hypovolemia/hypervolemia
▲ PC: Uremia

Nursing Diagnoses

▲ Risk for Infection related to access to peritoneal cavity, catheter exit site, and use of high-dextrose concentration in dialysis solution

* Risk for Injury to catheter site related to vulnerability

△ Risk for Ineffective Breathing Pattern related to immobility, pressure, and pain

△ Altered Comfort related to catheter insertion, instillation of dialysis solution, outflow, suction, and chemical irritation of peritoneum

---

▲ This diagnosis was reported to be monitored for or managed frequently (75%–100%).
△ This diagnosis was reported to be monitored for or managed often (50%–74%).
* This diagnosis was not included in the validation study.

△ Altered Nutrition: Less than body requirements related to anorexia
* Risk for Fluid Volume Excess related to fluid retention secondary to catheter problems (kinks, blockages) or position
△ Risk for Altered Family Processes related to the effects of interruptions of the treatment schedule on role responsibilities
△ Powerlessness related to chronic illness and the need for continuous treatment
* Impaired Home Maintenance Management related to insufficient knowledge of treatment procedure
△ Risk for Ineffective Management of Therapeutic Regimen related to insufficient knowledge of rationale for treatment, medications, home dialysis procedure, signs and symptoms of complications, community resources, and follow-up care

RADIATION THERAPY (External)

Postprocedure Period

Collaborative Problems

* *PC: Increased intracranial pressure*
▲ *PC: Myelosuppression*
△ *PC: Fluid/electrolyte imbalances*
△ *PC: Inflammation*

Nursing Diagnoses

▲ Anxiety related to prescribed radiation therapy and insufficient knowledge of treatments and self-care measures
△ Altered Comfort related to stimulation of the vomiting center and damage to the gastrointestinal mucosal cells secondary to radiation
▲ Fatigue related to systemic effects of radiation therapy
Altered Comfort related to damage to sebaceous and sweat glands secondary to radiation

---

▲ This diagnosis was reported to be monitored for or managed frequently (75%–100%).
△ This diagnosis was reported to be monitored for or managed often (50%–74%).
* This diagnosis was not included in the validation study.

△ Risk for Altered Oral Mucous Membrane related to dry mouth or inadequate oral hygiene
▲ Impaired Skin Integrity related to effects of radiation on epithelial and basal cells and effects of diarrhea on perineal area
▲ Altered Nutrition: Less than body requirements related to decreased oral intake, reduced salivation, mouth discomfort, dysphasia, nausea/vomiting, and increased metabolic rate
△ Self-Concept Disturbance related to alopecia, skin changes, weight loss, sterility, and changes in role, relationships, and lifestyle
△ Grieving related to changes in lifestyle, role, finances, functional capacity, body image, and health losses
△ Altered Family Processes related to imposed changes in family roles, relationships, and responsibilities
* Diarrhea related to increased peristalsis secondary to irradiation of abdomen/lower back
* Risk for Infection related to moist skin reaction
* Activity Intolerance related to fatigue secondary to treatments or transportation
* Risk for Ineffective Management of Therapeutic Regimen related to insufficient knowledge of skin care and signs of complications

TOTAL PARENTERAL NUTRITION
(Hyperalimentation Therapy)

Collaborative Problems

▲ *PC: Sepsis*
▲ *PC: Hyperglycemia*
△ *PC: Air embolism*
* *PC: Osmotic diuresis*
* *PC: Perforation*
△ *PC: Pneumothorax, hydrothorax, hemothorax*

▲ This diagnosis was reported to be monitored for or managed frequently (75%–100%).
△ This diagnosis was reported to be monitored for or managed often (50%–74%).
* This diagnosis was not included in the validation study.

Nursing Diagnoses

▲ Risk for Infection related to catheter's direct access to bloodstream

* Risk for Impaired Skin Integrity related to continuous skin surface irritation secondary to catheter and adhesive

* Risk for Altered Oral Mucous Membrane related to inability to ingest food/fluid

△ Risk for Ineffective Management of Therapeutic Regimen related to insufficient knowledge of home care, signs and symptoms of complications, catheter care, and follow-up care (laboratory studies)

TRACHEOSTOMY

Postoperative Period

Collaborative Problems

▲ *PC: Hypoxemia*
▲ *PC: Hemorrhage*
▲ *PC: Tracheal edema*

Nursing Diagnoses

▲ Risk for Ineffective Airway Clearance related to increased secretions secondary to tracheostomy, obstruction of inner cannula, or displacement of tracheostomy tube

▲ Risk for Infection related to excessive pooling of secretions and bypassing of upper respiratory defenses

▲ Impaired Verbal Communications related to inability to produce speech secondary to tracheostomy

Risk for Altered Sexuality Patterns related to change in appearance, fear of rejection

▲ Risk for Ineffective Management of Therapeutic Regimen related to insufficient knowledge of tracheostomy care, precautions, signs and symptoms of complications, emergency care, and follow-up care

---

▲ This diagnosis was reported to be monitored for or managed frequently (75%–100%).
△ This diagnosis was reported to be monitored for or managed often (50%–74%).
* This diagnosis was not included in the validation study.

TRACTION

See also *Fractures.*

Collaborative Problems

PC: Thrombophlebitis
PC: Renal calculi
PC: Urinary tract infection
PC: Neurovascular compromise

Nursing Diagnoses

Risk for Impaired Skin Integrity related to imposed immobility

Risk for Infection related to susceptibility to microorganism secondary to skeletal traction pins

Risk for Constipation related to decreased peristalsis secondary to immobility and analgesics

Risk for Altered Respiratory Function related to imposed immobility and pooling of respiratory secretions

References/Bibliography

Acute Pain Management Guideline Panel (1992). *Acute pain management in infants, children, and adolescents: Operative and medical procedures.* Quick Reference Guide for Clinicians. AHCRP Pub No. 92-0020. Rockville, Maryland: Agency for Health Care Policy and Research, Public Health Service, U.S. Department of Health and Human Services.

American Psychiatric Association (1994). *Diagnostic and statistical manual of mental disorders (4th ed.).* Washington, DC: Author.

Anetzberger, G. J. (1987). *The etiology of elder abuse by adult offsprings.* Springfield, IL: Charles C. Thomas.

Archer, S. E. (1983). Marketing public health nursing services. *Nursing Outlook*, *31*(6), 49–53.

Bandura, A. (1982). Self-efficacy mechanism in human agency. *American Psychology*, *37*(3), 122–147.

Blackburn, S. (1993). Assessment and management of neurologic dysfunction. In C. Kenner, A. Brueggemeyer, & L. Gunderson (Eds.), *Comprehensive neonatal nursing.* Philadelphia: W.B. Saunders.

Blackburn, S., & Vandenberg, K. (1993). Assessment and management of neonatal neurobehavioral development. In C. Kenner, A. Brueggemeyer, & L. Gunderson (Eds.), *Comprehensive neonatal nursing.* Philadelphia: W.B. Saunders.

Blair, K. (1986). The battered woman: Is she a silent partner? *Nurse Practitioner*, *11*(6), 38.

Boyd, M. A., & Nihart, M. A. (1998). *Psychiatric nursing: Contemporary practice.* Philadelphia: Lippincott Williams & Wilkins.

Bozzette, M. (1993). Observations of pain behavior in the NICU: An exploratory study. *Journal of Perinatal and Neonatal Nursing*, *7*(1), 76–87.

Brandt, P., Groth, G., Harman, E., Phillips, C., & Dunbar Jacob, J. (1997). Noncompliance. In M. Rantz & P. LeMone (Eds.), *Classification of nursing diagnosis.* Proceedings of the Twelfth Conference of North American Nursing Diagnosis Association. Glendale, CA: CINALI.

Breslin, E. (1992). Dyspnea-limited response in chronic obstructive pulmonary disease: Reduced unsupported arm activities. *Rehabilitation Nursing*, *17*(1), 13–20.

Burkle, N. (1988). Inadvertent hypothermia. *Journal of Gerontologic Nursing, 14*(6), 26–29.

Burnside, I., & Haight, B. (1994). Reminiscence and life review: Therapeutic interventions for older people. *Nurse Practitioner, 19*(4), 55–60.

Carscadden, J.S. (1993). On the cutting edge: A guide for working with people with people who self injure. (pp. 29–34).

Carson, V. B. (1989). *Spiritual dimensions of nursing practice.* Philadelphia: W.B. Saunders.

Collins, S. K., & Kuck, K. (1991). Music therapy in the neonatal intensive care unit. *Neonatal Network, 9*(6), 23–26.

Cooley, M. E., Yeomans, A. C., & Cobb, S. C. (1986). Sexual and reproductive issues for women with Hodgkin's disease. II. Application of PLISSIT model. *Cancer Nursing, 9*, 248–255.

Durham, R. (1983). Long-stay psychiatric patients in hospital. In S. Spence, & G. Shephard (Eds.), *Development in social skills training.* New York: Academic Press.

Eakes, G. (1995). Chronic sorrow: The lived experience of parents of chronically mentally ill individuals. *Archives of Psychiatric Nursing, 9*(2), 77–84.

Evans, L. K., Strumpf, N. E., & Williams, C. C. (1992). Limiting use of physical restraints: A prerequisite for independent functioning. In E. Calkins, A. Ford, & P. Katz (Eds.), *The practice of geriatrics* (2nd ed.). Philadelphia: W.B. Saunders.

Flandermyer, A. A. (1993). The drug exposed neonate. In C. Kenner, A. Brueggemeyer, & L. Gunderson (Eds.). *Comprehensive neonatal nursing.* Philadelphia: W. B. Saunders.

Gardner, D. L., & Campbell, B. (1991). Assessing postpartum fatigue. *Maternal Child Nursing Journal, 16*(5), 264–266.

Geisman, L. K. (1989). Advances in weaning from mechanical ventilation. *Critical Care Nursing Clinics of North America, 1*(4), 697–705.

Giger, J., & Davidhizar, R. (1995). *Transcultural nursing.* St. Louis: Mosby–Year Book.

Grainger, R. (1990). Anxiety interrupters. *American Journal of Nursing, 90*(2), 14–15.

Grunau, R., & Craig, K. (1987). Pain expression in neonates: Facial action and cry. *Pain, 28*(3), 395–410.

Hall, G. R. (1991). Altered thought processes: Dementia. In M. Maas, K. Buckwalter, & M. Hardy (Eds.), *Nursing diagnoses and interventions for the elderly.* Menlo Park, CA: Addison-Wesley Nursing.

Hall, G. R., & Buckwalter, K. C. (1987). Progressively lowered stress threshold: A conceptual model for care of adults with Alzheimer's disease. *Archives of Psychiatric Nursing, 1*(6), 399–406.

Harkulich, J., & Brugler, C. (1988). Nursing Diagnosis—translocation syndrome: Expert validation study. Partial funding granted by the Peg

Schiltz Fund, Delta Xi Chapter, Sigma Theta Tau International; Barnhouse, A. (1987). *Development of the nursing diagnosis of translocation syndrome with critical care patients.* Unpublished master's thesis. Kent, OH: Kent State University.

Heinrich, L. (1987). Care of the female rape victim. *Nurse Practitioner, 12*(11), 9.

Herman-Staab, B. (1994). Screening, management and appropriate referral for pediatric behavior problems. *Nurse Practitioner, 19*(7), 40–49.

Hilliker, N. A. (1998). Sleep disorders. In M. A. Boyd & M. A. Nihart. *Psychiatric nursing: Contemporary practice.* Philadelphia: Lippincott-Raven.

Hiltunen, E. (1987). *Diagnostic content validity of the nursing diagnosis: Decisional conflict.* Unpublished raw data.

Hinds, P. (1988) Adolescent hopefulness in illness and health. *Advances in Nursing Science, 10*(3), 79–88.

Holmstrom, L., & Burgess, A. W. (1975). Development of diagnostic categories: Sexual traumas. *American Journal of Nursing, 75,* 1288–1291.

Hootman, J. (1993). *Procedural manual of quality nursing intervention in school.* Portland, OR: Multnonah Education Service District

Jackson, D. B., & Saunders, R. B. (1993). *Child health nursing.* Philadelphia: J. B. Lippincott.

Janssen, J., & Giberson, D. (1988). Remotivation therapy. *Journal of Gerontological Nursing, 14*(6), 31–34.

Jenny, J. (1987). Knowledge deficit: Not a nursing diagnosis. *Image: Journal of Nursing Scholarship, 19*(4), 184–185.

Jenny, J., & Logan, J. (1991). Interventions for the nursing diagnosis Dysfunctional Ventilatory Weaning Response: A qualitative study. In R. M. Carroll-Johnson (Ed.), *Classification of nursing diagnoses.* Philadelphia: J.B. Lippincott.

Johnson, D. B., & Saunders, R. B. (1995). *Child health nursing.* Philadelphia: Lippincott-Raven.

Johnson-Crowley, N. (1993). Systematic assessment and home follow-up. In C. Kenner, A. Brueggemeyer, & L. Gunderson (Eds.), *Comprehensive neonatal nursing.* Philadelphia: W.B. Saunders.

Krieger, D. (1979). *The therapeutic touch: How to use your hands to help or to heal.* Englewood Cliffs, NJ: Prentice-Hall.

Levin, R. F., Krainovitch, B. C., Bahrenburg, E., & Mitchell, C. A. (1989). Diagnostic content validity of nursing diagnoses. *Image: Journal of Nursing Scholarship, 21*(1), 40–44.

Lindeman, M., Hokanson, J., & Batek, J. (1994). The alcoholic family. *Nursing Diagnosis, 5*(2), 65–73.

Little, D., Riddle, B., & Soule, C. (1994). The power in our hands: Integrating developmental care into neonatal transport. *Neonatal Network, 13*(7), 19–22.

Logan, J., & Jenny, J. (1991). Interventions for the nursing diagnosis dysfunctional ventilatory weaning response: A qualitative study. In R. M. Carroll-Johnson (Ed.), *Classification of nursing diagnoses: Proceedings of the ninth conference* (pp. 141–147). Philadelphia: J.B. Lippincott.

Lynch, C. S., & Phillips, M. W. (1989). Nursing diagnosis: Ineffective denial. In R. M. Carroll-Johnson (Ed.), *Classification of nursing diagnoses: Proceedings of the eighth conference.* Philadelphia: J.B. Lippincott.

Magnan, M. A. (1987). *Activity intolerance: Toward a nursing theory of activity.* Paper presented at the Fifth Annual Symposium of the Michigan Nursing Diagnosis Association, Detroit.

Mass, M., & Specht, J. (1990). Bowel incontinence. In M. Maas, K. Buckwalter, & M. Hardy (Eds.), *Nursing diagnoses and interventions for the elderly.* Redwood City, CA: Addison-Wesley Nursing.

Maresca, T. (1986). Assessment and management of acute diarrheal illness in adults. *Nurse Practitioner, 11*(11), 15–16.

May, K. A., & Mahlmeister, L. R. (1994). *Maternal and neonatal nursing family-centered care.* Philadelphia: Lippincott-Raven.

May, R. (1987). *The meaning of anxiety.* New York: W.W. Norton.

McFarland, G., & Wasli, E. (1993). Manipulation in nursing diagnosis and process. In B. S. Johnson (Ed.), *Psychiatric-mental health nursing* (3rd ed.) (p. 147). Philadelphia: J.B. Lippincott.

McLane, A., & McShane, R. (1986). Empirical validation of defining characteristics of constipation: A study of bowel elimination practices of healthy adults. In M. E. Hurley (Ed.), *Classification of nursing diagnoses: Proceedings of the sixth conference* (pp. 448–455). St. Louis: C.V. Mosby.

Meehan, T. G. (1991). Therpeutic touch. In G. Bulechek & J. McCloskey (Eds.). *Nursing interventions: Essential nursing treatments.* Philadelphia: W. B. Saunders.

Miller, C. (1999). *Nursing care of the older adult* (3nd ed.). Philadelphia: Lippincott, Williams & Wilkins

Mina, C. (1985). A program for helping grieving parents. *Maternal-Child Nursing Journal, 10,* 118–121.

Moon, J. L., & Humenick, S. S. (1989). Breast engorgement: Contributing variables and variables amenable to nursing interventions. *Journal of Obstetric, Gynecologic, and Neonatal Nursing, 18*(4), 309–315.

Newman, D. K., Lynch, K., Smith, D. A., & Cell, P. (1991). Restoring urinary continence. *American Journal of Nursing, 91*(1), 28–36.

Norris, J., & Kunes-Connell, M. (1987). Self-esteem disturbance: A clinical validation study. In A. McLane (Ed.), *Classification of nursing diagnoses: Proceedings of the seventh NANDA national conference.* St. Louis: C.V. Mosby.

North American Nursing Diagnosis Association (1990). *NANDA guidelines: Taxonomy 1 revised.* St. Louis: Author.

594

North American Nursing Diagnosis Association. (1992). *NANDA nursing diagnosis: Definitions and classifications*. Philadelphia: author.

Quinn, C. (1994). The four A's of restraint reduction: Attitude, assessment, anticipation, avoidance. *Orthopaedic Nursing, 13*(2), 11–19.

Rakel, B. A. (1992). Interventions related to teaching. In J. Bulechek & J. McCloskey (Eds.), Nursing intervention. *Nursing Clinics of North America, 27*(2), 397–423.

Rantz, M. (1991). Diversional activity deficit. In M. Maas, K. Buckwalter, & M. Hardy (Eds.), *Nursing diagnoses and interventions for the elderly*. Redwood City, CA: Addison-Wesley Nursing.

Reeder, S., Martin, L., & Koniak-Griffin, D. (1997). *Maternity nursing* (18th ed.). Philadelphia: Lippincott-Raven.

Rhoten, D. (1982). Fatigue and the postsurgical patient. In C. Norris (Ed.), *Concept clarification in nursing*. Rockville, MD: Aspen Systems.

Rolland, J. S. (1994). *Families, illness & disability*. New York: Basic Books.

Ross, D. (1991). Acute compartmental syndrome. *Orthopedic Nursing, 10*(2), 33–38.

Ruff, C., & Reaves, E. (1989). Diagnosing urinary incontinence in adults. *Nurse Practitioner, 14*(6), 10–17.

Shields, C. (1992). Family interaction and caregivers of Alzheimer's disease patients: Correlates of depression. *Family Process, 31*(3), 19–32.

Shrago, L., & Bocar, D. (1990). The infant's contribution to breastfeeding. *Journal of Obstetric, Gynecologic, and Neonatal Nursing, 19*(3), 209–211.

Smith, B. (1990). *Role of orientation therapy and reminiscence therapy, Alzheimer's disease* (pp. 180–187). St. Louis: C.V. Mosby.

Smith, L. S. (1987). Sexual assault: The nurse's role. *AD Nurse, 2*(2), 24–28.

Smith, S. (1990). The unique power of music therapy benefits Alzheimer's patients. *Activities, Adaptation and Aging, 14*, 49–63.

Stanley, M., & Beare, P. G. (1994). *Gerontological nursing*. Philadelphia: W.B. Saunders.

Stanley, M., & Beare, P. G. (1995). *Gerontological nursing*. Philadelphia: F.A. Davis.

Stone, R., Cafferata, G., & Sang, L. J. (1987). Caregivers of the frail elderly: A national profile. *Gerontologist, 27*(5), 616–626.

Thomas, K. A. (1989). How the NICU environment sounds to a preterm infant. *MCN: American Journal of Maternal Child Nursing, 14*(4), 249–251.

Thomas, S. P. (1998). Assessing and intervening with anger disorders. *Nursing Clinics of North America, 33*(1), 121–134.

Townsend, M. C. (1994). *Nursing diagnosis in psychiatric nursing* (3rd ed.). Philadelphia: F.A. Davis.

Vandenberg, K. (1990). The management of oral nippling in the sick neonate, the disorganized feeder. *Neonatal Network, 9*(1), 9–16.

Vincent, K. G. (1985). The validation of a nursing diagnosis. *Nursing Clinics of North America, 20*(4), 631–639.

Voith, A. M., Frank, A. M., & Pigg, J. S. (1987). Validations of fatigue as a nursing diagnosis. In A. McLane (Ed.), *Classification of nursing diagnoses: Proceedings of the seventh national conference* (p. 280). St. Louis: C.V. Mosby.

Wong, D. L. (1995). *Whaley & Wong's Essentials of Pediatric Nursing (3rd ed.).* St. Louis: C.V. Mosby.

Worden, J. (1982). *Grief counseling and grief therapy, a handbook for the mental health practitioner.* New York: Springer Publishing.

Williams, C. (1977). Community health nursing—what is it? *Nursing Outlook, 25*(4), 250–254.

Zerwich, J. (1992). Laying the groundwork for family self-help: Locating families, building trust and building strength. *Public Health Nursing, 9*(1), 15–21.

Appendix

Adult Screening Admission Assessment Guide

The screening admission assessment form directs the nurse to collect data to assess functional health patterns* of the individual and to screen for the presence of actual, risk, or possible nursing diagnoses. When the person has a medical problem, the nurse will also have to assess for data to collaborate with the physician in monitoring the problem.

As with any printed assessment tool, the nurse must determine whether to collect or defer collecting certain data.

The admission interview form can be structured to allow for deferring the collection of data. The following codes illustrate the defer options:

1 = N/A, not applicable: applies to sections that are not suitable

2 = Unable to acquire: applies to items or sections that need to be assessed but cannot be addressed at this time, for example, a confused patient who may be unable to provide the needed information

3 = Not a priority: applies to items or sections that are not appropriate at this time

4 = Other: applies to items or sections that are not assessed for reasons other than 2 or 3, for example, discontinuing the admission interview to transport the patient for emergency surgery. This option requires an explanatory note in the chart.

If desired, the admission assessment form can be marked to indicate selected items that must always be assessed unless, of course,

*The functional health patterns have been adapted from Gordon, M. (1982). *Nursing diagnosis: Application and process.* New York: McGraw-Hill.

the situation is an option 2—unable to acquire. An example of an admission assessment form appears on the following pages. The form contains several characteristics that facilitate its use for the defer options and has a format that allows one to check options, rather than write them. Some data collection is not facilitated by checking choices, such as support system, emotional status, and sexual concerns.

As the nurse interviews the person, significant data may surface. The nurse should then ask other questions (focus assessment) to determine the presence of a pattern. For further information, the reader is referred to Section II of *Nursing diagnosis: Application to clinical practice,* 8th ed., by Lynda Juall Carpenito (Philadelphia, Lippincott, Williams & Wilkins, 1999).

For example, the client reports during the initial interview that she has a problem with incontinence. The nurse should then ask specific questions using the focus assessment for Altered Patterns of Urinary Elimination to determine which diagnosis of incontinence is present. After the nurse has identified the related factors, the plan of care can be initiated.

NURSING ADMISSION
SCREENING ASSESSMENT

Date _____ Arrival Time _____ Contact Person _____ Phone _____
ADMITTED FROM: ____ Home alone   ____ Home with relative   ____ Long-term care
                ____ Homeless   ____ Home with _____   facility
                ____ ER   ____   (Specify)   ____ Other _____
MODE OF ARRIVAL: ____ Wheelchair   ____ Ambulance   ____ Stretcher
REASON FOR HOSPITALIZATION: _____
_____

LAST HOSPITAL ADMISSION: Date _____ Reason _____

PAST MEDICAL HISTORY: _____

MEDICATION (Prescription/Over-the-Counter)	DOSAGE	LAST DOSE	FREQUENCY

HEALTH PERCEPTION – MANAGEMENT PATTERN
USE OF:
Tobacco: ____ None ____ Quit (date) ____ Pipe ____ Cigar ____ <1 pk/day
                ____ 1–2 pks/day ____ >2 pks/day Pks/year history _____
Alcohol: ____ None ____ Type/amount ____ /day ____ /wk ____ /month
Other Drugs: ____ No ____ Yes Type _____ Use _____
Allergies (drugs, food, tape, dyes): _____ Reaction _____

ACTIVITY/EXERCISE PATTERN
SELF-CARE ABILITY:
  0 = Independent   1 = Assistive device   2 = Assistance from others
  3 = Assistance from person and equipment   4 = Totally dependent

	0	1	2	3	4
Eating/Drinking					
Bathing					
Dressing/Grooming					
Toileting					
Bed Mobility					
Transferring					
Ambulating					
Stair Climbing					
Shopping					
Cooking					
Home Maintenance					

ASSISTIVE DEVICES: ____ None ____ Crutches ____ Bedside commode ____ Walker
                   ____ Cane ____ Splint/Brace ____ Wheelchair ____ Other ____

CODE: (1) Non-applicable (2) Unable to acquire
      (3) Not a priority at this time (4) Other (specify in notes)

Side One

NUTRITION/METABOLIC PATTERN
Special Diet/Supplements _____
Previous Dietary Instruction: ____ Yes ____ No
Appetite: ____ Normal ____ Increased ____ Decreased ____ Decreased taste sensation
          ____ Nausea ____ Vomiting ____ Stomatitis
Weight Fluctuations Last 6 Months: ____ None _____ lbs. Gained/Lost
Swallowing Difficulty (Dysphagia): ____ None ____ Solids ____ Liquids
Dentures: ____ Upper (_ Partial _ Full) ____ Lower (_ Partial _ Full)
        With Patient ____ Yes ____ No
History of Skin/Healing Problems: ____ None ____ Abnormal Healing ____ Rash
                        ____ Dryness ____ Excess Perspiration

ELIMINATION PATTERN
Bowel Habits: ____ # BMs/day ____ Date of last BM ____ Within normal limits
              ____ Constipation ____ Diarrhea ____ Incontinence
              ____ Ostomy: Type ____ Appliance ____ Self-care ____ Yes ____ No
Bladder Habits: ____ WNL ____ Frequency ____ Dysuria ____ Nocturia ____ Urgency
              ____ Hematuria ____ Retention
Incontinency: ____ No ____ Yes ____ Total ____ Daytime ____ Nighttime
            ____ Occasional ____ Difficulty delaying voiding
            ____ Difficulty reaching toilet
Assistive Devices: ____ Intermittent catheterization
                ____ Indwelling catheter ____ External catheter
                ____ Incontinent briefs ____ Penile implant type _____

SLEEP/REST PATTERN
Habits: ____ hrs/night ____ AM nap ____ PM nap
      Feel rested after sleep ____ Yes ____ No
Problems: ____ None ____ Early waking ____ Insomnia ____ Nightmares

COGNITIVE–CONCEPTUAL PATTERN
Hearing: ____ WNL ____ Impaired (_ Right _ Left) ____ Deaf (_ Right _ Left)
        ____ Hearing Aid ____ Tinnitus
Vision: ____ WNL ____ Eyeglasses ____ Contact lens
       ____ Impaired ____ Right ____ Left
       ____ Blind ____ Right ____ Left
       ____ Cataract ____ Right ____ Left
       ____ Glaucoma
       ____ Prosthetis ____ Right ____ Left
Vertigo: ____ Yes ____ No
Discomfort/Pain: ____ None ____ Acute ____ Chronic ____ Description _____

Pain Management: _____

COPING STRESS TOLERANCE/SELF-PERCEPTION/SELF-CONCEPT PATTERN
Major concerns regarding hospitalization or illness (financial, self-care): _____

Major loss/change in past year: ____ No ____ Yes _____

Emotional State: _____

CODE: (1) Non-applicable (2) Unable to acquire
      (3) Not a priority at this time (4) Other (specify in notes)

Side Two

SEXUALITY/REPRODUCTIVE PATTERN

LMP: _____

Menstrual Problems: ____ Yes ____ No _____

Gravida _____ Para _____

Hx of STD _____ No, if Yes Specify _____

Last Pap Smear: _____ hx of Abnormal PAP_____Yes_____No

Monthly Self-Breast/Testicular Exam: ____ Yes ____ No

Sexual Concerns R/T Illness: _____

_____

ROLE-RELATIONSHIP PATTERN

Occupation: _____

Employment Status: ____ Employed ____ Short-term disability

_____ ____ Long-term disability ____ Unemployed

Support System: ____ Spouse ____ Neighbors/Friends ____ None

_____ ____ Family in same residence ____ Family in separate residence

_____ ____ Other _____

Family concerns regarding hospitalization: _____

_____

VALUE-BELIEF PATTERN

Religion: ____ Roman Catholic ____ Protestant ____ Jewish ____ Other

Religious Restrictions: ____ No ____ Yes (Specify) _____

Request Chaplain Visitation at This Time: ____ Yes ____ No

PHYSICAL ASSESSMENT (Objective)

1. CLINICAL DATA

Age _____ Height _____ Weight _____ (Actual/Approximate)

Temperature _____

Pulse: ____ Strong ____ Weak ____ Regular ____ Irregular

Blood Pressure: Right Arm ____ Left Arm ____ Sitting ____ Lying ____

General Appearance: Groomed ____ Unkempt ____ Thin ____Well-nourished _

_____ Obese ____

2. RESPIRATORY/CIRCULATORY

Rate _____

Quality: ____ WNL ____ Shallow ____ Rapid ____ Labored ____ Other _____

Cough: ____ No ____ Yes/Describe _____

Auscultation:

Upper rt lobes ____ WNL ____ Decreased ____ Absent ____ Abnormal sounds ____

Upper lt lobes ____ WNL ____ Decreased ____ Absent ____ Abnormal sounds ____

Lower rt lobes ____ WNL ____ Decreased ____ Absent ____ Abnormal sounds ____

Lower lt lobes ____ WNL ____ Decreased ____ Absent ____ Abnormal sounds ____

Right Pedal Pulse: ____ Strong ____ Weak ____ Absent

Left Pedal Pulse: ____ Strong ____ Weak ____ Absent

3. METABOLIC-INTEGUMENTARY

SKIN:

Color: ____ WNL ____ Pale ____ Cyanotic ____ Ashen ____ Jaundice ____ Other ____

Temperature: ____ WNL ____ Warm ____ Cool

Turgor: ____ WNL ____ Poor

Edema: ____ No ____ Yes/Description/location _____

Lesions: ____ None ____ Yes/Description/location _____

Bruises: ____ None ____ Yes/Description/location _____

Reddened: ____ No ____ Yes/Description/location _____

Pruritus: ____ No ____ Yes/Description/location _____

Tubes: Specify _____

MOUTH:

Gums: ____ WNL ____ White plaque ____ Lesions ____ Other _____

Teeth: ____ WNL ____ Other _____

ABDOMEN:

Bowel Sounds: ____ Present ____ Absent

Side Three

4. NEURO/SENSORY

Mental Status: ___ Alert ___ Receptive aphasia ___ Poor historian
        ___ Oriented ___ Confused ___ Combative ___ Unresponsive
Speech: ___ Normal ___ Slurred ___ Garbled ___ Expressive aphasia
        Spoken language_____ Interpreter _____
Pupils: ___ Equal ___ Unequal

Left: • • • • • ● ● ●

Right: • • • • • ● ● ●

Reactive to light:
  Left: ___ Yes ___ No/Specify _____
  Right: ___ Yes ___ No/Specify _____

Eyes: ___ Clear ___ Draining ___ Reddened ___ Other _____

5. MUSCULAR–SKELETAL

Range of Motion: ___ Full ___ Other _____
Balance and Gait: ___ Steady ___ Unsteady
Hand Grasps: ___ Equal ___ Strong ___ Weakness/Paralysis (_ Right _ Left)
Leg Muscles: ___ Equal ___ Strong ___ Weakness/Paralysis (_ Right _ Left)

DISCHARGE PLANNING

Lives: Alone ___ With _____ No known residence _____
Intended Destination Post Discharge: ___ Home ___ Undetermined ___ Other _____
Previous Utilization of Community Resources:
  ___ Home care/Hospice ___ Adult day care ___ Church groups ___ Other _____
  ___ Meals on Wheels ___ Homemaker/Home health aide ___ Community support group
Post-discharge Transportation:
  ___ Car ___ Ambulance ___ Bus/Taxi
  ___ Unable to determine at this time
Anticipated Financial Assistance Post-discharge?: ___ No ___ Yes _____
Anticipated Problems with Self-care Post-discharge?: ___ No ___ Yes _____
Assistive Devices Needed Post-discharge?: ___ No ___ Yes _____
Referrals: (record date)
  Discharge Coordinator _____ Home Health _____
  Social Service _____ V.N.A. _____
Other Comments: _____
     _____

SIGNATURE/TITLE _____ DATE _____

Side Four

602

How to Create a Priority Set of Diagnoses

1. Look up the diagnostic cluster in Section II for the primary condition for which the person was admitted.
2. Select the collaborative problems that are frequently monitored for or treated (those marked with a ▲).
3. Select those nursing diagnoses also marked with a ▲. Validate as actual or risk for this person.
4. Examine the remaining nursing diagnoses and collaborative problems. If you do not provide nursing interventions for them, will the client progress? Can these diagnoses be referred for treatment after discharge?
5. When using the data from a screening assessment, are there additional nursing diagnoses that require nursing interventions now (if not treated the client or family will not improve or functional status will be compromised)? Can these diagnoses be managed at a later time, *e.g.* after discharge by the client or by a referral?
6. Are there any coexisting medical conditions (*e.g.*, diabetes mellitus) or therapy not related to the primary condition, such as anticoagulant therapy, that could cause a physiological complication for which the nurse should monitor as a collaborative problem? Add to priority list.
7. Does the client or family have a problem that they desire nursing assistance with?

Index

Note: Page numbers followed by t indicate tables. Nursing diagnoses appear in **boldface**.